Essential Haematology

Companion website

This book has a companion website:

www.wiley.com/go/essentialhaematology

with:

- Figures and tables from the book for downloading
- Interactive multiple choice questions prepared by the authors

Essential Haematology

A. V. Hoffbrand

MA DM FRCP FRCPath FRCP(Edin) DSc FMedSci
Emeritus Professor of Haematology
University College London
Honorary Consultant Haematologist
Royal Free Hospital
London, UK

P. A. H. Moss

PhD MRCP FRCPath
Professor of Haematology
University of Birmingham
Birmingham, UK

Sixth Edition

WILEY-BLACKWELL

A John Wiley & Sons, Ltd., Publication

This edition first published 2011, © 1980, 1984, 1993, 2001, 2006, 2011 by AV Hoffbrand and PAH Moss

Blackwell Publishing was acquired by John Wiley & Sons in February 2007. Blackwell's publishing program has been merged with Wiley's global Scientific, Technical and Medical business to form Wiley-Blackwell.

Registered office: John Wiley & Sons Ltd, The Atrium, Southern Gate, Chichester, West Sussex, PO19 8SQ, UK

Editorial offices: 9600 Garsington Road, Oxford, OX4 2DQ, UK
The Atrium, Southern Gate, Chichester, West Sussex, PO19 8SQ, UK
111 River Street, Hoboken, NJ 07030-5774, USA

For details of our global editorial offices, for customer services and for information about how to apply for permission to reuse the copyright material in this book please see our website at www.wiley.com/wiley-blackwell

The right of the author to be identified as the author of this work has been asserted in accordance with the UK Copyright, Designs and Patents Act 1988.

First published 1980
Reprinted 1981, 1982, 1983 (twice)
Second edition 1984
Reprinted 1985
Reprinted with corrections 1985, 1988 (twice), 1989
German edition 1986 (reprinted 1990)
Japanese edition 1986
Spanish edition 1987 (reprinted twice)
Indonesian edition 1987
Third edition 1993
German 1996
Hungarian edition 1997
Chinese edition 1998
Reprinted with corrections 1993, 1994, 1995, 1996, 1997, 1998, 1999, 2000
Fourth edition 2001
German 2002
Indonesian 2005
Korean 2005
Portuguese 2005
Fifth edition 2006
Reprinted with Gaucher's disease 2008

Designations used by companies to distinguish their products are often claimed as trademarks. All brand names and product names used in this book are trade names, service marks, trademarks or registered trademarks of their respective owners. The publisher is not associated with any product or vendor mentioned in this book. This publication is designed to provide accurate and authoritative information in regard to the subject matter covered. It is sold on the understanding that the publisher is not engaged in rendering professional services. If professional advice or other expert assistance is required, the services of a competent professional should be sought.

The contents of this work are intended to further general scientific research, understanding, and discussion only and are not intended and should not be relied upon as recommending or promoting a specific method, diagnosis, or treatment by physicians for any particular patient. The publisher and the author make no representations or warranties with respect to the accuracy or completeness of the contents of this work and specifically disclaim all warranties, including without limitation any implied warranties of fitness for a particular purpose. In view of ongoing research, equipment modifications, changes in governmental regulations, and the constant flow of information relating to the use of medicines, equipment, and devices, the reader is urged to review and evaluate the information provided in the package insert or instructions for each medicine, equipment, or device for, among other things, any changes in the instructions or indication of usage and for added warnings and precautions. Readers should consult with a specialist where appropriate. The fact that an organization or Website is referred to in this work as a citation and/or a potential source of further information does not mean that the author or the publisher endorses the information the organization or Website may provide or recommendations it may make. Further, readers should be aware that Internet Websites listed in this work may have changed or disappeared between when this work was written and when it is read. No warranty may be created or extended by any promotional statements for this work. Neither the publisher nor the author shall be liable for any damages arising herefrom.

Library of Congress Cataloging-in-Publication Data

Hoffbrand, A. V.
Essential haematology / A.V. Hoffbrand, P.A.H. Moss, – 6th ed.
p. ; cm.
Includes bibliographical references and index.
ISBN 978-1-4051-9890-5
1. Blood–Diseases. 2. Hematology. I. Moss, P. A. H. II. Title.
[DNLM: 1. Hematologic Diseases. WH 120 H698e 2011]
RC633.H627 2011
616.1'5–dc22
2010024521

A catalogue record for this book is available from the British Library.

Set in 10/12pt Adobe Garamond Pro by Toppan Best-set Premedia Limited
Printed and bound in Singapore by Fabulous Printers Pte Ltd
1   2011

Contents

Companion website

This book has a companion website:

www.wiley.com/go/essentialhaematology

with:

• Figures and tables from the book for downloading
• Interactive multiple choice questions prepared by the authors

Preface to the Sixth Edition

Haematology has advanced more rapidly in the last ten years more than any branch of medicine. Current haematological literature is so prolific that it is increasing difficult for any one but a specialist to keep up to date.

The Anaemias by Janet Vaughan, 1st edition, Oxford Medical Publications, 1933

Almost 70 years later, haematology still continues to be at the forefront of medical advances. The increased understanding of blood diseases particularly their genetic basis and changes in their treatment is such that in writing this new edition, substantial changes have been necessary throughout. The classification of the neoplasms of the haemopoietic and lymphoid diseases has been revised by WHO (2008) and the names and definitions of many of these diseases have changed. Clinical features, genetics and immunophenotype are increasingly used to define biological entities. We have made changes in all the relevant chapters but, in a book intended primarily for undergraduates, we have simplified some of the classification tables and omitted detailed descriptions of rare diseases. On the other hand, some tests e.g. red cell survival and vitamin B_{12} absorption studies have become obsolete and are now omitted. As previously, we have used a colour line in the margin to indicate text that we consider more advanced than is needed for undergraduate medical students and more appropriate for postgraduates.

John Pettit, co-author on all five previous editions, has retired from authorship for this edition. Much of the success of the book when it first appeared 30 years ago and in all five previous editions has been due to John's ability to write clear, concise descriptions of the various diseases, and to produce first-class photomicrographs and line diagrams to illustrate the text. Many of these images appear in this latest edition.

The different aspects of iron overload are now merged into a new chapter and we have separated chapters on acute myeloid and acute lymphoblastic leukaemia. We have also introduced summary boxes at the *end* of each chapter to summarise the contents and added multiple choice questions to the website both at undergraduate and at a more advanced level to help in self-learning. The book's website will be updated annually.

We would like to thank Elsevier for the use of the following figures: 4.2, 11.14, 13.5b, 18.5, 18.6, 18.7, 20.13–16, 20.18, 21.2b, 22.3, 23.13, 26.7, 30.5 from Hoffbrand A.V., Pettit J.E. and Vyas P. (2010) *Color Atlas of Clinical Hematology*, 4th edition. Mosby Elsevier, Philadelphia. We would also like to thank Professor John W. Weisel for the use of the chapter title figure from Brown A.E.X., Nagaswami C., Litvionov R.I. and Weisel J.W. (2009) Focusing on fibrin. *Science* **327**: 741. The image shows colourised scanning electron micrograph of a thrombus taken from a patient with acute myocardial infarction. The thrombus is made up of a fibrin meshwork (brown) together with platelets (light purple). Erythrocytes (red) and leucocytes (green) are trapped in the network.

We wish to thank our many colleagues at the Royal Free Hospital and in Birmingham who have commented on the various chapters and made helpful suggestions for improvements. We are also indebted to our publishers, Wiley-Blackwell, and particularly to Rebecca Huxley who has provided tremendous skills throughout the assembly of this new edition, and Jane Fellows who has expertly drawn all the line diagrams.

A.V. Hoffbrand and P.A.H. Moss
November 2010

Preface to the First Edition

The major changes that have occurred in all fields of medicine over the last decade have been accompanied by an increased understanding of the biochemical, physiological and immunological processes involved in normal blood cell formation and function and the disturbances that may occur in different diseases. At the same time, the range of treatment available for patients with diseases of the blood and blood-forming organs has widened and improved substantially as understanding of the disease processes has increased and new drugs and means of support care have been introduced.

We hope the present book will enable the medical student of the 1980s to grasp the essential features of modern clinical and laboratory haematology and to achieve an understanding of how many of the manifestations of blood diseases can be explained with this new knowledge of the disease processes.

We would like to thank many colleagues and assistants who have helped with the preparation of the book. In particular, Dr H.G. Prentice cared for the patients whose haematological responses are illustrated in Figs 5.3 and 7.8 and Dr J. McLaughlin supplied Fig. 8.6. Dr S. Knowles reviewed critically the final manuscript and made many helpful suggestions. Any remaining errors are, however, our own. We also thank Mr J.B. Irwin and R.W. McPhee who drew many excellent diagrams, Mr Cedric Gilson for expert photomicrography, Mrs T. Charalambos, Mrs B. Elliot, Mrs M. Evans and Miss J. Allaway for typing the manuscript, and Mr Tony Russell of Blackwell Scientific Publications for his invaluable help and patience.

AVH, JEP
1980

How to get the best out of your textbook

Welcome to the new edition of *Essential Haematology*. Over the next two pages you will be shown how to make the most of the learning features included in the textbook

An interactive textbook ▶

For the first time, your textbook gives you free access to a Wiley Desktop Edition – a digital, interactive version of this textbook. You can view your book on a PC, Mac, laptop and Apple mobile device, and it allows you to:

Search: Save time by finding terms and topics instantly in your book, your notes, even your whole library (once you've downloaded more textbooks)

Note and Highlight: Colour code highlights and make digital notes right in the text so you can find them quickly and easily

Organize: Keep books, notes and class materials organized in folders inside the application

Share: Exchange notes and highlights with friends, classmates and study groups

Upgrade: Your textbook can be transferred when you need to change or upgrade your computer or device

Link: Link directly from the page of your interactive textbook to all of the material contained on the companion website

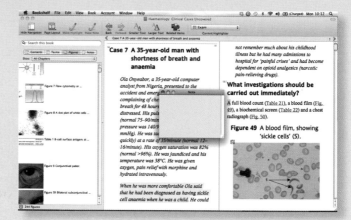

Simply find your unique Wiley Desktop Edition product code on the inside front cover of this textbook and carefully scratch away the top coating on the label, then visit **http://www.vitalsource.com/software/bookshelf/downloads/** to get started

Full support is available at **http://support.vitalsource.com/**

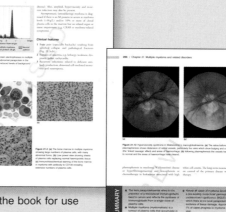

A companion website

Your textbook is also accompanied by a FREE companion website that contains:

- Self-assessment material consisting of multiple choice questions and answers
- All of the illustrations and photographs contained in the book for use in assignments and presentations
- References and further reading suggestions

Log on to **www.wiley.com/go/essentialhaematology** to find out more

Features contained within your textbook

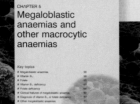

◀ Every chapter has its own chapter-opening page that offers a list of key topics contained within the chapter

Throughout your textbook you will find a series of icons outlining the learning features in the book:
▼

The coloured line in the margin indicates text that we consider more advanced than is needed for undergraduate medical students and more appropriate for postgraduates

Self-assessment multiple choice questions and answers are available on the companion website: **www.wiley.com/go/essentialhaematology**. You can also access these questions by clicking on this icon in your Desktop Edition

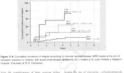

◀ Your textbook is full of useful photographs, illustrations and tables. The Desktop Edition version of your textbook will allow you to copy and paste any photograph or illustration into assignments, presentations and your own notes. The photographs and illustrations are also available to download from the companion website
▼

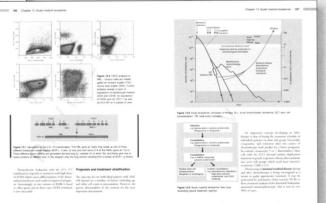

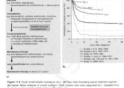
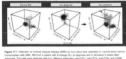

▲
Every chapter ends with a chapter summary which can be used for both study and revision purposes

We hope you enjoy using your new textbook. Good luck with your studies!

CHAPTER 1
Haemopoiesis

Key topics

Essential Haematology, 6th Edition. © A. V. Hoffbrand and P. A. H. Moss. Published 2011 by Blackwell Publishing Ltd.

This first chapter is concerned with the general aspects of blood cell formation (haemopoiesis). The processes that regulate haemopoiesis and the early stages of formation of red cells (erythropoiesis), granulocytes and monocytes (myelopoiesis) and platelets (thrombopoiesis) are also discussed.

Site of haemopoiesis

In the first few weeks of gestation the yolk sac is the main site of haemopoiesis. However, definitive haemopoiesis derives from a population of stem cells first observed on the dorsal aorta termed the AGM (aorta-gonads-mesonephros) region. These common precursors of endothelial and haemopoietic cells (haemangioblasts) are believed to seed the liver, spleen and bone marrow and from 6 weeks until 6–7 months of fetal life the liver and spleen are the major haemopoietic organs and continue to produce blood cells until about 2 weeks after birth (Table 1.1; see Fig. 7.1b). The bone marrow is the most important site from 6 to 7 months of fetal life. During normal childhood and adult life the marrow is the only source of new blood cells. The developing cells are situated outside the bone marrow sinuses; mature cells are released into the sinus spaces, the marrow microcirculation and so into the general circulation.

In infancy all the bone marrow is haemopoietic but during childhood there is progressive fatty replacement of marrow throughout the long bones so that in adult life haemopoietic marrow is confined to the central skeleton and proximal ends of the femurs and humeri (Table 1.1). Even in these haemopoietic areas, approximately 50% of the marrow consists of fat (Fig. 1.1). The remaining fatty marrow is capable of reversion to haemopoiesis and in many diseases there is also expansion of haemopoiesis down the long bones. Moreover, the liver and spleen can resume their fetal haemopoietic role ('extramedullary haemopoiesis').

Haemopoietic stem and progenitor cells

Haemopoiesis starts with a pluripotential stem cell that can self-renew but also give rise to the separate cell lineages. These cells are able to repopulate a bone marrow from which all stem cells have been eliminated by lethal irradiation or chemotherapy. This **haemopoietic stem cell** is rare, perhaps 1 in every 20 million nucleated cells in bone marrow. Although its exact phenotype is unknown, on immunological testing it is $CD34^+$ $CD38^-$ and negative for lineage markers (Lin^-) and has the appearance of a small or medium-sized lymphocyte (see Fig. 23.3). The cells reside in specialized 'niches'. Cell differentiation occurs from the stem cell via committed **haemopoietic progenitors** which are restricted in their developmental potential (Fig. 1.2). The existence of the separate progenitor cells can be demonstrated by *in vitro* culture techniques. Very early progenitors are assayed by culture on bone marrow stroma as long-term culture initiating cells whereas late progenitors are generally assayed

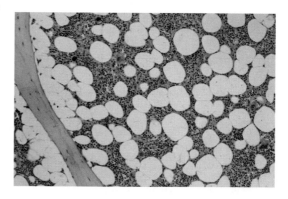

Figure 1.1 A normal bone marrow trephine biopsy (posterior iliac crest). Haematoxylin and eosin stain; approximately 50% of the intertrabecular tissue is haemopoietic tissue and 50% is fat.

Table 1.1 Sites of haemopoiesis.	
Fetus	0–2 months (yolk sac)
	2–7 months (liver, spleen)
	5–9 months (bone marrow)
Infants	Bone marrow (practically all bones)
Adults	Vertebrae, ribs, sternum, skull, sacrum and pelvis, proximal ends of femur

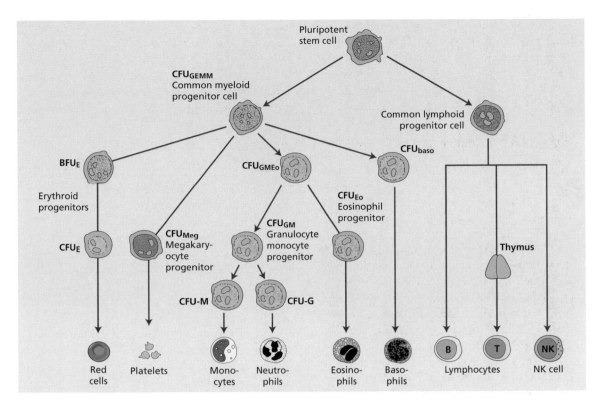

Figure 1.2 Diagrammatic representation of the bone marrow pluripotent stem cell and the cell lines that arise from it. Various progenitor cells can be identified by culture in semi-solid medium by the type of colony they form. It is possible that an erythroid/megakaryocytic progenitor may be formed before the common lymphoid progenitor diverges from the mixed granulocytic/monocyte/eosinophil myeloid progenitor. Baso, basophil; BFU, burst-forming unit; CFU, colony-forming unit; E, erythroid; Eo, eosinophil; GEMM, granulocyte, erythroid, monocyte and megakaryocyte; GM, granulocyte, monocyte; Meg, megakaryocyte; NK, natural killer.

in semi-solid media. An example is the earliest detectable mixed myeloid precursor which gives rise to granulocytes, erythrocytes, monocytes and megakaryocytes and is termed CFU (colony-forming unit)-GEMM (Fig. 1.2). The bone marrow is also the primary site of origin of lymphocytes (see Chapter 9) which differentiate from a common lymphoid precursor.

The stem cell has the capability for *self-renewal* (Fig. 1.3) so that marrow cellularity remains constant in a normal healthy steady state. There is considerable amplification in the system: one stem cell is capable of producing about 10^6 mature blood cells after 20 cell divisions (Fig. 1.3). The precursor

cells are, however, capable of responding to haemopoietic growth factors with increased production of one or other cell line when the need arises. The development of the *mature cells* (red cells, granulocytes, monocytes, megakaryocytes and lymphocytes) is considered further in other sections of this book.

Bone marrow stroma

The bone marrow forms a suitable environment for stem cell survival, self-renewal and formation of differentiated progenitor cells. It is composed of stromal cells and a microvascular network (Fig. 1.4).

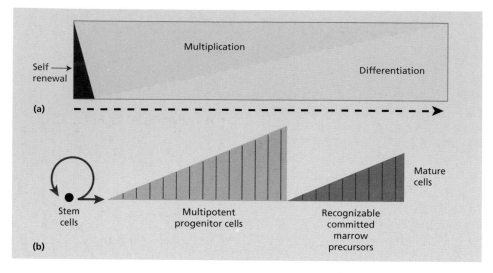

Figure 1.3 (a) Bone marrow cells are increasingly differentiated and lose the capacity for self-renewal as they mature. **(b)** A single stem cell gives rise, after multiple cell divisions (shown by vertical lines), to >10⁶ mature cells.

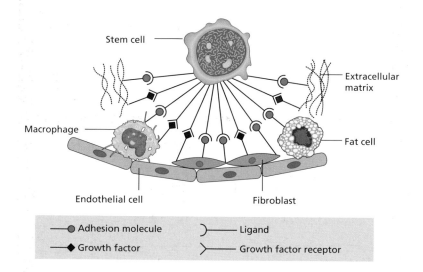

Figure 1.4 Haemopoiesis occurs in a suitable microenvironment ('niche') provided by a stromal matrix on which stem cells grow and divide. There are specific recognition and adhesion sites (see p. 13); extracellular glycoproteins and other compounds are involved in the binding.

The stromal cells include adipocytes, fibroblasts, osteoblasts, endothelial cells and macrophages and they secrete extracellular molecules such as collagen, glycoproteins (fibronectin and thrombospondin) and glycosaminoglycans (hyaluronic acid and chondroitin derivatives) to form an extracellular matrix.

In addition, stromal cells secrete several growth factors necessary for stem cell survival.

Mesenchymal stem cells, also called multipotent mesenchymal stromal cells or adherent stromal cells, are critical in stromal cell formation. Together with osteoblasts they form niches and provide the growth factors, adhesion molecules and cytokines which support stem cells, e.g. the protein jagged, on stromal cells binds to a receptor NOTCH1 on stem cells which then becomes a transcription factor involved in the cell cycle.

Stem cells are able to traffic around the body and are found in peripheral blood in low numbers. In order to exit the bone marrow, cells must cross the blood vessel endothelium and this process of **mobilization** is enhanced by administration of growth factors such as granulocyte colony-stimulating factor (G-CSF) (see p. 6). The reverse process of stem cell **homing** appears to depend on a chemokine gradient in which the stromal-derived factor 1 (SDF-1) is critical. Several critical interac-

tions maintain stem cell viability and production in the stroma including stem cell factor (SCF) and jagged proteins expressed on stroma and their respective receptors KIT and NOTCH expressed on stem cell.

Tissue-specific stem cells

Stem cells are present in many different organs. These are **pluripotent** and can generate various types of tissue, e.g. epithelial cells, nerve cells (Fig. 1.5). Studies in patients and animals who have received haemopoietic stem cell transplants (see Chapter 23) have suggested that donor haemopoietic cells may contribute to tissues such as neurons,

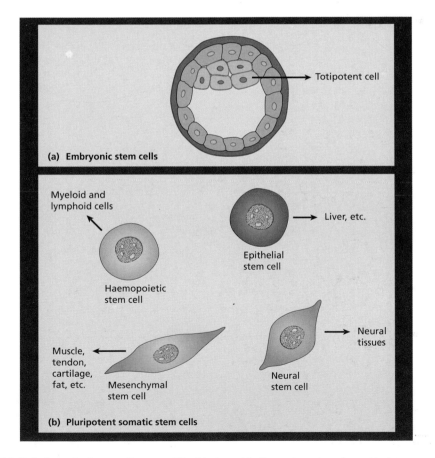

Figure 1.5 **(a)** Cells from the inner cell mass of the blastocyst in the early embryo are able to generate all the tissues of the body and are known as totipotent. **(b)** Specialized adult stem cells of the bone marrow, nervous tissue, epithelial and other tissues give rise to differentiated cells of the same tissue.

liver and muscle. The contribution of adult donor haemopoietic cells to non-haemopoietic tissues is at most very small. The persistence of pluripotential stem cells in postnatal life, the presence of mesenchymal stem cells in bone marrow and fusion of transplanted cells with host cells have all been proposed to explain many of the findings suggesting stem cell 'plasticity'.

The regulation of haemopoiesis

Haemopoiesis starts with stem cell division in which one cell replaces the stem cell (***self-renewal***) and the other is committed to differentiation. These early committed progenitors express low levels of transcription factors that may commit them to discrete cell lineages. Which cell lineage is selected for differentiation may depend both on chance and on the external signals received by progenitor cells. Several transcription factors (see p. 13) regulate survival of stem cells (e.g. SCL, GATA-2, NOTCH-1) whereas others are involved in differentiation along the major cell lineages. For instance, PU.1 and the CEBP family commit cells to the myeloid lineage whereas GATA-1 and FOG-1 have an essential roles in erythropoietic and megakaryocytic differentiation.

Table 1.2 General characteristics of myeloid and lymphoid growth factors.

Glycoproteins that act at very low concentrations
Act hierarchically
Usually produced by many cell types
Usually affect more than one lineage
Usually active on stem/progenitor cells and on functional end cells
Usually show synergistic or additive interactions with other growth factors
Often act on the neoplastic equivalent of a normal cell
Multiple actions: proliferation, differentiation, maturation, functional activation, prevention of apoptosis of progenitor cells

Haemopoietic growth factors

The haemopoietic growth factors are glycoprotein hormones that regulate the proliferation and differentiation of haemopoietic progenitor cells and the function of mature blood cells. They may act locally at the site where they are produced by cell–cell contact or circulate in plasma. They also bind to the extracellular matrix to form niches to which stem and progenitor cells adhere. The growth factors may cause cell proliferation but can also stimulate differentiation, maturation, prevent apoptosis and affect the function of mature cells (Fig. 1.6).

They share a number of common properties (Table 1.2) and act at different stages of haemopoiesis (Table 1.3; Fig. 1.7). Stromal cells are the major

Table 1.3 Haemopoietic growth factors.

Act on stromal cells
IL-1
TNF
Act on pluripotential stem cells
SCF
FLT3-L
VEGF
Act on multipotential progenitor cells
IL-3
GM-CSF
IL-6
G-CSF
Thrombopoietin
Act on committed progenitor cells
G-CSF*
M-CSF
IL-5 (eosinophil-CSF)
Erythropoietin
Thrombopoietin*

CSF, colony-stimulating factor; FLT3-L, FLT3 ligand; G-CSF, granulocyte colony-stimulating factor; GM-CSF, granulocyte–macrophage colony-stimulating factor; IL, interleukin; M-CSF, macrophage colony-stimulating factor; SCF, stem cell factor; TNF, tumour necrosis factor; VEGF, vascular endothelial growth factor.
*These also act synergistically with early acting factors on pluripotential progenitors.

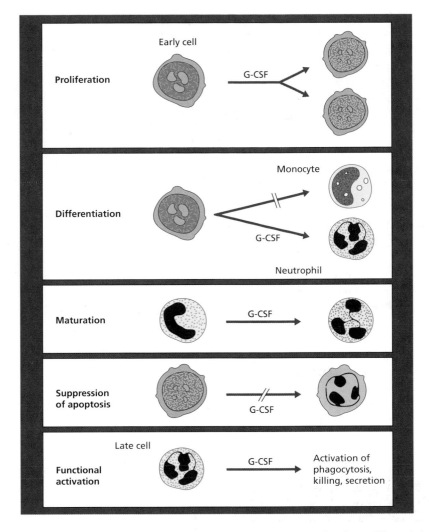

Figure 1.6 Growth factors may stimulate proliferation of early bone marrow cells, direct differentiation to one or other cell type, stimulate cell maturation, suppress apoptosis or affect the function of mature non-dividing cells, as illustrated here for granulocyte colony-stimulating factor (G-CSF) for an early myeloid progenitor and a neutrophil.

source of growth factors except for erythropoietin, 90% of which is synthesized in the kidney, and thrombopoietin, made largely in the liver. An important feature of growth factor action is that two or more factors may synergize in stimulating a particular cell to proliferate or differentiate. Moreover, the action of one growth factor on a cell may stimulate production of another growth factor or growth factor receptor. SCF and FLT ligand (FLT-L) act locally on the pluripotential stem cells and on early

myeloid and lymphoid progenitors (Fig. 1.7). Interleukin-3 (IL-3) and granuloctye–macrophage colony-stimulating factor (GM-CSF) are multipotential growth factors with overlapping activities. G-CSF and thrombopoietin enhance the effects of SCF, FLT-L, IL-3 and GM-CSF on survival and differentiation of the early haemopoietic cells.

These factors maintain a pool of haemopoietic stem and progenitor cells on which later acting factors erythropoietin, G-CSF, macrophage colony-

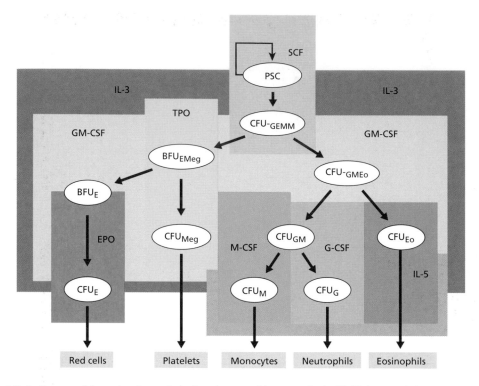

Figure 1.7 A diagram of the role of growth factors in normal haemopoiesis. Multiple growth factors act on the earlier marrow stem and progenitor cells. EPO, erythropoietin; PSC, pluripotential stem cell; SCF, stem cell factor; TPO, thrombopoietin. For other abbreviations see Fig. 1.2.

stimulating factor (M-CSF), IL-5 and thrombopoietin act to increase production of one or other cell lineage in response to the body's need. Granulocyte and monocyte formation, for example, can be stimulated by infection or inflammation through release of IL-1 and tumour necrosis factor (TNF) which then stimulate stromal cells to produce growth factors in an interacting network (see Fig. 8.4). In contrast, cytokines such as transforming growth factor-β (TGF-β) and γ-interferon (IFN-γ) can exert a negative effect on haemopoiesis and may have a role in the development of aplastic anaemia (see p. 290).

Growth factor receptors and signal transduction

The biological effects of growth factors are mediated through specific receptors on target cells. Many receptors (e.g. erythropoietin (epo) receptor (R), GMCSF-R) are from the ***haematopoietin receptor superfamily*** which dimerize after binding their ligand.

Dimerization of the receptor leads to activation of a complex series of intracellular signal transduction pathways of which the three major ones are the JAK/STAT, the mitogen-activated protein (MAP) kinase and the phosphatidylinositol 3 (PI3) kinase pathways (Fig. 1.8; see Fig. 15.2). The Janus-associated kinase (JAK) proteins are a family of four tyrosine-specific protein kinases that associate with the intracellular domains of the growth factor receptors (Fig. 1.8). A growth factor molecule binds simultaneously to the extracellular domains of two or three receptor molecules, resulting in their aggregation. Receptor aggregation induces activation of the JAKs which now phosphorylate members of the signal transducer and activator of transcription (STAT) family of transcription factors. This results

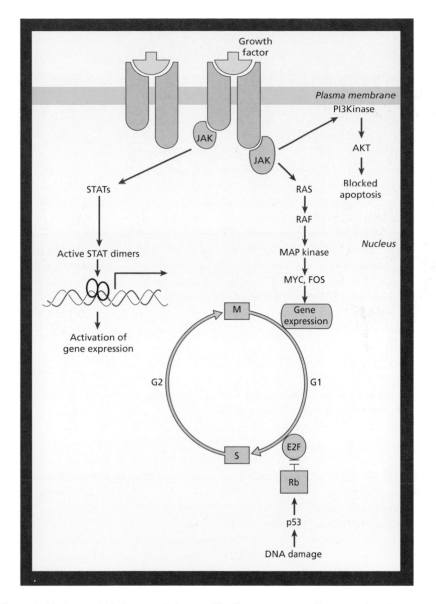

Figure 1.8 Control of haemopoiesis by growth factors. The factors act on cells expressing the corresponding receptors. Binding of a growth factor to its receptor activates the JAK/STAT, MAPK and phosphatidyl-inositol 3-kinase (PI3K) pathways (see Fig. 15.2) which leads to transcriptional activation of specific genes. E2F is a transcription factor needed for cell transition from G1 to S phase. E2F is inhibited by the tumour suppressor gene *Rb* (retinoblastoma) which can be indirectly activated by p53. The synthesis and degradation of different cyclins (Fig. 1.10) stimulates the cell to pass through the different phases of the cell cycle. The growth factors may also suppress apoptosis by activating AKT (protein kinase B).

in their dimerization and translocation from the cell cytoplasm across the nuclear membrane to the cell nucleus. Within the nucleus STAT dimers activate transcription of specific genes. A model for control of gene expression by a transcription factor is shown in Fig. 1.9. The clinical importance of this pathway is revealed by the finding of an activating mutation of the *JAK2* gene as the cause of polycythaemia rubra vera (see p. 201).

JAK can also activate the MAPK pathway which is regulated by Ras and controls proliferation. PI3 kinases phophorylate inositol lipids which have a wide range of downstream effects including activation of AKT leading to block of apoptosis and other actions (Fig. 1.8; see Fig. 15.2). Different domains of the intracellular receptor protein may signal for the different processes (e.g. proliferation or suppression of apoptosis) mediated by growth factors.

A second smaller group of growth factors, including SCF, FLT-3L and M-CSF (Table 1.3), bind to receptors that have an extracellular immunoglobulin-like domain linked via a transmembrane bridge to a cytoplasmic tyrosine kinase domain. Growth factor binding results in dimerization of these receptors and consequent activation of the tyrosine kinase domain. Phosphorylation of tyrosine residues in the receptor itself generates binding sites for signalling proteins which initiate

complex cascades of biochemical events resulting in changes in gene expression, cell proliferation and prevention of apoptosis.

The cell cycle

The cell division cycle, generally known simply as the **cell cycle**, is a complex process that lies at the heart of haemopoiesis. Dysregulation of cell proliferation is also the key to the development of malignant disease. The duration of the cell cycle is variable between different tissues but the basic principles remain constant. The cycle is divided into the mitotic phase (**M phase**), during which the cell physically divides, and **interphase** during which the chromosomes are duplicated and cell growth occurs prior to division (Fig. 1.10). The M phase is further partitioned into classical **mitosis** in which nuclear division is accomplished, and **cytokinesis** in which cell fission occurs.

Interphase is divided into three main stages: a G_1 **phase** in which the cell begins to commit to replication, an **S phase** during which DNA content doubles (Fig. 1.10b) and the chromosomes replicate and the G_2 **phase** in which the cell organelles are copied and cytoplasmic volume is increased. If cells rest prior to division they enter a G_0 state where they can remain for long periods of time. The number of cells at each stage of the cell cycle can

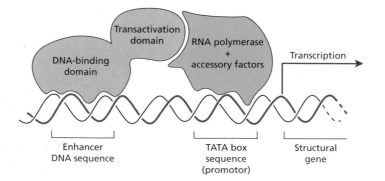

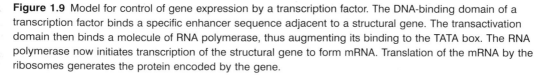

Figure 1.9 Model for control of gene expression by a transcription factor. The DNA-binding domain of a transcription factor binds a specific enhancer sequence adjacent to a structural gene. The transactivation domain then binds a molecule of RNA polymerase, thus augmenting its binding to the TATA box. The RNA polymerase now initiates transcription of the structural gene to form mRNA. Translation of the mRNA by the ribosomes generates the protein encoded by the gene.

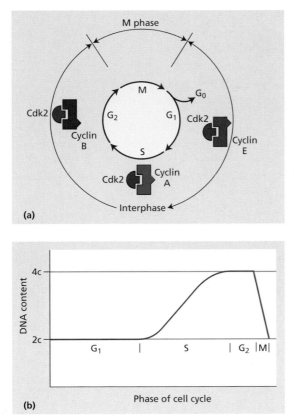

(a)

(b)

Figure 1.10 (a) The stages of the cell cycle. Progression through cell cycle is regulated by specific combinations of cyclin-dependent protein kinases (Cdk) and cyclin proteins. The synthesis and degradation of different cyclins stimulates the cell to pass through the different phases of the cell cycle.
(b) Relationship between the DNA content of a cell expressed in arbitrary units as 2c increasing to 4c and its position in the cell cycle. (Adapted from Wickramasinghe S.N. (1975) *Human Bone Marrow*, Blackwell Scientific, Oxford, p. 13.)

be assessed by exposing cells to a chemical or radiolabel that gets incorporated into newly generated DNA or by flow cytometry.

The cell cycle is controlled by two **checkpoints** which act as brakes to coordinate the division process at the end of the G_1 and G_2 phases. Two major classes of molecules control these checkpoints, **cyclin-dependent protein kinases** (Cdk)

which phosophorylate downstream protein targets and **cyclins** which bind to Cdks and regulate their activity. An example of the importance of these systems is demonstrated by mantle cell lymphoma which results from the constitutive activation of cyclin D1 as a result of a chromosomal translocation (see p. 267).

Apoptosis

Apoptosis (programmed cell death) is a regulated process of physiological cell death in which individual cells are triggered to activate intracellular proteins that lead to the death of the cell. Morphologically it is characterized by cell shrinkage, condensation of the nuclear chromatin, fragmentation of the nucleus and cleavage of DNA at internucleosomal sites. It is an important process for maintaining tissue homeostasis in haemopoiesis and lymphocyte development.

Apoptosis results from the action of intracellular cysteine proteases called **caspases** which are activated following cleavage and lead to endonuclease digestion of DNA and disintegration of the cell skeleton (Fig. 1.11). There are two major pathways by which caspases can be activated. The first is by signalling through membrane proteins such as Fas or TNF receptor via their intracellular death domain. An example of this mechanism is shown by activated cytotoxic T cells expressing FAS ligand which induce apoptosis in target cells. The second pathway is via the release of cytochrome c from mitochondria. Cytochrome c binds to APAF-1 which then activates caspases. DNA damage induced by irradiation or chemotherapy may act through this pathway. The protein p53 has an important role in sensing DNA damage. It activates apoptosis by raising the cell level of BAX which then increases cytochrome c release (Fig. 1.11). P53 also shuts down the cell cycle to stop the damaged cell from dividing (Fig. 1.8). The cellular level of p53 is rigidly controlled by a second protein MDM2. Following death, apoptotic cells display molecules that lead to their ingestion by macrophages.

As well as molecules that mediate apoptosis there are several intracellular proteins that protect

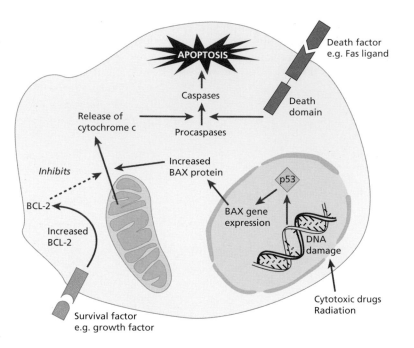

Figure 1.11 Representation of apoptosis. Apoptosis is initiated via two main stimuli: (i) signalling through cell membrane receptors such as FAS or tumour necrosis factor (TNF) receptor; or (ii) release of cytochrome c from mitochondria. Membrane receptors signal apoptosis through an intracellular death domain leading to activation of caspases which digest DNA. Cytochrome c binds to the cytoplasmic protein Apaf-1 leading to activation of caspases. The intracellular ratio of pro-apoptotic (e.g. BAX) or anti-apoptotic (e.g. BCL-2) members of the BCL-2 family may influence mitochondrial cytochrome c release. Growth factors raise the level of BCL-2 inhibiting cytochrome c release whereas DNA damage, by activating p53, raises the level of BAX which enhances cytochrome c release.

cells from apoptosis. The best characterized example is BCL-2. BCL-2 is the prototype of a family of related proteins, some of which are anti-apoptotic and some, like BAX, pro-apoptotic. The intracellular ratio of BAX and BCL-2 determines the relative susceptibility of cells to apoptosis (e.g. determines the lifespan of platelets) and may act through regulation of cytochrome c release from mitochondria.

Many of the genetic changes associated with malignant disease lead to a reduced rate of apoptosis and hence prolonged cell survival. The clearest example is the translocation of the *BCL-2* gene to the immunoglobulin heavy chain locus in the t(14; 18) translocation in follicular lymphoma.

Overexpression of the BCL-2 protein makes the malignant B cells less susceptible to apoptosis. Apoptosis is the normal fate for most B cells undergoing selection in the lymphoid germinal centres.

Several translocations leading to the generation of fusion proteins such as t(9; 22), t(1; 14) and t(15; 17) also result in inhibition of apoptosis (see Chapter 11). In addition, genes encoding proteins that are involved in mediating apoptosis following DNA damage, such as p53 and ATM, are also frequently mutated and therefore inactivated in haemopoietic malignancies.

Necrosis is death of cells and adjacent cells due to ischemia, chemical trauma or hyperthermia. The cells swell, the plasma membrane loses integrity. There is usually an inflammatory infiltrate in response to spillage of cell contents. Autophagy is the digestion of cell organelles by lysosomes. It may be involved in cell death but in some situations also in maintaining cell survival by recycling nutrients.

Transcription factors

Transcription factors regulate gene expression by controlling the transcription of specific genes or gene families. Typically, they contain at least two domains: a *DNA-binding domain* such as a leucine zipper or helix-loop-helix motif which binds to a specific DNA sequence, and an *activation domain* which contributes to assembly of the transcription complex at a gene promoter (Fig. 1.9). Mutation, deletion or translocation of transcription factors underlie many cases of haematological neoplasms.

Adhesion molecules

A large family of glycoprotein molecules termed adhesion molecules mediate the attachment of marrow precursors, leucocytes and platelets to various components of the extracellular matrix, to endothelium, to other surfaces and to each other. The adhesion molecules on the surface of leucocytes are termed receptors and these interact with molecules (termed ligands) on the surface of potential target cells. Three main families exist:

1 *Immunoglobulin superfamily* This includes receptors that react with antigens (the T-cell receptors and the immunoglobulins) and antigen-independent surface adhesion molecules.
2 *Selectins* These are mainly involved in leucocyte and platelet adhesion to endothelium during inflammation and coagulation.
3 *Integrins* These are involved in cell adhesion to extracellular matrix (e.g. to collagen in wound healing and in leucocyte and platelet adhesion).

The adhesion molecules are thus important in the development and maintenance of inflammatory and immune responses, and in platelet–vessel wall and leucocyte–vessel wall interactions. Expression of adhesion molecules can be modifed by extracellular and intracellular factors and this alteration of expression may be quantitative or functional. IL-1, TNF, IFN-γ, T-cell activation, adhesion to extracellular proteins and viral infection may all up-regulate expression of these molecules.

The pattern of expression of adhesion molecules on tumour cells may determine their mode of spread and tissue localization (e.g. the pattern of metastasis of carcinoma cells or non-Hodgkin lymphoma cells into a follicular or diffuse pattern). The adhesion molecules may also determine whether or not cells circulate in the bloodstream or remain fixed in tissues. They may also partly determine whether or not tumour cells are susceptible to the body's immune defences.

SUMMARY

- Haemopoiesis (blood cell formation) arises from pluripotent stem cells in the bone marrow. Stem cells give rise to progenitor cells which, after cell divisions and differentiation, form red cells, granulocytes (neutrophils, eosinophils and basophils), monocytes, platelets and B and T lymphocytes.
- Haemopoetic tissue occupies about 50% of the marrow space in normal adult marrow. Haemopoiesis in adults is confined to the central skeleton but in infants and young children haemopoietic tissue extends down the long bones of the arms and legs.
- Stem cells reside in the bone marrow in niches formed by stromal cells and circulate in the blood.
- Growth factors attach to specific cell receptors and produce a cascade of phosphorylation events to the cell nucleus. Transcription factors carry the message to those genes that are to be 'switched on', to stimulate cell division,

(Continued)

differentiation, functional activity or suppress apoptosis.

■ Transcription factors are molecules that bind to DNA and control the transcription of specific genes or gene families.

■ Apoptosis is a physiological process of cell death resulting from activation of caspases. The intracellular ratio of pro-apoptotic proteins (e.g. BAX) to anti-apoptotic proteins (e.g. BCL-2) determines the cell susceptibility to apoptosis.

■ Adhesion molecules are a large family of glycoproteins that mediate attachment of marrow precursors and mature leucocytes and platelets to extracellular matrix, endothelium and to each other.

Now visit www.wiley.com/go/essentialhaematology to test yourself on this chapter.

CHAPTER 2
Erythropoiesis and general aspects of anaemia

Key topics

Essential Haematology, 6th Edition. © A. V. Hoffbrand and P. A. H. Moss. Published 2011 by Blackwell Publishing Ltd.

We each make approximately 10^{12} new erythrocytes (red cells) each day by the complex and finely regulated process of erythropoiesis. Erythropoiesis passes from the stem cell through the progenitor cells colony-forming unit granulocyte, erythroid, monocyte and megakaryocyte (CFU_{GEMM}), burst-forming unit erythroid (BFU_E) and erythroid CFU (CFU_E) (Fig. 2.2) to the first recognizable erythrocyte precursor in the bone marrow, the pronormoblast. This is a large cell with dark blue cytoplasm, a central nucleus with nucleoli and slightly clumped chromatin (Fig. 2.1). The pronormoblast gives rise to a series of progressively smaller normoblasts by a number of cell divisions. They also contain progressively more haemoglobin (which stains pink) in the cytoplasm; the cytoplasm stains paler blue as it loses its RNA and protein synthetic apparatus while nuclear chromatin becomes more condensed (Figs 2.1 and 2.2). The nucleus is finally extruded from the late normoblast within the marrow and a reticulocyte stage results which still contains some ribosomal RNA and is still able to synthesize haemoglobin (Fig. 2.3). This cell is slightly larger than a mature red cell, spends 1–2 days in the marrow and also circulates in the peripheral blood for 1–2 days before maturing, when RNA is completely lost. A completely pink-staining mature erythrocyte results which is a non-nucleated biconcave disc. A single

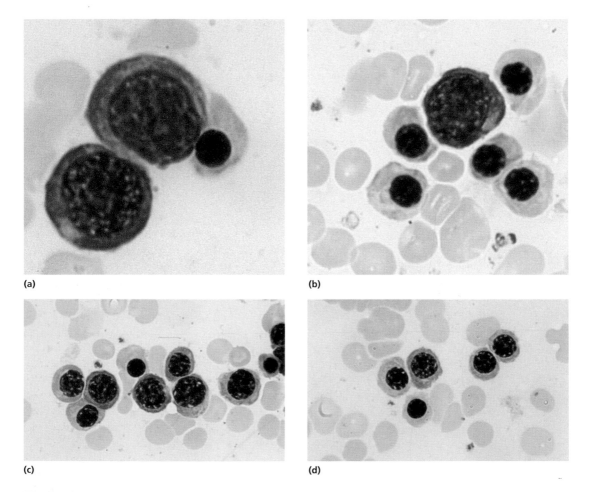

(a)

(b)

(c)

(d)

Figure 2.1 Erythroblasts (normoblasts) at varying stages of development. The earlier cells are larger, with more basophilic cytoplasm and a more open nuclear chromatin pattern. The cytoplasm of the later cells is more eosinophilic as a result of haemoglobin formation.

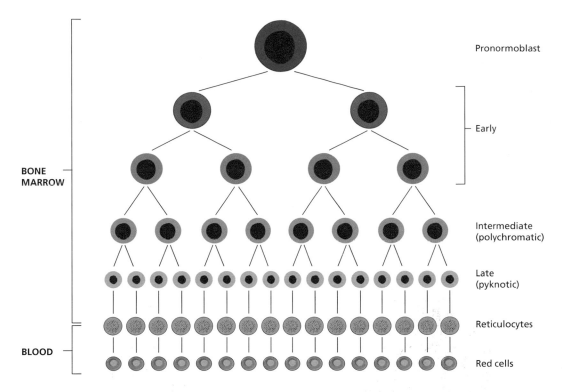

Figure 2.2 The amplification and maturation sequence in the development of mature red cells from the pronormoblast.

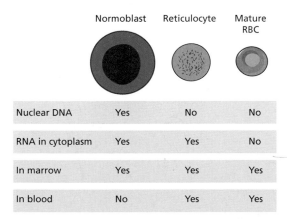

	Normoblast	Reticulocyte	Mature RBC
Nuclear DNA	Yes	No	No
RNA in cytoplasm	Yes	Yes	No
In marrow	Yes	Yes	Yes
In blood	No	Yes	Yes

Figure 2.3 Comparison of the DNA and RNA content, and marrow and peripheral blood distribution, of the erythroblast (normoblast), reticulocyte and mature red blood cell (RBC).

pronormoblast usually gives rise to 16 mature red cells (Fig. 2.2). Nucleated red cells (normoblasts) are not present in normal human peripheral blood. They appear in the blood if erythropoiesis is occurring outside the marrow (extramedullary erythropoiesis) and also with some marrow diseases.

Erythropoietin

Erythropoiesis is regulated by the hormone erythropoietin. Erythropoietin is a heavily glycosylated polypeptide of 165 amino acids with a molecular weight of 34 kDa. Normally, 90% of the hormone is produced in the peritubular interstitial cells of the kidney and 10% in the liver and elsewhere. There are no preformed stores and the stimulus to erythropoietin production is the oxygen (O_2) tension in the tissues of the kidney (Fig. 2.4). Hypoxia induces hypoxia-inducible factors (HIF-2α and β) which

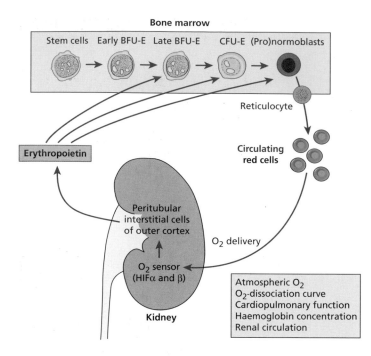

Figure 2.4 The production of erythropoietin by the kidney in response to its oxygen (O₂) supply. Erythropoietin stimulates erythropoiesis and so increases O₂ delivery. BFU$_E$, erythroid burst-forming unit; CFU$_E$, erythroid colony-forming unit. Hypoxia induces hypoxia inducible factors (HIFs) α and β, which stimulate erythropoietin production. Von-Hippel–Lindau (VHL) protein breaks down HIFs. PHD2 (prolyl hydroxylase) hydroxylates HIF-2α allowing VHL binding to HIFs. Mutations in VHL, PHD2 or HIF-2α underlie congenital polycythaemia (see p. 208).

stimulate erythropoietin production. The erythropoietin gene contains a Hif response element at its 3′ end. Erythropoietin production therefore increases in anaemia, when haemoglobin for some metabolic or structural reason is unable to give up O₂ normally, when atmospheric O₂ is low or when defective cardiac or pulmonary function or damage to the renal circulation affects O₂ delivery to the kidney.

Erythropoietin stimulates erythropoiesis by increasing the number of progenitor cells committed to erythropoiesis. The transcription factors GATA-1 and FOG-1 are activated by erythropoietin receptor stimulation and are important in enhancing expression of erythroid-specific genes (e.g. haem biosynthetic and red cell membrane proteins) and also enhancing expression of anti-apoptotic genes and of the transferrin receptor (CD71). Late BFU$_E$ and CFU$_E$, which have erythropoietin receptors, are stimulated to proliferate, differentiate and produce haemoglobin. The proportion of erythroid cells in the marrow increases and, in the chronic state, there is anatomical expansion of erythropoiesis into fatty marrow and sometimes into extramedullary sites. In infants, the marrow cavity may expand into cortical bone resulting in bone deformities with frontal bossing and protrusion of the maxilla (see p. 95).

Conversely, increased O₂ supply to the tissues (because of an increased red cell mass or because haemoglobin is able to release its O₂ more readily than normal) reduces the erythropoietin drive. Tissue hypoxia also stimulates new blood vessel formation by vascular endothelial growth factor (VEGF) and reduces transferrin but lowers hepcidin synthesis (see p. 38).

Plasma erythropoietin levels can be valuable in clinical diagnosis. They are high if a tumour-secreting erythropoietin is causing polycythaemia but low in severe renal disease or polycythaemia vera (Fig. 2.5).

Indications for erythropoietin therapy

Recombinant erythropoietin is of great value in treating anaemia resulting from renal disease or from various other causes. It is given subcutaneously either 3 times weekly or once every 1–2 weeks or every 4 weeks depending on the indication and on the preparation used (erythropoietin alpha or beta, darbepoetin alpha, a heavily glycosylated longer acting form, or Micera the longest acting prepara-

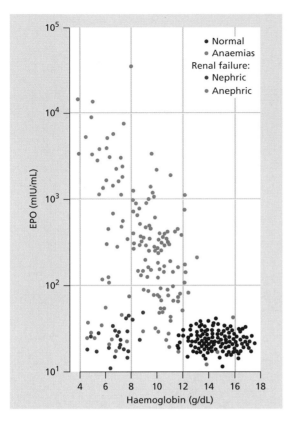

Figure 2.5 The relation between erythropoietin (EPO) in plasma and haemoglobin concentration. Anaemias exclude conditions shown to be associated with impaired production of EPO. (From M. Pippard *et al.* (1992) *B J Haematol* **82**: 445, with permission.)

Table 2.1 Clinical uses of erythropoietin.

Anaemia of chronic renal disease

Myelodysplastic syndrome

Anaemia associated with malignancy and chemotherapy

Anaemia of chronic diseases, e.g. rheumatoid arthritis

Anaemia of prematurity

Perioperative uses

Table 2.2 Normal haemoglobins in adult blood.

	Hb A	Hb F	Hb A$_2$
Structure	$\alpha_2\beta_2$	$\alpha_2\gamma_2$	$\alpha_2\delta_2$
Normal (%)	96–98	0.5–0.8	1.5–3.2

folate, vitamin C, vitamin E, vitamin B$_6$, thiamine and riboflavin) and hormones such as androgens and thyroxine. Deficiency in any of these may be associated with anaemia.

Haemoglobin

Haemoglobin synthesis

The main function of red cells is to carry O$_2$ to the tissues and to return carbon dioxide (CO$_2$) from the tissues to the lungs. In order to achieve this gaseous exchange they contain the specialized protein haemoglobin. Each red cell contains approximately 640 million haemoglobin molecules. Each molecule of normal adult haemoglobin A (Hb A) (the dominant haemoglobin in blood after the age of 3–6 months) consists of four polypeptide chains, $\alpha_2\beta_2$, each with its own haem group. The molecular weight of Hb A is 68 000. Normal adult blood also contains small quantities of two other haemoglobins: Hb F and Hb A$_2$. These also contain α chains, but with γ and δ chains, respectively, instead of β (Table 2.2). The synthesis of the various globin

tion). The main indication is end-stage renal disease (with or without dialysis). Other uses are listed in Table 2.1. In these conditions, higher doses are often needed. The haemoglobin level and quality of life may be improved (see Chapter 12). A low serum erythropoietin level prior to treatment is valuable in predicting an effective response. Oral or parenteral iron is often needed to maximize the response to erythropoietin therapy. Side-effects include a rise in blood pressure, thrombosis and local injection site reactions. It has been associated with progression of some tumours.

The marrow requires many other precursors for effective erythropoiesis. These include metals such as iron or cobalt, vitamins (especially vitamin B$_{12}$,

chains in the fetus and adult is discussed in more detail in Chapter 7. The major switch from fetal to adult haemoglobin occurs 3–6 months after birth (Table 2.2; see Fig. 7.1b).

Haem synthesis occurs largely in the mitochondria by a series of biochemical reactions commencing with the condensation of glycine and succinyl coenzyme A under the action of the key rate limiting enzyme δ-aminolaevulinic acid (ALA) synthase (Fig. 2.6). Pyridoxal phosphate (vitamin B_6) is a coenzyme for this reaction which is stimulated by erythropoietin. Ultimately, protoporphyrin combines with iron in the ferrous (Fe^{2+}) state to form haem (Fig. 2.7), each molecule of which combines with a globin chain made on the polyribosomes (Fig. 2.6). A tetramer of four globin chains each with its own haem group in a 'pocket' is then formed to make up a haemoglobin molecule (Fig. 2.8).

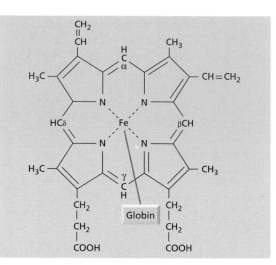

Figure 2.7 The structure of haem.

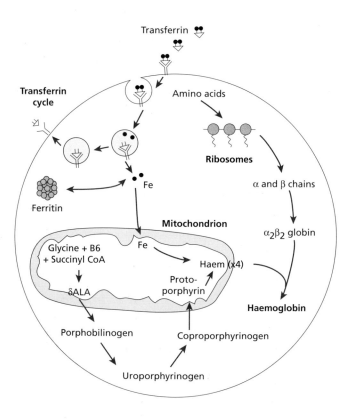

Figure 2.6 Haemoglobin synthesis in the developing red cell. The mitochondria are the main sites of protoporphyrin synthesis, iron (Fe) is supplied from circulating transferrin; globin chains are synthesized on ribosomes. δ-ALA, δ-aminolaevulinic acid; CoA, coenzyme A.

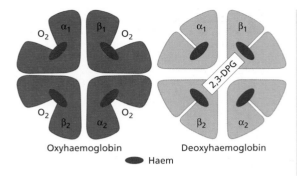

Figure 2.8 The oxygenated and deoxygenated haemoglobin molecule. α, β, globin chains of normal adult haemoglobin (Hb A). 2,3-DPG, 2,3-diphosphoglycerate.

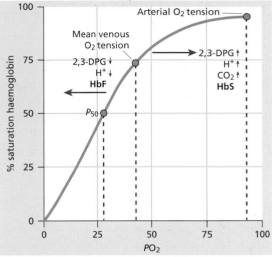

Figure 2.9 The haemoglobin oxygen (O_2) dissociation curve. 2,3-DPG, 2,3-diphosphoglycerate.

Haemoglobin function

The red cells in systemic arterial blood carry O_2 from the lungs to the tissues and return in venous blood with CO_2 to the lungs. As the haemoglobin molecule loads and unloads O_2 the individual globin chains in the haemoglobin molecule move on each other (Fig. 2.8). The $\alpha_1\beta_1$ and $\alpha_2\beta_2$ contacts stabilize the molecule. The β chains slide on the $\alpha_1\beta_2$ and $\alpha_2\beta_1$ contacts during oxygenation and deoxygenation. When O_2 is unloaded the β chains are pulled apart, permitting entry of the metabolite 2,3-diphosphoglycerate (2,3-DPG) resulting in a lower affinity of the molecule for O_2. This movement is responsible for the sigmoid form of the haemoglobin O_2 dissociation curve (Fig. 2.9). The P_{50} (i.e. the partial pressure of O_2 at which haemoglobin is half saturated with O_2) of normal blood is 26.6 mmHg. With increased affinity for O_2, the curve shifts to the left (i.e. the P_{50} falls) while with decreased affinity for O_2, the curve shifts to the right (i.e. the P_{50} rises).

Normally, *in vivo*, O_2 exchange operates between 95% saturation (arterial blood) with a mean arterial O_2 tension of 95 mmHg and 70% saturation (venous blood) with a mean venous O_2 tension of 40 mmHg (Fig. 2.9).

The normal position of the curve depends on the concentration of 2,3-DPG, H^+ ions and CO_2 in the red cell and on the structure of the haemoglobin molecule. High concentrations of 2,3-DPG, H^+ or CO_2, and the presence of certain haemoglobins, e.g. sickle haemoglobin (Hb S), shift the curve to the right (oxygen is given up more easily) whereas fetal haemoglobin (Hb F) – which is unable to bind 2,3-DPG – and certain rare abnormal haemoglobins associated with polycythaemia shift the curve to the left because they give up O_2 less readily than normal.

Methaemoglobinaemia

This is a clinical state in which circulating haemoglobin is present with iron in the oxidized (Fe^{3+}) instead of the usual Fe^{2+} state. It may arise because of a hereditary deficiency of methaemoglobin reductase deficiency or inheritance of a structurally abnormal haemoglobin (Hb M). Hb Ms contain an amino acid substitution affecting the haem pocket of the globin chain. Toxic methaemoglobinaemia (and/or sulphaemoglobinaemia) occurs when a drug or other toxic substance oxidizes haemoglobin. In all these states, the patient is likely to show cyanosis.

The red cell

In order to carry haemoglobin into close contact with the tissues and for successful gaseous exchange, the red cell, 8 μm in diameter, must be able: to pass repeatedly through the microcirculation whose minimum diameter is 3.5 μm, to maintain haemoglobin in a reduced (ferrous) state and to maintain osmotic equilibrium despite the high concentration of protein (haemoglobin) in the cell. Its total journey throughout its 120-day lifespan has been estimated to be 480 km (300 miles). To fulfil these functions, the cell is a flexible biconcave disc with an ability to generate energy as adenosine triphosphate (ATP) by the anaerobic glycolytic (Embden–Meyerhof) pathway (Fig. 2.10) and to generate reducing power as NADH by this pathway and as reduced nicotinamide adenine dinucleotide phosphate (NADPH) by the hexose monophosphate shunt (Fig. 2.11).

Red cell metabolism

Embden–Meyerhof pathway

In this series of biochemical reactions, glucose that enters the red cell from plasma by facilitated transfer is metabolized to lactate (Fig. 2.10a). For each molecule of glucose used, two molecules of ATP and thus two high-energy phosphate bonds are generated. This ATP provides energy for maintenance of red cell volume, shape and flexibility. The red cell has an osmotic pressure five times that of plasma and an inherent weakness of the membrane results in continual Na^+ and K^+ movement. A membrane ATPase sodium pump is needed, and this uses one molecule of ATP to move three sodium ions out and two potassium ions into the cell.

The Embden–Meyerhof pathway also generates NADH which is needed by the enzyme methaemoglobin reductase to reduce functionally dead methaemoglobin (oxidized haemoglobin) containing ferric iron (produced by oxidation of approximately 3% of haemoglobin each day) to functionally active, reduced haemoglobin. The Luebering–Rapoport shunt, or side arm, of this pathway (Fig. 2.10b) generates 2,3-DPG which forms a 1:1 complex

with haemoglobin and, as mentioned above, is important in the regulation of haemoglobin's oxygen affinity.

Hexose monophosphate (pentose phosphate) pathway

Approximately 10% of glycolysis occurs by this oxidative pathway in which glucose-6-phosphate is converted to 6-phosphogluconate and so to ribulose-5-phosphate (Fig. 2.11). NADPH is generated and is linked with glutathione which maintains sulphydril (SH) groups intact in the cell including those in haemoglobin and the red cell membrane. NADPH is also used by another methaemoglobin reductase to maintain haemoglobin iron in the functionally active Fe^{2+} state. In one of the most common inherited abnormalities of red cells, glucose-6-phosphate dehydrogenase (G6PD) deficiency, the red cells are extremely susceptible to oxidant stress (see p. 79).

Red cell membrane

The red cell membrane comprises a lipid bilayer, integral membrane proteins and a membrane skeleton (Fig. 2.12). Approximately 50% of the membrane is protein, 20% phospholipids, 20% cholesterol molecules and up to 10% is carbohydrate. Carbohydrates occur only on the external surface while proteins are either peripheral or integral, penetrating the lipid bilayer. Several red cell proteins have been numbered according to their mobility on polyacrylamide gel electrophoresis (PAGE), e.g. band 3, proteins 4.1, 4.2 (Fig. 2.12).

The membrane skeleton is formed by structural proteins that include α and β spectrin, ankyrin, protein 4.1 and actin. These proteins form a horizontal lattice on the internal side of the red cell membrane and are important in maintaining the biconcave shape. Spectrin is the most abundant and consists of two chains, α and β, wound around each other to form heterodimers which then self-associate head-to-head to form tetramers. These tetramers are linked at the tail end to actin and are attached to protein band 4.1. At the head end, the β spectrin chains attach to ankyrin which connects to band 3,

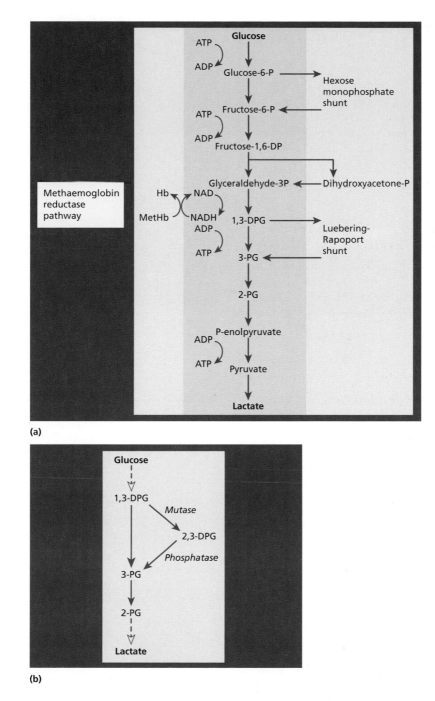

(a)

(b)

Figure 2.10 (a) The Embden–Meyerhof glycolytic pathway. **(b)** The Luebering–Rapoport shunt which regulates the concentration of 2,3-diphosphoglycerate (2,3-DPG) in the red cell. ADP, adenosine diphosphate; ATP, adenosine triphosphate; Hb, haemoglobin; NAD, NADH, nicotinamide adenine dinucleotide; PG, phosphoglycerate.

the transmembrane protein that acts as an anion channel ('vertical connections') (Fig. 2.12). Protein 4.2 enhances this interaction.

Defects of the proteins may explain some of the abnormalities of shape of the red cell membrane (e.g. hereditary spherocytosis and elliptocytosis) (see Chapter 6) while alterations in lipid composition because of congenital or acquired abnormalities in plasma cholesterol or phospholipid may be associated with other membrane abnormalities (e.g. in liver disease).

Anaemia

This is defined as a reduction in the haemoglobin concentration of the blood below normal for age and sex (Table 2.3). Although normal values can vary between laboratories, typical values would be less than 13.5 g/dL in adult males and less than 11.5 g/dL in adult females (Fig. 2.13). From the age of 2 years to puberty, less than 11.0 g/dL indicates anaemia. As newborn infants have a high haemoglobin level, 14.0 g/dL is taken as the lower limit at birth (Fig. 2.13). Reduction of haemoglobin is usually accompanied by a fall in red cell count and packed cell volume (PCV) but these may be normal in some patients with subnormal haemoglobin levels (and therefore by definition anaemic). Alterations in total circulating plasma volume as well as of total circulating haemoglobin mass determine the haemoglobin concentration. Reduction in plasma volume (as in dehydration) may mask anaemia or even cause (apparent, pseudo) poly-

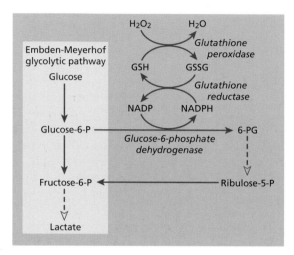

Figure 2.11 The hexose monophosphate shunt pathway. GSH, GSSG, glutathione; NADP, NADPH, nicotinamide adenine dinucleotide phosphate; P, phosphate; PG, phosphoglycerate.

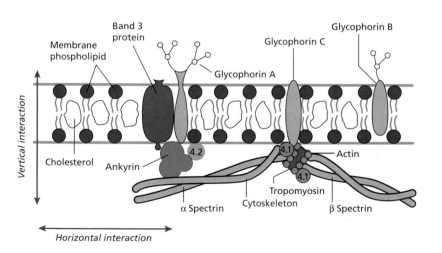

Figure 2.12 The structure of the red cell membrane. Some of the penetrating and integral proteins carry carbohydrate antigens; other antigens are attached directly to the lipid layer.

Table 2.3 Normal adult red cell values.

	Male	Female
Haemoglobin (g/dL)	13.5–17.5	11.5–15.5
Haematocrit (PCV) (%)	40–52	36–48
Red cell count (×10^{12}/L)	4.5–6.5	3.9–5.6
Mean cell haemoglobin (MCH) (pg)	27–34	
Mean cell volume (MCV) (fL)	80–95	
Mean cell haemoglobin concentration (g/dL)	30–35	
Reticulocyte count (×10^9/L)	50–150	

PCV, packed cell volume.

cythaemia (see p. 208); conversely, an increase in plasma volume (as with splenomegaly or pregnancy) may cause anaemia even with a normal total circulating red cell and haemoglobin mass.

After acute major blood loss, anaemia is not immediately apparent because the total blood volume is reduced. It takes up to a day for the plasma volume to be replaced and so for the degree of anaemia to become apparent (see p. 412). Regeneration of the haemoglobin mass takes substantially longer. The initial clinical features of major blood loss are therefore a result of reduction in blood volume rather than of anaemia.

Clinical features of anaemia

The major adaptations to anaemia are in the cardiovascular system (with increased stroke volume and tachycardia) and in the haemoglobin O_2 dissociation curve. In some patients with quite severe anaemia there may be no symptoms or signs, whereas others with mild anaemia may be severely incapacitated. The presence or absence of clinical features can be considered under four major headings.

1 *Speed of onset* Rapidly progressive anaemia causes more symptoms than anaemia of slow onset because there is less time for adaptation in the cardiovascular system and in the O_2 dissociation curve of haemoglobin.

2 *Severity* Mild anaemia often produces no symptoms or signs but these are usually present when the haemoglobin is less than 9–10 g/dL. Even severe anaemia (haemoglobin concentration as low as 6.0 g/dL) may produce remarkably few symptoms, however, when there is very gradual onset in a young subject who is otherwise healthy.

3 *Age* The elderly tolerate anaemia less well than the young because of the effect of lack of oxygen on organs when normal cardiovascular compensation (increased cardiac output caused by increased stroke volume and tachycardia) is impaired.

4 *Haemoglobin O_2 dissociation curve* Anaemia, in general, is associated with a rise in 2,3-DPG in the red cells and a shift in the O_2 dissociation curve to the right so that oxygen is given up more readily to tissues. This adaptation is particularly marked in some anaemias that either affect red cell metaboism directly (e.g. pyruvate kinase deficiency which causes a rise in 2,3-DPG concentration in the red cells) or that are associated with a low affinity haemoglobin (e.g. Hb S) (Fig. 2.9).

Symptoms

If the patient does have symptoms these are usually shortness of breath, particularly on exercise, weakness, lethargy, palpitation and headaches. In older subjects, symptoms of cardiac failure, angina pectoris or intermittent claudication or confusion may be present. Visual disturbances because of retinal haemorrhages may complicate very severe anaemia, particularly of rapid onset.

Signs

These may be divided into general and specific. General signs include pallor of mucous membranes which occurs if the haemoglobin level is less than

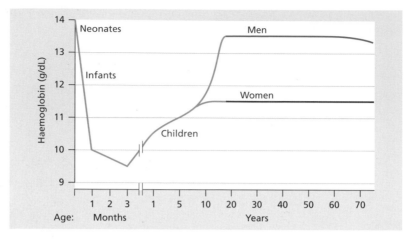

Figure 2.13 The lower limit of normal blood haemoglobin concentration in men, women and children of various ages.

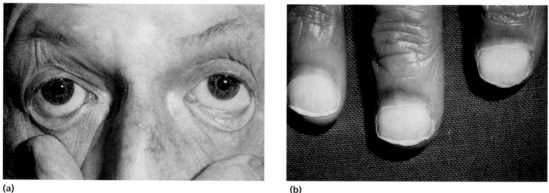

(a)   (b)

Figure 2.14 Pallor of the conjunctival mucosa **(a)** and of the nail bed **(b)** in two patients with severe anaemia (haemoglobin 6.0 g/dL).

9–10 g/dL (Fig. 2.14). Conversely, skin colour is not a reliable sign. A hyperdynamic circulation may be present with tachycardia, a bounding pulse, cardiomegaly and a systolic flow murmur especially at the apex. Particularly in the elderly, features of congestive heart failure may be present. Retinal haemorrhages are unusual (Fig. 2.15).

Specific signs are associated with particular types of anaemia, e.g. koilonychia (spoon nails) with iron deficiency, jaundice with haemolytic or megaloblastic anaemias, leg ulcers with sickle cell and other haemolytic anaemias, bone deformities with thalassaemia major.

The association of features of anaemia with excess infections or spontaneous bruising suggest that neutropenia or thrombocytopenia may be present, possibly as a result of bone marrow failure.

Classification and laboratory findings in anaemia

Red cell indices

The most useful classification is that based on red cell indices (Table 2.3) and divides the anaemia into microcytic, normocytic and macrocytic (Table 2.4).

As well as suggesting the nature of the primary defect, this approach may also indicate an underlying abnormality before overt anaemia has developed.

In two common physiological situations the mean corpuscular volume (MCV) may be outside the normal adult range. In the newborn for a few weeks the MCV is high but in infancy it is low (e.g. 70 fL at 1 year of age) and rises slowly throughout childhood to the normal adult range. In normal pregnancy there is a slight rise in MCV, even in the

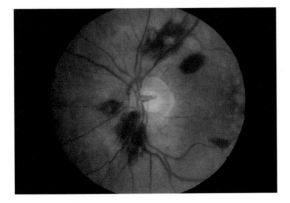

Figure 2.15 Retinal haemorrhages in a patient with severe anaemia (haemoglobin 2.5 g/dL) caused by severe chronic haemorrhage.

absence of other causes of macrocytosis (e.g. folate deficiency).

Other laboratory findings

Although the red cell indices will indicate the type of anaemia, further useful information can be obtained from the initial blood sample.

Leucocyte and platelet counts

Measurement of these helps to distinguish 'pure' anaemia from 'pancytopenia' (subnormal levels of red cells, neutrophils and platelets) which suggests a more general marrow defect (e.g. caused by marrow hypoplasia or infiltration) or general destruction of cells (e.g. hypersplenism). In anaemias caused by haemolysis or haemorrhage, the neutrophil and platelet counts are often raised; in infections and leukaemias, the leucocyte count is also often raised and there may be abnormal leucocytes or neutrophil precursors present.

Reticulocyte count

The normal percentage is 0.5–2.5%, and the absolute count 50–150×10^9/L. This should rise in

Table 2.4 Classification of anaemia.

Microcytic, hypochromic	Normocytic, normochromic	Macrocytic
MCV <80 fL MCH <27 pg	MCV 80–95 fL MCH ≥27 pg	MCV >95 fL
Iron deficiency Thalassaemia Anaemia of chronic disease (some cases) Lead poisoning Sideroblastic anaemia (some cases)	Many haemolytic anaemias Anaemia of chronic disease (some cases) After acute blood loss Renal disease Mixed deficiencies Bone marrow failure (e.g. post-chemotherapy, infiltration by carcinoma, etc.)	Megaloblastic: vitamin B$_{12}$ or folate deficiency Non-megaloblastic: alcohol, liver disease, myelodysplasia, aplastic anaemia, etc. (see Table 5.10)

MCH, mean corpuscular haemoglobin; MCV, mean corpuscular volume.

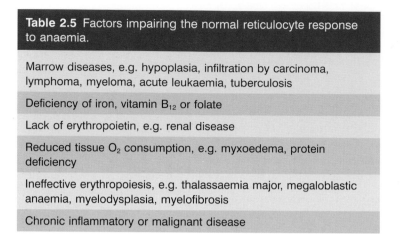

Table 2.5 Factors impairing the normal reticulocyte response to anaemia.

Marrow diseases, e.g. hypoplasia, infiltration by carcinoma, lymphoma, myeloma, acute leukaemia, tuberculosis

Deficiency of iron, vitamin B_{12} or folate

Lack of erythropoietin, e.g. renal disease

Reduced tissue O_2 consumption, e.g. myxoedema, protein deficiency

Ineffective erythropoiesis, e.g. thalassaemia major, megaloblastic anaemia, myelodysplasia, myelofibrosis

Chronic inflammatory or malignant disease

anaemia because of erythropoietin increase and be higher the more severe the anaemia. This is particularly so when there has been time for erythroid hyperplasia to develop in the marrow as in chronic haemolysis. After an acute major haemorrhage there is an erythropoietin response in 6 hours, the reticulocyte count rises within 2–3 days, reaches a maximum in 6–10 days and remains raised until the haemoglobin returns to the normal level. If the reticulocyte count is not raised in an anaemic patient this suggests impaired marrow function or lack of erythropoietin stimulus (Table 2.5).

Blood film

It is essential to examine the blood film in all cases of anaemia. Abnormal red cell morphology (Fig. 2.16) or red cell inclusions (Fig. 2.17) may suggest a particular diagnosis. When causes of both microcytosis and macrocytosis are present (e.g. mixed iron and folate or B_{12} deficiency) the indices may be normal but the blood film reveals a 'dimorphic' appearance (a dual population of large well-haemoglobinized cells and small hypochromic cells). During the blood film examination white cell abnormalities are sought and platelet number and morphology are assessed and the presence or absence of abnormal cells (e.g. normoblasts, granulocyte precursors or blast cells) is noted.

Bone marrow examination

This may be performed by aspiration or trephine biopsy (Fig. 2.18). During bone marrow aspiration a needle is inserted into the marrow and a liquid sample of marrow is sucked into a syringe. This is then spread on a slide for microscopy and stained by the usual Romanowsky technique. The detail of the developing cells can be examined (e.g. normoblastic or megaloblastic), the proportion of the different cell lines assessed (myeloid : erythroid ratio) and the presence of cells foreign to the marrow (e.g. secondary carcinoma) observed. The cellularity of the marrow can also be viewed provided fragments are obtained. An iron stain is performed routinely so that the amount of iron in reticuloendothelial stores (macrophages) and as fine granules ('siderotic' granules) in the developing erythroblasts can be assessed (see Fig. 3.10).

An aspirate sample may also be used for a number of other specialized investigations (Table 2.6).

A trephine biopsy provides a solid core of bone including marrow and is examined as a histological specimen after fixation in formalin, decalcification and sectioning. Usually immunohistology is performed depending on the diagnosis suspected. It is less valuable than aspiration when individual cell detail is to be examined but provides a panoramic view of the marrow from which overall marrow

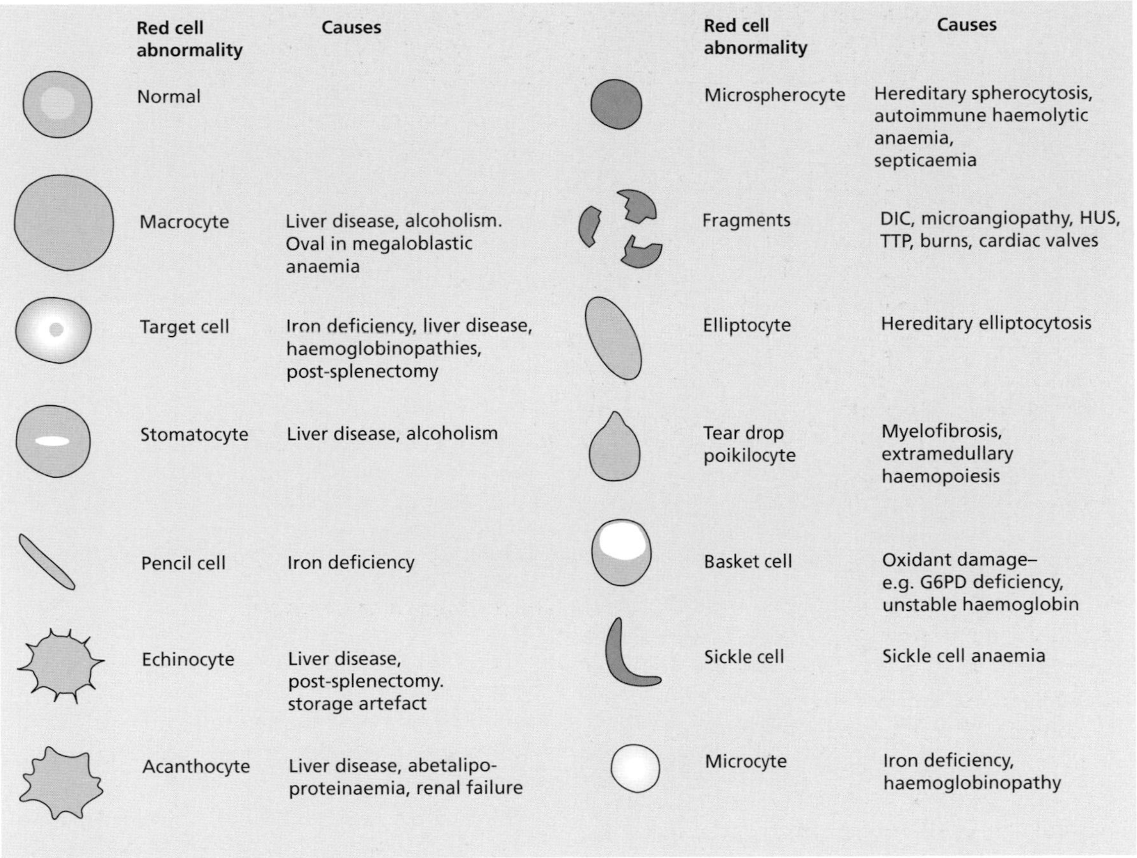

Red cell abnormality	Causes		Red cell abnormality	Causes
Normal			Microspherocyte	Hereditary spherocytosis, autoimmune haemolytic anaemia, septicaemia
Macrocyte	Liver disease, alcoholism. Oval in megaloblastic anaemia		Fragments	DIC, microangiopathy, HUS, TTP, burns, cardiac valves
Target cell	Iron deficiency, liver disease, haemoglobinopathies, post-splenectomy		Elliptocyte	Hereditary elliptocytosis
Stomatocyte	Liver disease, alcoholism		Tear drop poikilocyte	Myelofibrosis, extramedullary haemopoiesis
Pencil cell	Iron deficiency		Basket cell	Oxidant damage– e.g. G6PD deficiency, unstable haemoglobin
Echinocyte	Liver disease, post-splenectomy. storage artefact		Sickle cell	Sickle cell anaemia
Acanthocyte	Liver disease, abetalipo-proteinaemia, renal failure		Microcyte	Iron deficiency, haemoglobinopathy

Figure 2.16 Some of the more frequent variations in size (anisocytosis) and shape (poikilocytosis) that may be found in different anaemias. DIC, disseminated intravascular coagulopathy; G6PD, glucose-6-phosphate dehydrogenase; HUS, haemolytic uraemic syndrome; TTP, thrombotic thrombocytopenic purpura.

architecture, cellularity and presence of fibrosis or abnormal infiltrates can be reliably determined.

Ineffective erythropoiesis

Erythropoiesis is not entirely efficient because approximately 10–15% of developing erythroblasts die within the marrow without producing mature cells. This is termed ineffective erythropoiesis and it is substantially increased in a number of chronic anaemias (Fig. 2.19). The serum unconjugated bilirubin (derived from breaking down haemoglobin) and lactate dehydrogenase (LDH, derived from breaking down cells) are usually raised when ineffective erythropoiesis is marked. The reticulocyte count is low in relation to the degree of anaemia and to the proportion of erythroblasts in the marrow.

Assessment of erythropoiesis

Total erythropoiesis and the amount of erythropoiesis that is effective in producing circulating red cells can be assessed by examining the bone marrow, haemoglobin level and reticulocyte count.

Total erythropoiesis is assessed from the marrow cellularity and the myeloid:erythroid ratio (i.e. the proportion of granulocyte precursors to red cell

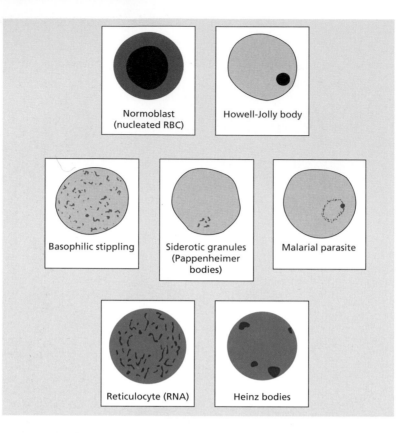

Figure 2.17 Red blood cell (RBC) inclusions which may be seen in the peripheral blood film in various conditions. The reticulocyte RNA and Heinz bodies are only demonstrated by supravital staining (e.g. with new methylene blue). Heinz bodies are oxidized denatured haemoglobin. Siderotic granules (Pappenheimer bodies) contain iron. They are purple on conventional staining but blue with Perls' stain. The Howell–Jolly body is a DNA remnant. Basophilic stippling is denatured RNA.

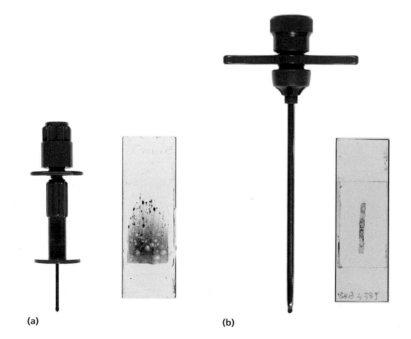

(a)

(b)

Figure 2.18 **(a)** The bone marrow aspiration needle and a smear made from a bone marrow aspirate. **(b)** The bone marrow trephine (biopsy) needle and normal trephine section.

Table 2.6 Comparison of bone marrow aspiration and trephine biopsy.

	Aspiration	Trephine
Site	Posterior iliac crest or sternum (tibia in infants)	Posterior iliac crest
Stains	Romanowsky; Perls' reaction (for iron)	Haematoxylin and eosin; reticulin (silver stain)
Result available	1–2 hours	1–7 days (according to decalcification method)
Main indications	Investigation of anaemia, pancytopenia, suspected leukaemia or myeloma, neutropenia, thrombocytopenia, etc.	Indications for additional trephine: suspicion of leukaemia, myeloproliferative disorders, myelodysplasia, aplastic anaemia, malignant lymphoma, myeloma amyloid, secondary carcinoma, cases of splenomegaly or pyrexia of undetermined cause. Any case where aspiration gives a 'dry' tap
Special tests	Cytogenetics, FISH (see p. 160), microbiological culture, biochemical analysis, flow cytometry, cytochemical markers, DNA or RNA analysis for gene abnormalities, microarrays (see p. 160), progenitor cell culture	Immunohistological staining

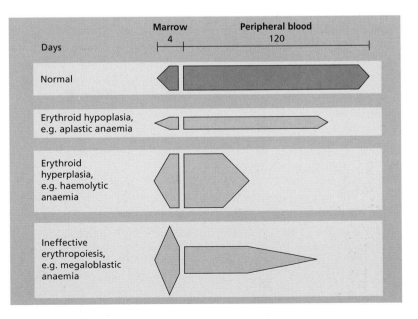

Figure 2.19 The relative proportions of marrow erythroblastic activity, circulating red cell mass and red cell lifespan in normal subjects and in three types of anaemia.

precursors in the bone marrow, normally 2.5 : 1 to 12 : 1). This ratio falls and may be reversed when total erythropoiesis is selectively increased.

Effective erythropoiesis is assessed by the reticulocyte count. This is raised in proportion to the degree of anaemia when erythropoiesis is effective, but is low when there is ineffective erythropoiesis or an abnormality preventing normal marrow response (Table 2.5).

SUMMARY

- Erythropoiesis (red cell production) is regulated by erythropoietin, which is secreted by the kidney in response to hypoxia. Erythropoiesis occurs from mixed progenitor cells through a series of nucleated red cell precursors (normoblasts) to a reticulocyte stage, containing RNA but not DNA.
- Various short or long-acting manifestations of erythropoietin are used clinically to treat anaemia in renal failure and other diseases.
- Haemoglobin is the main protein in red cells. It consists of four polypeptide (globin) chains, in adults 2α and 2β, each containing an iron atom bound to protoporphyrin to form haem.
- The red cell has two biochemical pathways for metabolizing glucose, the Embden–Meyerhof which generates ATP and NADH and the hexose monophosphate pathway which generates NADPH, important for maintaining glutathione which keeps cell proteins in the reduced state.
- The red cell membrane consists of a lipid bilayer with a membrane skeleton of penetrating and integral proteins and carbohydrate surface antigens.
- Anaemia is defined as a haemoglobin level in blood below the normal level for age and sex. It is classified according to the size of the red cells into macrocytic, normocytic and microcytic. The reticulocyte count, morphology of the red cells and changes in the white cell and/or platelet count help in the diagnosis of the cause of anaemia.
- The general clinical features of anaemia include shortness of breath on exertion, pallor of mucous membranes, tachycardia.
- Other features relate to particular types of anaemia, e.g. jaundice, leg ulcers.
- Bone marrow examination by aspiration or trephine biopsy may be important in the investigation of anaemia as well as of many other haematological diseases.

Now visit www.wiley.com/go/essentialhaematology to test yourself on this chapter.

CHAPTER 3
Hypochromic anaemias

Key topics

Essential Haematology, 6th Edition. © A. V. Hoffbrand and P. A. H. Moss. Published 2011 by Blackwell Publishing Ltd.

Iron deficiency is the most common cause of anaemia in every country of the world. It is the most important cause of a microcytic hypochromic anaemia, in which the two red cell indices, mean corpuscular volume (MCV) and mean corpuscular haemoglobin (MCH), are reduced and the blood film shows small (microcytic) and pale (hypochromic) red cells. This appearance is caused by a defect in haemoglobin synthesis (Fig. 3.1). The major differential diagnosis in microcytic hypochromic anaemia is thalassaemia which is considered in Chapter 7 and anaemia of chronic disease which is dealt with in this chapter.

Nutritional and metabolic aspects of iron

Iron is one of the most common elements in the Earth's crust, yet iron deficiency is the most common cause of anaemia, affecting about 500 million people worldwide. This is because the body has a limited ability to absorb iron and excess loss of iron as a result of haemorrhage is frequent. Also, in many developing countries, dietary intake is inadequate from childhood.

Body iron distribution and transport

The transport and storage of iron is largely mediated by three proteins: transferrin, transferrin receptor 1 (TfR1) and ferritin.

Transferrin can contain up to two atoms of iron. It delivers iron to tissues that have transferrin receptors, especially erythroblasts in the bone marrow which incorporate the iron into haemoglobin (Fig. 3.2). The transferrin is then reutilized. At the end of their life, red cells are broken down in the macrophages of the reticuloendothelial system and the iron is released from haemoglobin, enters the plasma and provides most of the iron on transferrin. Only a small proportion of plasma transferrin iron comes from dietary iron, absorbed through the duodenum and jejunum.

Some iron is stored in the macrophages as ferritin and haemosiderin, the amount varying widely according to overall body iron status. Ferritin is a water-soluble protein–iron complex of molecular weight 465 000. It is made up of an outer protein shell, apoferritin, consisting of 22 subunits and an iron–phosphate–hydroxide core. It contains up to 20% of its weight as iron and is not visible by light microscopy. Each molecule of apoferritin may bind up to 4000–5000 atoms of iron.

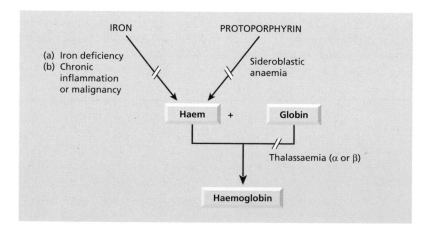

Figure 3.1 The causes of a hypochromic microcytic anaemia. These include lack of iron (iron deficiency) or of iron release from macrophages to serum (anaemia of chronic inflammation or malignancy), failure of protoporphyrin synthesis (sideroblastic anaemia) or of globin synthesis (α- or β-thalassaemia). Lead also inhibits haem and globin synthesis.

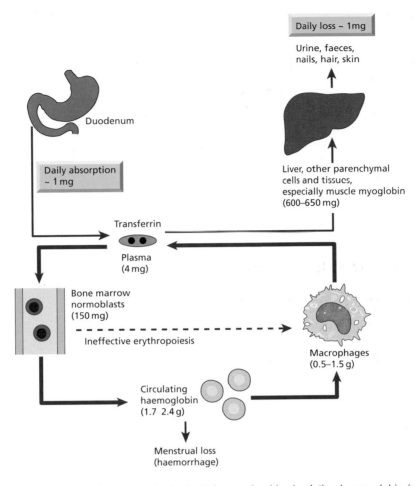

Figure 3.2 Daily iron cycle. Most of the iron in the body is contained in circulating haemoglobin (see Table 3.1) and is reutilized for haemoglobin synthesis after the red cells die. Iron is transferred from macrophages to plasma transferrin and so to bone marrow erythroblasts. Iron absorption is normally just sufficient to make up for iron loss. The dashed line indicates ineffective erythropoiesis.

Haemosiderin is an insoluble protein–iron complex of varying composition containing approximately 37% iron by weight. It is derived from partial lysosomal digestion of aggregates of ferritin molecules and is visible in macrophages and other cells by light microscopy after staining by Perls' (Prussian blue) reaction. Iron in ferritin and haemosiderin is in the ferric form. It is mobilized after reduction to the ferrous form, vitamin C being involved. A copper-containing enzyme, caeruloplasmin, catalyses oxidation of the iron to the ferric form for binding to plasma transferrin.

Iron is also present in muscle as myoglobin and in most cells of the body in iron-containing enzymes (e.g. cytochromes, succinic dehydrogenase, catalase) (Table 3.1). This tissue iron is less likely to become depleted than haemosiderin, ferritin and haemoglobin in states of iron deficiency, but some reduction of haem-containing enzymes may occur.

Regulation of ferritin and transferrin receptor 1 synthesis

The levels of ferritin, TfR1, δ-aminolevulinic acid synthase (ALA-S) and divalent metal transporter 1

Table 3.1 The distribution of body iron.

Amount of iron in average adult	Male (g)	Female (g)	Percentage of total
Haemoglobin	2.4	1.7	65
Ferritin and haemosiderin	1.0 (0.3–1.5)	0.3 (0–1.0)	30
Myoglobin	0.15	0.12	3.5
Haem enzymes (e.g. cytochromes, catalase, peroxidases, flavoproteins)	0.02	0.015	0.5
Transferrin-bound iron	0.004	0.003	0.1

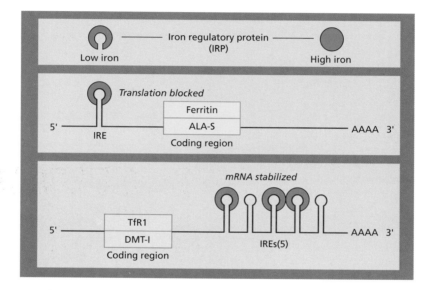

Figure 3.3 Regulation of transferrin receptor 1 (TfR1), divalent metal transporter 1 (DMT-1) and ferritin expression by iron regulatory protein (IRP) sensing of intracellular iron levels. IRPs are able to bind to stem-loop structures called iron response elements (IREs). IRP binding to the IRE within the 3′ untranslated region of TfR1 and DMT-1 leads to stabilization of the mRNA and increased protein synthesis, whereas IRP binding to the IRE within the 5′ untranslated region of ferritin and δ-aminolevulinic acid synthase (ALA-S) mRNA reduces translation. IRPs can exist in two states: at times of high iron levels the IRP binds iron and exhibits a reduced affinity for the IREs whereas when iron levels are low the binding of IRPs to IREs is increased. In this way synthesis of TfR, ALA-S, DMT-1 and ferritin is coordinated to physiological requirements. IRP, iron regulatory protein.

(DMT-1) are linked to iron status so that iron overload causes a rise in tissue ferritin and a fall in TfR1 and DMT-1 whereas in iron deficiency ferritin and ALA-S are low and TfR1 increased. This linkage arises through the binding of an iron regulatory protein (IRP) to iron response elements (IREs) on the ferritin, TfR1, ALA-S and DMT-1 mRNA molecules. Iron deficiency increases the ability of IRP to bind to the IREs whereas iron overload reduces the binding. The site of IRP binding to IREs, whether upstream (5′) or downstream (3′) from the coding gene, determines whether the amount of mRNA and so protein produced is increased or decreased (Fig. 3.3). Upstream binding reduces translation whereas downstream binding stabilizes the mRNA, increasing translation and so protein synthesis.

When plasma iron is raised and transferrin is saturated the amount of iron transferred to parenchymal cells (e.g. those of the liver, endocrine organs, pancreas and heart) is increased and this is the basis of the pathological changes associated with iron loading conditions. There may also be free iron in plasma which is toxic to different organs.

Hepcidin

Hepcidin is a 25-amino acid polypeptide produced by liver cells. It is the major hormonal regulator of iron homeostasis (Fig. 3.4). It inhibits iron release from macrophages and intestinal epithelial cells by its interaction with the transmembrane iron exporter ferroportin, accelerating degradation of ferroportin mRNA. Raised hepcidin levels therefore reduce iron absorption and iron release from macrophages.

Control of hepcidin expression

Membrane bound hemojuvelin (HJV) is a co-receptor with bone morphogenetic protein (BMP) which stimulates hepcidin expression. A complex between HFE and transferrin receptor 2 (TfR2) promotes HJV binding to BMP. The amount of HFE–TfR2 complex is determined by the degree of iron saturation of transferrin as follows. Diferric transferrin competes with TfR1 for binding to HFE. The more diferric transferrin, the less TfR1 is bound to HFE and more HFE is available to bind to TfR2 with consequently increased hepcidin synthesis. Low concentrations of diferric transferrin, as in iron deficiency, allow HFE binding to TfR1, reducing the amount of HFE able to bind TfR2 and thus reducing hepcidin secretion.

Matriptase 2 digests membrane-bound HJV. In iron deficiency, increased matriptase activity therefore results in decreased hepcidin synthesis. Erythroblasts secrete two proteins, GDF 15 and TWSG1, which suppress hepcidin secretion. In conditions with increased numbers of early erythroblasts in the marrow (e.g. conditions of ineffective erythropoiesis such as thalassaemia major), iron absorption is increased because of suppression of hepcidin secretion by these two proteins. Hypoxia also suppresses hepcidin synthesis whereas in inflammation interleukin 6 (IL-6) and other cytokines increase hepcidin synthesis (Fig. 3.4).

Dietary iron

Iron is present in food as ferric hydroxides, ferric–protein and haem–protein complexes. Both the iron content and the proportion of iron absorbed differ from food to food; in general, meat – in particular liver – is a better source than vegetables, eggs or dairy foods. The average Western diet contains 10–15 mg iron daily from which only 5–10% is normally absorbed. The proportion can be increased to 20–30% in iron deficiency or pregnancy (Table 3.2) but even in these situations most dietary iron remains unabsorbed.

Iron absorption

Organic dietary iron is partly absorbed as haem and partly broken down in the gut to inorganic

Table 3.2 Iron absorption.

Factors favouring absorption	Factors reducing absorption
Haem iron	Inorganic iron
Ferrous form (Fe^{2+})	Ferric form (Fe^{3+})
Acids (HCl, vitamin C)	Alkalis – antacids, pancreatic secretions
Solubilizing agents (e.g. sugars, amino acids)	Precipitating agents – phytates, phosphates, tea
Reduced serum hepcidin, e.g. iron deficiency	Increased serum hepcidin, e.g. iron excess
Ineffective erythropoiesis	Decreased erythropoiesis
Pregnancy	Inflammation
Hereditary haemochromatosis	
Increased expression of DMT-1 in duodenal enterocytes	Decreased expression of DMT-1 in duodenal enterocytes

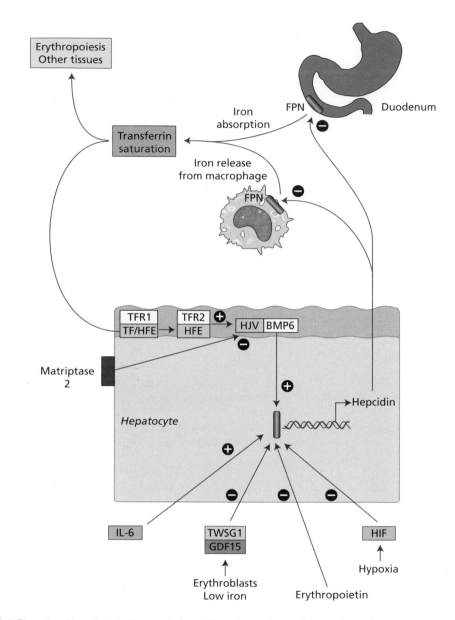

Figure 3.4 The role of hepcidin in the regulation of iron absorption and iron release from macrophages. BMP, bone morphogenetic protein; FPN, ferroportin; HJV, hemojuvelin; IL-6, interleukin 6; TF, transferrin, transcription factor Smad4 which stimulates hepcidin synthesis.

iron. Absorption occurs through the duodenum. Haem is absorbed through a receptor, yet to be identified, on the apical membrane of the duodenal enterocyte. Haem is then digested to release iron. Inorganic iron absorption is favoured by factors such as acid and reducing agents that keep

iron in the gut lumen in the Fe^{2+} rather than the Fe^{3+} state (Table 3.2). The protein DMT-1 is involved in transfer of iron from the lumen of the gut across the enterocyte microvilli (Fig. 3.5). Ferroportin at the basolateral surface controls exit of iron from the cell into portal plasma. The

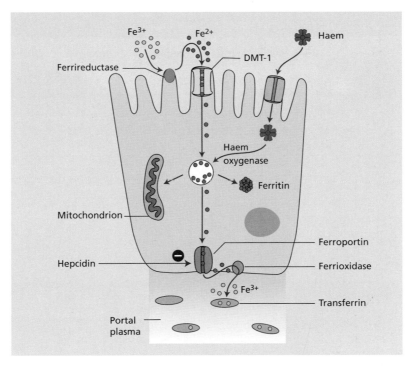

Figure 3.5 The regulation of iron absorption. Dietary ferric (Fe^{3+}) iron is reduced to Fe^{2+} and its entry to the enterocyte is through the divalent cation binder DMT-1. Its export into portal plasma is controlled by ferroportin. It is oxidized before binding to transferrin in plasma. Haem is absorbed after binding to its receptor protein.

amount of iron absorbed is regulated according to the body's needs by changing the levels of DMT-1 and ferroportin. For DMT-1 this occurs by the same mechanism (IRP/IRE binding) by which transferrin receptor is increased in iron deficiency (Fig. 3.3). Hepcidin is a major regulator by affecting ferroportin concentration. Low hepcidin levels in iron deficiency allow increased ferroportin levels and so more iron to enter portal plasma.

Ferrireductase present at the apical surface converts iron from the Fe^{3+} to Fe^{2+} state and another enzyme, hephaestin (ferrioxidase) (which contains copper), converts Fe^{2+} to Fe^{3+} at the basal surface prior to binding to transferrin.

Iron requirements

The amount of iron required each day to compensate for losses from the body and for growth varies with age and sex; it is highest in pregnancy, adolescent and menstruating females (Table 3.3). Therefore these groups are particularly likely to develop iron deficiency if there is additional iron loss or prolonged reduced intake.

Iron deficiency

Clinical features

When iron deficiency is developing, the reticuloendothelial stores (haemosiderin and ferritin) become completely depleted before anaemia occurs (Fig. 3.6). As the condition develops the patient may show the general symptoms and signs of anaemia (see p. 25) and also a painless glossitis, angular stomatitis, brittle, ridged or spoon nails (koilonychia), dysphagia as a result of pharyngeal webs (Paterson–Kelly or Plummer–Vinson syndrome) (Fig. 3.7) and

Table 3.3 Estimated daily iron requirements. Units are mg/day.					
	Urine, sweat, faeces	**Menses**	**Pregnancy**	**Growth**	**Total**
Adult male	0.5–1				0.5–1
Postmenopausal female	0.5–1				0.5–1
Menstruating female*	0.5–1	0.5–1			1–2
Pregnant female*	0.5–1		1–2		1.5–3
Children (average)	0.5			0.6	1.1
Female (age 12–15)*	0.5–1	0.5–1		0.6	1.6–2.6

*These groups are more likely to develop iron deficiency.

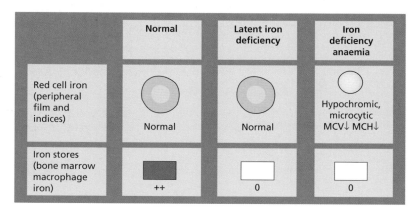

Figure 3.6 The development of iron deficiency anaemia. Reticuloendothelial (macrophage) stores are lost completely before anaemia develops. MCH, mean corpuscular haemoglobin; MCV, mean corpuscular volume.

unusual dietary cravings (pica). The cause of the epithelial cell changes is not clear but may be related to reduction of iron in iron-containing enzymes. In children, iron deficiency is particularly significant as it can cause irritability, poor cognitive function and a decline in psychomotor development.

Causes of iron deficiency

In developed countries, chronic blood loss, especially uterine or from the gastrointestinal tract, is the dominant cause (Table 3.4) and dietary deficiency is rarely a cause on its own. Half a litre of whole blood contains approximately 250 mg iron

and, despite the increased absorption of food iron at an early stage of iron deficiency, negative iron balance is usual in chronic blood loss.

Increased demands during infancy, adolescence, pregnancy, lactation and in menstruating women account for the high risk of iron deficiency anaemia in these particular clinical groups. Newborn infants have a store of iron derived from delayed clamping of the cord and the breakdown of excess red cells. From 3 to 6 months there is a tendency for negative iron balance because of growth. From 6 months, supplemented formula milk and mixed feeding, particularly with iron-fortified foods, prevents iron deficiency.

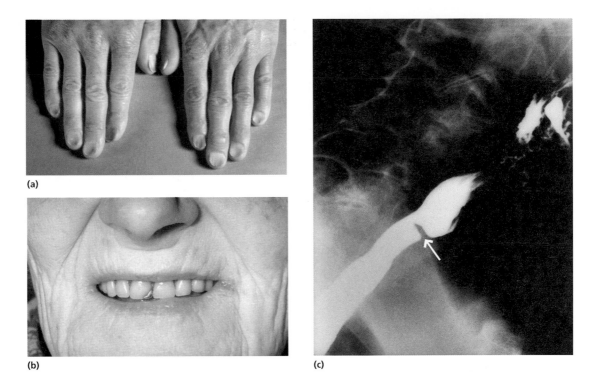

Figure 3.7 Iron deficiency anaemia. **(a)** Koilonychia: typical 'spoon' nails. **(b)** Angular cheilosis: fissuring and ulceration of the corner of the mouth. **(c)** Paterson–Kelly (Plummer–Vinson) syndrome: barium swallow X-ray showing a filling defect (arrow) caused by a post-cricoid web.

In pregnancy increased iron is needed for an increased maternal red cell mass of approximately 35%, transfer of 300 mg of iron to the fetus and because of blood loss at delivery. Although iron absorption is also increased, iron therapy is often needed if the haemoglobin (Hb) falls below 10 g/dL or the mean cell volume (MCV) is below 82 fL in the third trimester.

Menorrhagia (a loss of 80 mL or more of blood at each cycle) is difficult to assess clinically, although the loss of clots, the use of large numbers of pads or tampons or prolonged periods all suggest excessive loss.

It takes about 8 years for a normal adult male to develop iron deficiency anaemia solely as a result of a poor diet or malabsorption resulting in no iron intake at all. In developed countries inadequate intake or malabsorption are only rarely the sole cause of iron deficiency anaemia. Gluten-induced enteropathy, partial or total gastrectomy and atrophic gastritis (often autoimmune and with *Helicobacter pylori* infection) may, however, predispose to iron deficiency. In developing countries, iron deficiency may occur as a result of a life-long poor diet, consisting mainly of cereals and vegetables. Hookworm may aggravate iron deficiency, as may repeated pregnancies or growth and menorrhagia in young females.

Laboratory findings

These are summarized and contrasted with those in other hypochromic anaemias in Table 3.7.

Red cell indices and blood film

Even before anaemia occurs, the red cell indices fall and they fall progressively as the anaemia becomes more severe. The blood film shows hypochromic microcytic cells with occasional target cells and

Table 3.4 Causes of iron deficiency.

Chronic blood loss
Uterine
Gastrointestinal, e.g. peptic ulcer, oesophageal
varices, aspirin (or other non-steroidal anti-
inflammatory drugs) ingestion, partial
gastrectomy, carcinoma of the stomach,
caecum, colon or rectum, hookworm,
angiodysplasia, colitis, piles, diverticulosis
Rarely, haematuria, haemoglobinuria, pulmonary
haemosiderosis, self-inflicted blood loss

Increased demands (see also Table 3.3)
Prematurity
Growth
Pregnancy
Erythropoietin therapy

Malabsorption
Gluten-induced enteropathy, gastrectomy,
autoimmune gastritis

Poor diet
A major factor in many developing countries but
rarely the sole cause in developed countries

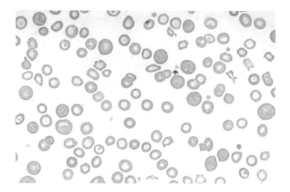

Figure 3.9 Dimorphic blood film in iron deficiency anaemia responding to iron therapy. Two populations of red cells are present: one microcytic and hypochromic, the other normocytic and well haemoglobinized.

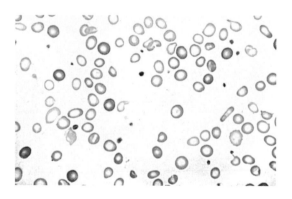

Figure 3.8 The peripheral blood film in severe iron deficiency anaemia. The cells are microcytic and hypochromic with occasional target cells.

pencil-shaped poikilocytes (Fig. 3.8). The reticulo-cyte count is low in relation to the degree of anaemia. When iron deficiency is associated with severe folate or vitamin B_{12} deficiency a 'dimorphic' film occurs with a dual population of red cells of which one is macrocytic and the other microcytic and hypochromic; the indices may be normal. A dimorphic blood film is also seen in patients with iron deficiency anaemia who have received recent iron therapy and produced a population of new haemoglobinized normal-sized red cells (Fig. 3.9) and when the patient has been transfused. The platelet count is often moderately raised in iron deficiency, particularly when haemorrhage is continuing.

Bone marrow iron

Bone marrow examination is not essential to assess iron stores except in complicated cases. In iron deficiency anaemia there is a complete absence of iron from stores (macrophages) and from developing erythroblasts (Fig. 3.10). The erythroblasts are small and have a ragged cytoplasm.

Serum iron and total iron-binding capacity

The serum iron falls and total iron-binding capacity (TIBC) rises so that the TIBC is less than 20% saturated (Fig. 3.11). This contrasts both with the anaemia of chronic disorders (see below) when the serum iron and the TIBC are both reduced and with other hypochromic anaemias where the serum iron is normal or even raised.

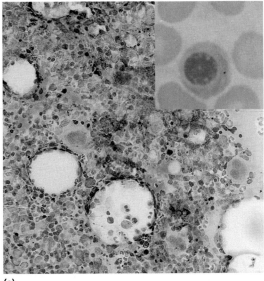
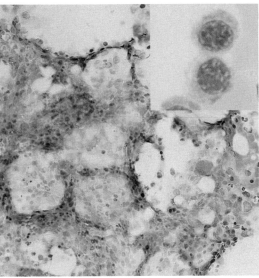

(a)

(b)

Figure 3.10 Bone marrow iron assessed by Perls' stain. **(a)** Normal iron stores indicated by blue staining in the macrophages. Inset: normal siderotic granule in erythroblast. **(b)** Absence of blue staining (absence of haemosiderin) in iron deficiency. Inset: absence of siderotic granules in erythroblasts.

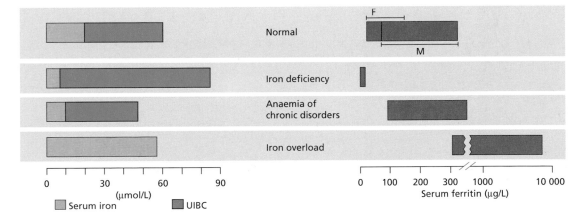

Figure 3.11 The serum iron, unsaturated serum iron-binding capacity (UIBC) and serum ferritin in normal subjects and in those with iron deficiency, anaemia of chronic disorders and iron overload. The total iron-binding capacity (TIBC) is made up of the serum iron and the UIBC. In some laboratories, the transferrin content of serum is measured directly by immunodiffusion, rather than by its ability to bind iron, and is expressed in g/L. Normal serum contains 2–4 g/L transferrin (1 g/L transferrin = 20 μmol/L binding capacity). Normal ranges for serum iron are 10–30 μmol/L; for TIBC, 40–75 μmol/L; for serum ferritin, male, 40–340 μg/L; female, 14–150 μg/L.

Serum ferritin

A small fraction of body ferritin circulates in the serum, the concentration being related to tissue, particularly reticuloendothelial, iron stores. The normal range in men is higher than in women (Fig. 3.11). In iron deficiency anaemia the serum ferritin is very low while a raised serum ferritin indicates iron overload or excess release of ferritin from damaged tissues or an acute phase response (e.g. in inflammation). The serum ferritin is normal or raised in the anaemia of chronic disorders.

Investigation of the cause of iron deficiency (Fig. 3.12)

In premenopausal women, menorrhagia and/or repeated pregnancies are the usual causes of the deficiency. If these are not present other causes must be sought. In some patients with menorrhagia a clotting or platelet abnormality (e.g. von Willebrand disease) is present. In men and postmenopausal women, gastrointestinal blood loss is the main cause of iron deficiency and the exact site is sought from the clinical history, physical and rectal examination, by occult blood tests, and by appropriate use of

upper and lower gastrointestinal endoscopy and/or radiology (e.g. computed tomography (CT) of the pneumocolon) or virtual colonscopy using the 3D colon system (Figs 3.12 and 3.13). Tests for parietal

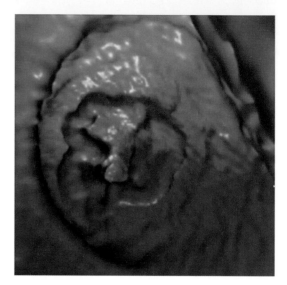

Figure 3.13 Virtual colonoscopy to show carcinoma of colon causing colonic obstruction and iron deficiency.

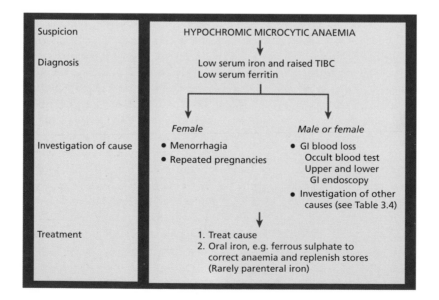

Figure 3.12 Investigation and management of iron deficiency anaemia. GI, gastrointestinal; TIBC, total iron-binding capacity.

cell antibodies, *Helicobacter* infection and serum gastrin level may help to diagnose autoimmune gastritis. In difficult cases a camera in a capsule can be swallowed which relays pictures of the gastrointestinal tract electronically. Tests for transglutaminase antibodies and duodenal biopsy to look for gluten-induced enteropathy can be valuable. Hookworm ova are sought in stools of subjects from areas where this infestation occurs. Rarely, a coeliac axis angiogram is needed to demonstrate angiodysplasia.

If gastrointestinal blood loss is excluded, loss of iron in the urine as haematuria or haemosiderinuria (resulting from chronic intravascular haemolysis) is considered. A normal chest X-ray excludes the rare condition of pulmonary haemosiderosis. Rarely, patients bleed themselves producing iron deficiency.

Treatment

The underlying cause is treated as far as possible. In addition, iron is given to correct the anaemia and replenish iron stores.

Oral iron

The best preparation is ferrous sulphate which is cheap, contains 67 mg iron in each 200-mg tablet and is best given on an empty stomach in doses spaced by at least 6 hours. If side-effects occur (e.g. nausea, abdominal pain, constipation or diarrhoea), these can be reduced by giving iron with food or by using a preparation of lower iron content (e.g. ferrous gluconate which contains less iron (37 mg) per 300-mg tablet). An elixir is available for children. Slow-release preparations should not be used.

Oral iron therapy should be given for long enough both to correct the anaemia and to replenish body iron stores, which usually means for at least 6 months. The haemoglobin should rise at the rate of approximately 2 g/dL every 3 weeks. Failure of response to oral iron has several possible causes (Table 3.5) which should all be considered before parenteral iron is used.

Iron fortification of the diet in infants in Africa reduces the incidence of anaemia but increases suceptibility to malaria.

Table 3.5 Failure of response to oral iron.

Continuing haemorrhage
Failure to take tablets
Wrong diagnosis – especially thalassaemia trait, sideroblastic anaemia
Mixed deficiency – associated folate or vitamin B_{12} deficiency
Another cause for anaemia (e.g. malignancy, inflammation)
Malabsorption – coeliac disease, atrophic gastritis, *Helicobacter* infection
Use of slow-release preparation

Parenteral iron

Three preparations are available in the UK. The dose is calculated according to body weight and degree of anaemia. Ferric hydroxide-sucrose (Venofer®) is administered by slow intravenous injection or infusion, usually 200 mg iron in each infusion. Iron dextran (CosmoFer®) can be given as slow intravenous injection or infusion either in small single doses or as a total dose infusion given in one day. Ferric carboxymaltose (Ferinject®) is also given by slow intravenous injection or infusion. In the USA, ferumoxytol (Feraheme®) is also licensed for chronic renal failure. There may be hypersensitivity or anaphylactoid reactions so parenteral iron is only given when there are high iron requirements as in gastrointestinal bleeding, severe menorrhagia, chronic haemodialysis, with erythropoietin therapy, and when oral iron is ineffective (e.g. iron malabsorption resulting from gluten-induced enteropathy or atrophic gastritis) or impractical (e.g. active Crohn's disease). The haematological response to parenteral iron is no faster than to adequate dosage of oral iron but the stores are replenished faster. Intravenous iron has also been found to increase functional capacity and quality of life in some patients with congestive heart failure, even in the absence of anaemia (see p. 387).

Iron refractory iron deficency anaemia (IRIDA)

Rare auosomal recessive cases of hypochromic microcytic anaemia have been described caused by inherited mutations of matriptase 2 or DMT-1 genes (Figs 3.4 and 3.5). There may be a haematological response to intravenous but not oral iron.

Anaemia of chronic disorders

One of the most common anaemias occurs in patients with a variety of chronic inflammatory and malignant diseases (Table 3.6). The characteristic features are:

1 Normochromic, normocytic or mildly hypochromic (MCV rarely <75 fL) indices and red cell morphology.
2 Mild and non-progressive anaemia (haemoglobin rarely <9.0 g/dL) – the severity being related to the severity of the disease.
3 Both the serum iron and TIBC are reduced.
4 The serum ferritin is normal or raised.

5 Bone marrow storage (reticuloendothelial) iron is normal but erythroblast iron is reduced (Table 3.7).

The pathogenesis of this anaemia appears to be related to decreased release of iron from macrophages to plasma because of raised serum hepcidin levels, reduced red cell lifespan and an inadequate

Table 3.6 Causes of the anaemia of chronic disorders.

Chronic inflammatory diseases
Infections (e.g. pulmonary abscess, tuberculosis, osteomyelitis, pneumonia, bacterial endocarditis)
Non-infectious (e.g. rheumatoid arthritis, systemic lupus erythematosus and other connective tissue diseases, sarcoidosis, Crohn's disease, Gaucher's disease)

Malignant diseases
Carcinoma, lymphoma, sarcoma

Table 3.7 Laboratory diagnosis of a hypochromic anaemia.

	Iron deficiency	Chronic inflammation or malignancy	Thalassaemia trait (α or β)	Sideroblastic anaemia
MCV/ MCH	Reduced in relation to severity of anaemia	Normal or mild reduction	Reduced; very low for degree of anaemia	Usually low in congenital type but MCV usually raised in acquired type
Serum iron	Reduced	Reduced	Normal	Raised
TIBC	Raised	Reduced	Normal	Normal
Serum ferritin	Reduced	Normal or raised	Normal	Raised
Bone marrow iron stores	Absent	Present	Present	Present
Erythroblast iron	Absent	Absent	Present	Ring forms
Haemoglobin electrophoresis	Normal	Normal	Hb A$_2$ raised in β form	Normal

MCH, mean corpuscular haemoglobin; MCV, mean corpuscular volume; TIBC, total iron-binding capacity.

erythropoietin response to anaemia caused by the effects of cytokines such as IL-1 and tumour necrosis factor (TNF) on erythropoiesis.

The anaemia is corrected by successful treatment of the underlying disease and does not respond to iron therapy. Erythropoietin injections improves the anaemia in some cases. In many conditions this anaemia is complicated by anaemia resulting from other causes (e.g. iron, vitamin B_{12} or folate deficiency, renal failure, bone marrow failure, hypersplenism, endocrine abnormality, leucoerythroblastic anaemia) and these are discussed in Chapter 28.

Sideroblastic anaemia

This is a refractory anaemia defined by the presence of many pathological ring sideroblasts in the bone marrow (Fig. 3.14). These are abnormal erythroblasts containing numerous iron granules arranged in a ring or collar around the nucleus instead of the few randomly distributed iron granules seen when normal erythroblasts are stained for iron. Sideroblastic anaemia is diagnosed when 15% or more of marrow erythroblasts are ring sideroblasts. They can be found at lower numbers in a variety of haematological conditions.

Sideroblastic anaemia is classified into different types (Table 3.8) and the common link is a defect in haem synthesis. In the **hereditary forms** the anaemia is usually characterized by a markedly hypochromic and microcytic blood picture. The most common mutations are in the ALA-S gene which is on the X chromosome. Pyridoxal-6-phosphate is a coenzyme for ALA-S. Other rare types include an X-linked disease with spinocerebellar degeneration and ataxia mitochondrial defects (Pearson's syndrome), thiamine-responsive and other autosomal defects. The much more common **primary acquired form** is a subtype of myelodysplasia. It is termed 'refractory anaemia with ring sideroblasts'. This condition is discussed together with the other types of myelodysplasia in Chapter 16.

In some patients, particularly with the hereditary type, there is a response to pyridoxine therapy. Folate deficiency may occur and folic acid therapy may also be tried. Other treatments, e.g. erythropoietin, may be tried in the primary acquired form (Chapter 16). In many severe cases, however, repeated blood transfusions are the only method of maintaining a satisfactory haemoglobin concentration and transfusional iron overload requiring iron chelation therapy becomes a major problem.

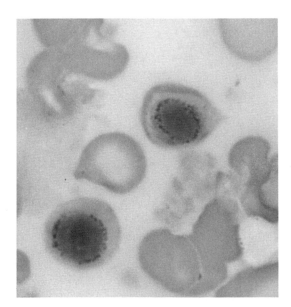

Figure 3.14 Ring sideroblasts with a perinuclear ring of iron granules in sideroblastic anaemia.

Table 3.8 Classification of sideroblastic anaemia.

Hereditary

X chromosome linked ALA-S mutation or rarely with spinocerebellar degeneration and ataxia

Usually occurs in males, transmitted by females; also occurs rarely in females

Other rare types (see text)

Acquired

Primary

Myelodysplasia (refractory anaemia with ring sideroblasts) (see p. 215)

N.B. Ring sideroblast formation (<15% of erythroblasts) may also occur in the bone marrow in:

other malignant diseases of the marrow (e.g. other types of myelodysplasia, myelofibrosis, myeloid leukaemia, myeloma)

drugs, e.g. antituberculous (isoniazid, cycloserine), alcohol, lead

other benign conditions (e.g. haemolytic anaemia, megaloblastic anaemia, malabsorption, rheumatoid arthritis)

ALA-S, δ-aminolevulinic acid synthase.

Lead poisoning

Lead inhibits both haem and globin synthesis at a number of points. In addition it interferes with the breakdown of RNA by inhibiting the enzyme pyrimidine 5′ nucleotidase, causing accumulation of denatured RNA in red cells, the RNA giving an appearance called basophilic stippling on the ordinary (Romanowsky) stain (see Fig. 2.17). The anaemia may be hypochromic or predominantly haemolytic, and the bone marrow may show ring sideroblasts. Free erythrocyte protoporphyrin is raised.

Differential diagnosis of hypochromic anaemia

Table 3.7 lists the laboratory investigations that may be necessary. The clinical history is particularly important as the source of the haemorrhage leading to iron deficiency or the presence of a chronic disease may be revealed. The country of origin and the family history may suggest a possible diagnosis of thalassaemia or other genetic defect of haemoglobin. Physical examination may also be helpful in determining a site of haemorrhage, features of a chronic inflammatory or malignant disease, koilonychia or, in some haemoglobinopathies, an enlarged spleen or bony deformities.

In thalassaemia trait the red cells tend to be small, often with an MCV of 70 fL or less, even when anaemia is mild or absent; the red cell count is usually over 5.5×10^{12}/L. Conversely, in iron deficiency anaemia the indices fall progressively with the degree of anaemia and when anaemia is mild the indices are normal or only just reduced below normal (e.g. MCV 75–80 fL). In the anaemia of chronic disorders the indices are also not markedly low, an MCV in the range 75–82 fL being usual.

It is usual to perform a serum iron and TIBC measurement, or alternatively serum ferritin estimation, to confirm a diagnosis of iron deficiency. Haemoglobin high-performance liquid chromatography (HPLC) or electrophoresis with an estimation of Hb A_2 and Hb F is carried out in all patients suspected of thalassaemia or other genetic defect of haemoglobin, because of the family history, country of origin, red cell indices and blood film. Iron deficiency or the anaemia of chronic disorders may also occur in these subjects. β-Thalassaemia trait is characterized by a raised Hb A_2 above 3.5%, but in α-thalassaemia trait there is no abnormality on simple haemoglobin studies so the diagnosis is usually made by exclusion of all other causes of hypochromic red cells and by the presence of a red cell count $>5.5 \times 10^{12}$/L. DNA studies can be used to confirm the diagnosis. In some α-thalassaemia patients, however, occasional red cells show deposits of Hb H (β_4) in reticulocyte preparations (Chapter 7).

Bone marrow examination is essential if a diagnosis of sideroblastic anaemia is suspected but is not usually needed in diagnosis of the other hypochromic anaemias.

SUMMARY

- Iron is present in the body in haemoglobin, myoglobin, haemosiderin and ferritin, and in iron-containing enzymes. Transferrin is the main transport protein in blood and hepcidin the main regulator of iron absorption and iron release from macrophages.
- Iron metabolism is regulated according to iron status by intracellular iron regulatory proteins and by control of hepcidin synthesis.
- Iron deficiency is the most common cause of anaemia throughout the world. The serum ferritin, serum iron and saturation of the iron binding capacity are reduced.
- In Western countries, it is usually caused by haemorrhage from the gastrointestinal or the female genital tract. Dietary intake is important particularly in underdeveloped countries.
- The red cells are hypochromic and microcytic. It is treated by oral or parenteral iron and by treating, as far as possible, the underlying cause.
- Other frequent causes of a hypochromic, microcytic anaemia are the anaemia of chronic disorders, which occurs in patients with chronic inflammatory or malignant diseases, and α- or β-thalassaemia. Less frequent causes include sideroblastic anaemia (some cases) and lead poisoning.
- Sideroblastic anaemias are characterised by frequent ring sideroblasts in the marrow. The most frequent is a sub-type of myelodysplasia.

Now visit www.wiley.com/go/essentialhaematology to test yourself on this chapter.

CHAPTER 4
Iron overload

Key topics

Essential Haematology, 6th Edition. © A. V. Hoffbrand and P. A. H. Moss. Published 2011 by Blackwell Publishing Ltd.

There is no physiological mechanism for eliminating excess iron from the body and so iron absorption is normally carefully regulated to avoid accumulation. Iron overload (haemosiderosis) occurs in disorders associated with excessive absorption or may result from repeated blood transfusions in patients with severe chronic anaemias. Excessive iron deposition in tissues can cause serious damage to organs (haemochromatosis), particularly the heart, liver and endocrine organs. The causes of iron overload are listed in Table 4.1 and of genetic haemochromatosis in Table 4.2.

Assessment of iron status

The tests that can be performed to assess iron overload are listed in Table 4.3. Tests may also be carried out to determine the degree of organ damage caused by iron (Table 4.3). The serum ferritin is the most widely used test and this and the percentage saturation of transferrin (iron-binding capacity) are useful screening tests for iron overload and for monitoring its treatment. Liver biopsy with staining for iron and chemical analysis of iron content is useful for assessing both parenchymal iron (hepatic cells) and reticuloendothelial iron in Kupffer cells. Magnetic resonance imaging (MRI), particularly the T2* technique, is the best non-invasive guide to liver and cardiac iron.

Hereditary (genetic, primary) haemochromatosis

This is a group of diseases in which there is excessive absorption of iron from the gastrointestinal tract leading to iron overload of the parenchymal cells of the liver (Fig. 4.1), of the endocrine organs and, in severe cases, of the heart.

The most common gene involved is *HFE* and most patients are homozygous for a missense mutation (845 G to A) which leads to insertion of a tyrosine residue rather than cysteine in the mature protein (C282Y). This allele has a prevalence of approximately 1 in 300 within the white North European population. The *HFE* gene is situated close to the major histocompatibility complex (MHC) locus on chromosome 6. The abnormal allele is associated with HLA-A3 and -B8. Only a

Table 4.1 The causes of iron overload.

Increased iron absorption	Hereditary (primary) haemochromatosis Ineffective erythropoiesis, e.g. thalassaemia intermedia, sideroblastic anaemia Chronic liver disease
Increased iron intake	African siderosis (dietary and genetic)
Repeated red cell transfusions	Transfusional siderosis

Table 4.2 Genetic causes of haemochromatosis and hyperferritinaemia.

Type	Inheritance	Clinical condition	Gene defect
I	AR	Classical hereditary haemochromatosis	HFE
II	AR	Juvenile haemochromatosis	Hemojuvelin Hepcidin
III	AR	Hereditary haemochromatosis	Transferrin receptor 2
IV	AD	Marked increase in RE iron, less hepatic iron	Ferroportin 1
	AD	Hereditary hyperferritinaemia – cataract syndrome (no iron deposition)	Ferritin

AD, autosomal dominant; AR, autosomal recessive; RE, reticuloendothelial.

Table 4.3 Assessment of iron overload.		
Assessment of iron stores		
Serum ferritin		
Serum iron and percentage saturation of transferrin (iron-binding capacity)		
Serum non-transferrin bound iron		
Bone marrow biopsy (Perls' stain) for reticuloendothelial stores		
Liver biopsy (parenchymal and reticuloendothelial stores)		
Liver CT scan or MRI		
Cardiac MRI (T2* technique)		
Deferoxamine or deferiprone urine iron excretion test (chelatable iron)		
Repeated phlebotomy until iron deficiency occurs		
Assessment of tissue damage caused by iron overload		
Cardiac	Clinical; chest X-ray; ECG; 24-hour monitor; echocardiography; radionuclide (MUGA) scan to check left ventricular ejection fraction at rest and with stress	
Liver	Liver function tests; liver biopsy; CT scan or MRI	
Endocrine	Clinical examination (growth and sexual development); glucose tolerance test; pituitary gonadotrophin release tests; thyroid, parathyroid, gonadal, adrenal function, growth hormone assays; radiology for bone age; isotopic bone density study	

CT, computed tomography; ECG, electrocardiography; MRI, magnetic resonance imaging; MUGA, multiple gated acquisition.

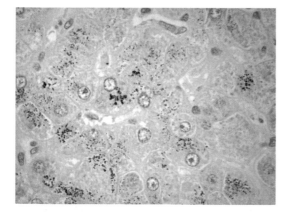

Figure 4.1 Liver biopsy. Iron loading of hepatic parenchymal cells (Perls' stain). (Courtesy of Professor A.P. Dhillon)

small proportion of those homozygous for the mutation present with clinical features of the disease and these usually show a serum ferritin >1000 μg/L. A second mutation resulting in a histidine to aspartic acid substitution H63D is found with the C282Y mutation in approximately 5% of patients but homozygotes for the H63D mutation do not have the disease.

Serum hepcidin levels are low in patients with mutated *HFE* because *HFE* is involved in hepcidin synthesis or secretion (see Fig. 3.4). Low serum hepcidin levels lead to high levels of ferroportin on the basolateral surface of the duodenal enterocyte and so lead to increased iron absorption and increased release of iron from macrophages.

The consequent iron overload damages parenchymal cells and patients may present in adult life with hepatic disease, endocrine disturbances such as diabetes mellitus or impotence, melanin skin pigmentation (Fig. 4.2) and arthropathy (resulting from pyrophosphate deposition). In some severe cases there is cardiac failure or arrhythmia. Diagnosis is suspected by increased serum iron, increased serum transferrin saturation and ferritin. It is confirmed by testing for the *HFE* mutation. Liver biopsy may quantify the degree of iron overload and assess liver damage. MRI can also be used to measure liver and cardiac iron.

Treatment is with regular venesection, initially at 1–2 week intervals, each unit of blood lost removing 200–250 mg iron. There are differences of opinion whether patients without evidence of organ dysfunction from iron overload should be treated but most do venesect if the serum ferritin is raised, whatever the organ status. Venesection is monitored by serum iron, total iron-binding capacity (TIBC), serum ferritin and by tests of organ function. The aim is to restore serum ferritin to normal, although some venesect until the serum ferritin is low (20–50 μg/L).

Rarer forms of genetic haemochromatosis are caused by mutations in the genes for hemojuvelin, transferrin receptor 2 and hepcidin (Table 4.2). All three are associated with low levels of hepcidin in serum. They often present as severe iron overload with cardiomyopathy in children, adolescents or young adults. However, ferroportin mutations usually cause reticuloendothelial but not parenchymal cell iron overload but may rarely cause parenchymal overload, depending on the site of the mutation in ferroportin gene.

Mutations of the ferritin light chain gene cause a raised monoclonal serum ferritin with cataracts resulting from ferritin deposition in the eye but no tissue iron overload. Gaucher's disease, an autosomal recessive condition, leads to iron storage in Gaucher cells (lipid-engorged enlarged tissue macrophages); serum ferritin levels are increased in Gaucher's disease.

African iron overload

This occurs in sub-Saharan African through a combination of increased iron absorption because of a genetic defect, possibly in the ferroportin gene, and a dietary increased iron overload caused by consumption of beverages of high iron content because of the use of iron cooking pots. Both reticuloendothelial and parenchymal iron are increased.

Transfusional iron overload

This develops in patients with refractory anaemias, most frequently thalassaemia major, who are sustained by blood transfusions. Iron overload is inevitable unless iron chelation therapy is given (Table 4.4). Each 450 mL of transfused blood contains

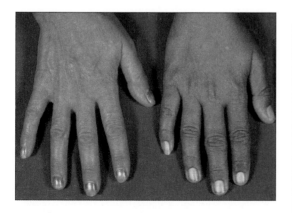

Figure 4.2 Melanin skin pigmentation. The right hand is of a teenager with iron overload caused by thalassaemia major. The left hand is of her mother who has normal iron status.

Table 4.4 Causes of refractory anaemia that may lead to transfusional iron overload.

Congenital	Acquired
β-Thalassaemia major	Myelodysplasia
β-Thalassaemia/Hb E disease	Red cell aplasia
Sickle cell anaemia (some cases)	Aplastic anaemia
Red cell aplasia (Diamond–Blackfan)	Primary myelofibrosis
Sideroblastic anaemia	
Dyserythropoietic anaemia	

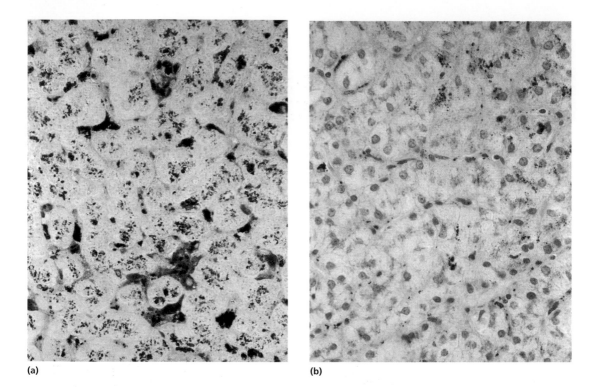

(a)   (b)

Figure 4.3 β-Thalassaemia major: needle biopsy of liver. **(a)** Grade IV siderosis with iron deposition in the hepatic parenchymal cells, bile duct epithelium, macrophages and fibroblasts (Perls' stain). **(b)** Reduction of iron excess in liver after intensive chelation therapy.

approximately 200–250 mg iron. To make matters worse, iron absorption from food is *increased* in β-thalassaemia major and many other anaemias secondary to ineffective erythropoiesis due to inappropriately low serum hepcidin levels. These are due to release of GDF 15 and TWSG1 from early erythroblasts (see Fig. 3.4). Iron damages the liver (Fig. 4.3) and the endocrine organs with failure of growth, delayed or absent puberty, diabetes mellitus, hypothyroidism and hypoparathyroidism.

Skin pigmentation as a result of excess melanin and haemosiderin gives a slate grey appearance at an early stage of iron overload (Fig. 4.2).

Most importantly, iron damages the heart. In the absence of intensive iron chelation, death occurs in the second or third decade in thalassaemia major, usually from congestive heart failure or cardiac arrhythmias. T2* MRI is a valuable measure of cardiac (or liver) iron (Fig. 4.4). It can detect increased cardiac iron before sensitive tests detect impaired cardiac function. The lower limit of normal is 20 ms relaxation time and a relaxation time <10 ms correlates with patients showing symptoms and clinical evidence of cardiac failure or arrhythmia. Serum ferritin and liver iron show poor correlation with cardiac iron estimated by T2* MRI (Fig. 4.4).

Treatment

Iron chelation therapy is used to treat iron overload. The most established drug, **deferoxamine**, is inactive orally. It is usually given by subcutaneous infusion 40 mg/kg over 8–12 hours, 5–7 days weekly. It is commenced in infants with thalassamia major after 10–15 units of blood have been transfused.

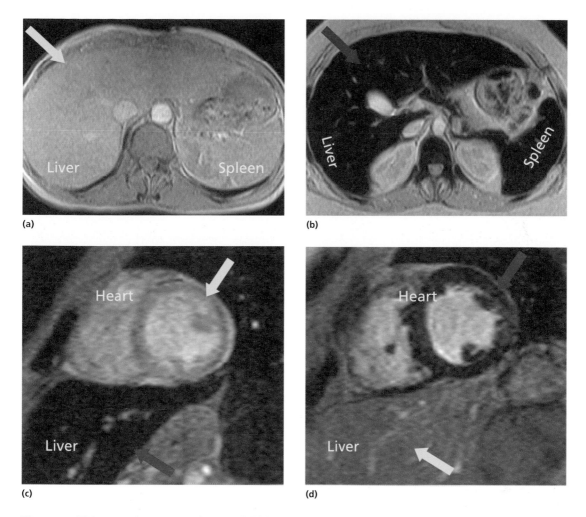

Figure 4.4 T2* magnetic resonance images (MRIs) showing tissue appearance in iron overload: **(a)** normal volunteer, **(b)** severe iron overload. Green arrow, normal appearance; red arrow, iron overload. Lack of correlation: liver and cardiac iron in two cases of thalassaemia major **(c)** and **(d)**. (Courtesy of Professor D.J. Pennell.)

Iron chelated by deferoxamine is mainly excreted in the urine but up to one-third is also excreted in the stools. Vitamin C 200 mg/day is given to increase iron excretion. Deferoxamine can also be given intravascularly via a separate bag at the time of blood transfusion. If patients comply with this intensive iron chelation regimen, life expectancy for patients with thalassaemia major and other chronic refractory anaemias receiving regular blood transfusion (Table 4.4) improves considerably. The drug more rapidly chelates liver compared to cardiac iron but in some cases intensive continuous chelation therapy with intravenous deferoxamine alone or combined with oral deferiprone can reverse heart damage caused by iron overload. However, lack of compliance is frequent and the drug is costly. In addition, deferoxamine may have side-effects, especially in children with relatively low serum ferritin levels. These include high tone deafness, retinal damage, bone abnormalities and growth retardation. Patients should have auditory and fundoscopic examinations at regular intervals.

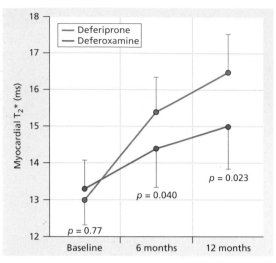

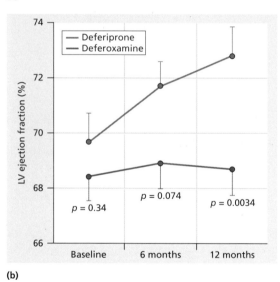

(a)

(b)

Figure 4.5 (a) Reduction in cardiac iron assessed by T2* MRI is greater in patients treated with deferiprone than with deferoxamine. **(b)** Improvement in left ventricular (LV) ejection factor is greater with deferiprone than with deferoxamine. (From Pennell D.J. *et al.* (2006) *Blood* **107**, 3738–44, with permission.)

It is usual to attempt to keep the ferritin level between 1000 and 1500 µg/L, when the body iron stores are approximately 5–10 times normal. However, the serum ferritin correlates poorly with cardiac iron and is raised in relation to iron status in viral hepatitis and other inflammatory disorders and should therefore be interpreted in conjunction with other tests such as T2* MRI assessment of cardiac iron, liver biopsy iron (Fig. 4.5) and urine excretion of iron in response to deferoxamine or deferiprone. The serum ferritin is most useful in monitoring changes in iron stores because it gives some indication of whether the stores are falling, steady or rising. The function of the heart, liver and endocrine organs are also needed to determine the efficacy of chelation therapy (Table 4.3).

Deferiprone is an orally active iron chelator which causes predominantly urinary iron excretion. It is usually given 75 mg/kg in three doses daily. It is licensed in 61 countries but not in the USA or Canada. It may be used alone or in combination with deferoxamine. The drugs have an additive or even synergistic effect on iron excretion. Deferiprone is more effective than deferoxamine at removing cardiac iron (Fig. 4.5). Compliance is also better. Side-effects include an arthropathy, agranulocytosis (in about 1%), neutropenia, gastrointestinal disturbance and zinc deficiency. Monitoring of the blood count, initially weekly, is needed in all patients receiving deferiprone.

Deferasirox (Exjade®) is the newest oral chelator. It is given once daily 20–40 mg/kg having a prolonged plasma half-life and causes faecal iron excretion only. Skin rashes and transient changes in liver enzymes and a rise in serum creatinine have been reported. The ease of administration and its lack of major side-effects have resulted in its widespread use.

Life expectancy has improved dramatically for thalassaemia major and other transfusion dependent patients with the introduction of subcutaneous deferoxamine and more recently the two orally active chelators. There is evidence that they can in many cases reverse liver and cardiac damage caused by iron overload, and may also improve endocrine status (e.g. diabetes mellitus). With good compliance, serious organ damage from iron overload should be avoided.

- Iron overload is caused by excessive absorption of iron from food (genetic haemochromatosis) or by repeated blood transfusions in patients with refractory anaemias. Each unit of blood contains 200–250 mg of iron.
- Excess iron absorbed from the gastrointestinal tract accumulates in the parenchymal cells of the liver, endocrine organs and, in severe cases, the heart.
- Transfusional iron overload causes damage to these organs and also iron accumulation in macrophages of the reticuloendothelial system.
- Genetic haemochromatosis is usually caused by homozygous mutation (845G $\rightarrow$ A) of the *HFE* gene causing a low serum hepcidin level. Rarer forms exist caused by mutations of other genes coding for proteins (hemojuvelin, hepcidin,

transferrin receptor 2 and ferroportin). Repeated venesections are used to reduce the body iron burden.
- Transfusional iron overload most frequently occurs in thalassaemia major but also in other transfusion dependent refractory anaemias (e.g. some cases of myelodysplasia, sickle cell anaemia, primary myelofibrosis, red cell aplasia and aplastic anaemia).
- Cardiac failure or arrhythmia caused by cardiac siderosis, best detected by MRI, is the most frequent cause of death from transfusional iron overload.
- Treatment is with iron chelating drugs: deferoxamine (given subcutaneously or intravenously), deferiprone or deferasirox (which are both active by mouth). Combinations of chelators are also employed.

Now visit www.wiley.com/go/essentialhaematology to test yourself on this chapter.

CHAPTER 5
Megaloblastic anaemias and other macrocytic anaemias

Key topics

Essential Haematology, 6th Edition. © A. V. Hoffbrand and P. A. H. Moss. Published 2011 by Blackwell Publishing Ltd.

Introduction to macrocytic anaemia

In macrocytic anaemia the red cells are abnormally large (mean corpuscular volume, MCV >98 fL). There are several causes (see Table 2.4) but they can be broadly subdivided into megaloblastic and non-megaloblastic (Table 5.10), based on the appearance of developing erythroblasts in the bone marrow.

Megaloblastic anaemias

This is a group of anaemias in which the erythroblasts in the bone marrow show a characteristic abnormality – maturation of the nucleus being delayed relative to that of the cytoplasm. The underlying defect accounting for the asynchronous maturation of the nucleus is defective DNA synthesis and this is usually caused by deficiency of vitamin B_{12} or folate. Less commonly, abnormalities of metabolism of these vitamins or other lesions in DNA synthesis may cause an identical haematological appearance (Table 5.1).

Vitamin B_{12} (B_{12}, cobalamin)

This vitamin is synthesized in nature by microorganisms; animals acquire it by eating other animal foods, by internal production from intestinal bacteria (not in humans) or by eating bacterially con-taminated foods. The vitamin consists of a small group of compounds, the cobalamins, which have the same basic structure, with a cobalt atom at the centre of a corrin ring which is attached to a nucleotide portion (Fig. 5.1). The vitamin is found in foods of animal origin such as liver, meat, fish and dairy produce but does not occur in fruit, cereals or vegetables. Table 5.2 compares nutritional aspects of B_{12} and folate.

Absorption

A normal diet contains a large excess of B_{12} compared with daily needs (Table 5.2). B_{12} is released from protein-binding in food and is combined with the glycoprotein intrinsic factor (IF) (molecular weight 45 000) which is synthesized by the gastric parietal cells. The IF–B_{12} complex can then bind to a specific surface receptor for IF, cubilin, which then binds to a second protein, amnionless, which directs endocytosis of the cubilin IF–B_{12} complex in the

Table 5.1 Causes of megaloblastic anaemia.

Vitamin B_{12} deficiency

Folate deficiency

Abnormalities of vitamin B_{12} or folate metabolism (e.g. transcobalamin deficiency, nitrous oxide, antifolate drugs)

Other defects of DNA synthesis
  Congenital enzyme deficiencies (e.g. orotic aciduria)
  Acquired enzyme deficiencies (e.g. alcohol, therapy with hydroxyurea, cytosine arabinoside)

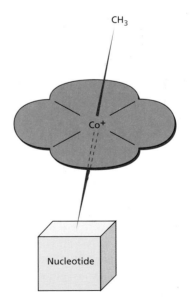

Figure 5.1 The structure of methylcobalamin (methyl B_{12}), the main form of vitamin B_{12} in human plasma. Other forms include deoxyadenosylcobalamin (ado B_{12}), the main form in human tissues; hydroxocobalamin (hydroxo B_{12}), the main form in treatment.

Table 5.2 Vitamin B_{12} and folate: nutritional aspects.

	Vitamin B_{12}	Folate
Normal daily dietary intake	7–30 µg	200–250 µg
Main foods	Animal produce only	Most, especially liver, greens and yeast
Cooking	Little effect	Easily destroyed
Minimal adult daily requirement	1–2 µg	100–150 µg
Body stores	2–3 mg (sufficient for 2–4 years)	10–12 mg (sufficient for 4 months)

Absorption
  Site
  Mechanism
 	
  Limit
	Ileum
	Intrinsic factor
	
	2–3 µg/day
		Duodenum and jejunum
		Conversion to
		  methyltetrahydrofolate
		50–80% of dietary content

Enterohepatic circulation	5–10 µg/day	90 µg/day
Transport in plasma	Most bound to haptocorrin; TC essential for cell uptake	Weakly bound to albumin
Major intracellular physiological forms	Methyl- and deoxyadenosylcobalamin	Reduced polyglutamate derivatives
Usual therapeutic form	Hydroxocobalamin	Folic (pteroylglutamic) acid

TC, transcobalamin; haptocorrin = transcobalamin 1.

distal ileum where B_{12} is absorbed and IF destroyed (Fig. 5.2).

Transport: the transcobalamins

Vitamin B_{12} is absorbed into portal blood where it becomes attached to the plasma-binding protein transcobalamin (TC, previously called transcobalamin II) which delivers B_{12} to bone marrow and other tissues. Although TC is the essential plasma protein for transferring B_{12} into the cells of the body, the amount of B_{12} on TC is normally very low (<50 ng/L). TC deficiency causes megaloblastic anaemia because of failure of B_{12} to enter marrow (and other cells) from plasma but the serum B_{12} level in TC deficiency is normal. This is because most B_{12} in plasma is bound to another transport protein, haptocorrin (previously called transcobalamin I). This is a glycoprotein largely synthesized by granulocytes and macrophages. In myeloprolifera-

tive diseases where granulocyte production is greatly increased, the haptocorrin and B_{12} levels in serum both rise considerably. B_{12} bound to haptocorrin does not transfer to marrow; it appears to be functionally 'dead'. Closely related glycoproteins to plasma haptocorrin are present in gastric juice, milk and other body fluids.

Biochemical function

Vitamin B_{12} is a coenzyme for two biochemical reactions in the body: first, as methyl B_{12} it is a cofactor for methionine synthase, the enzyme responsible for methylation of homocysteine to methionine using methyl tetrahydrofolate (methyl THF) as methyl donor (Fig. 5.3a); and, secondly, as deoxyadenosyl B_{12} (ado B_{12}) it assists in conversion of methylmalonyl coenzyme A (CoA) to succinyl CoA (Fig. 5.3b). Assays of homocysteine and methylmalonic acid in plasma are used in

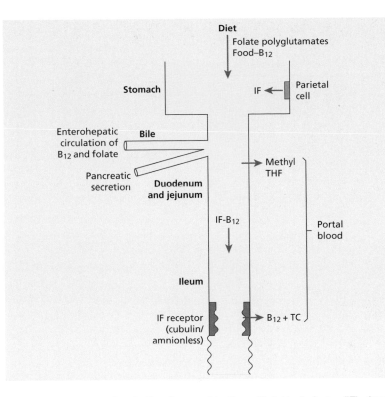

Figure 5.2 The absorption of dietary vitamin B_{12} after combination with intrinsic factor (IF), through the ileum. Folate absorption occurs through the duodenum and jejunum after conversion of all dietary forms to methyl-tetrahydrofolate (methyl THF). TC, transcobalamin.

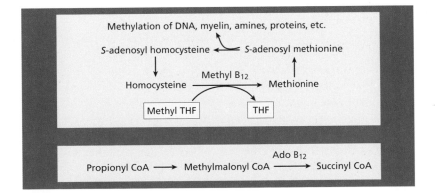

Figure 5.3 The biochemical reactions of vitamin B_{12} in humans. Ado B_{12}, deoxyadenosylcobalamin; CoA, coenzyme A; THF, tetrahydrofolate.

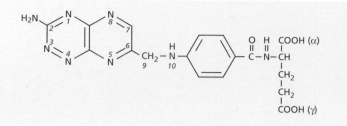

Figure 5.4 The structure of folic (pteroylglutamic) acid. Dietary folates may contain: (a) additional hydrogen atoms at positions 7 and 8 (dihydrofolate) or 5, 6, 7 and 8 (tetrahydrofolate); (b) a formyl group at N_5 or N_{10}, a methyl group at N_5 or other 1-carbon groups; and (c) additional glutamate moiety attached to the γ-carboxyl group of the glutamate moiety.

some laboratories as tests for B_{12} deficiency (see p. 69).

Folate

Folic (pteroylglutamic) acid is the parent compound of a large group of compounds, the folates, that are derived from it (Fig. 5.4). Humans are unable to synthesize the folate structure and thus require preformed folate as a vitamin.

Absorption, transport and function

Dietary folates are converted to methyl THF (which, like folic acid, contains only one glutamate moiety) during absorption through the upper small intestine. Once inside the cell they are converted to folate polyglutamates (Fig. 5.5). Folate binding proteins are present on cell surfaces including the enterocyte and facilitate entry of reduced folates into cells. There is no specific plasma protein that enhances cellular folate uptake.

Folates are needed in a variety of biochemical reactions in the body involving single carbon unit transfer, in amino acid interconversions (e.g. homocysteine conversion to methionine) (Figs 5.3, 5.5) and serine to glycine or in synthesis of purine precursors of DNA.

Biochemical basis for megaloblastic anaemia (Fig. 5.5)

DNA is formed by polymerization of the four deoxyribonucleoside triphosphates. Folate defi-

ciency is thought to cause megaloblastic anaemia by inhibiting thymidylate synthesis, a rate-limiting step in DNA synthesis in which thymidine monophosphate (dTMP) is synthesized. This reaction needs 5,10-methylene THF polyglutamate as coenzyme.

All body cells, including those of the bone marrow, receive folate from plasma as methyl THF. B_{12} is needed in the conversion of this methyl THF to THF, a reaction in which homocysteine is methylated to methionine. THF (but not methyl THF) is a substrate for folate polyglutamate synthesis inside cells. The folate polyglutamates act as intracellular folate coenzymes, including 5,10-methylene THF polyglutamate, the coenzyme form of folate involved in the synthesis of dTMP and of dTTP (Fig. 5.5). Lack of B_{12} prevents the demethylation of methyl THF, thus depriving cells of THF of 5,10-methylene THF polyglutamate and so of dTMP and dTTP (Fig. 5.5).

Other congenital or acquired causes of megaloblastic anaemia (e.g. antimetabolite drug therapy) inhibit purine or pyrimidine synthesis at one or other step. The result is a reduced supply of one or other of the four precursors needed for DNA synthesis.

Folate reduction

During the synthesis of dTMP, the folate polyglutamate coenzyme becomes oxidized from the THF state to dihydrofolate (DHF) (Fig. 5.5). Regeneration of active THF requires the enzyme DHF reductase. Inhibitors of this enzyme (e.g. methotrexate) there-

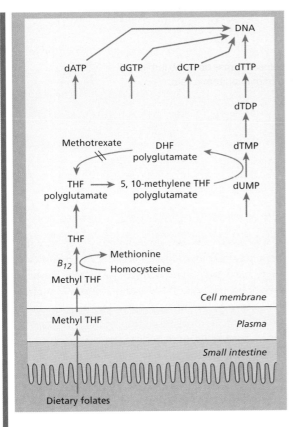

Figure 5.5 The biochemical basis of megaloblastic anaemia caused by vitamin B_{12} or folate deficiency. Folate is required in one of its coenzyme forms, 5,10-methylene tetrahydrofolate (THF) polyglutamate, in the synthesis of thymidine monophosphate from its precursor deoxyuridine monophosphate. Vitamin B_{12} is needed to convert methyl THF, which enters the cells from plasma, to THF, from which polyglutamate forms of folate are synthesized. Dietary folates are all converted to methyl THF (a monoglutamate) by the small intestine. A, adenine; C, cytosine; d, deoxyribose; DHF, dihydrofolate; DP, diphosphate; G, guanine; MP, monophosphate; T, thymine; TP, triphosphate; U, uracil.

Table 5.3 Causes of severe vitamin B_{12} deficiency.

Nutritional
Especially vegans

Malabsorption
Gastric causes
Pernicious anaemia
Congenital lack or abnormality of intrinsic factor
Total or partial gastrectomy

Intestinal causes
Intestinal stagnant loop syndrome – jejunal diverticulosis, blind-loop, stricture, etc.
Chronic tropical sprue
Ileal resection and Crohn's disease
Congenital selective malabsorption with proteinuria (autosomal recessive megaloblastic anaemia)
Fish tapeworm

Causes of mild vitamin B_{12} deficiency; other causes of malabsorption of vitamin B_{12} (e.g. malabsorption of food B_{12}, in the elderly, atrophic gastritis, severe pancreatitis, gluten-induced enteropathy, HIV infection or therapy with metformin): These conditions do not usually lead to vitamin B_{12} deficiency sufficient to cause anaemia or neuropathy.

fore inhibit all folate coenzyme reactions, and so DNA synthesis (Fig. 5.5). Methotrexate is a useful drug, mainly in the treatment of malignant or inflammatory disease (e.g. of the skin) with excessive cell turnover. The weaker antagonist, pyrimethamine, is used primarily against malaria. Trimethoprim, active against bacterial DHF reduct-ase but only very weakly against the human enzyme, is used alone or in combination with a sulphona-mide, as co-trimoxazole. Toxicity caused by methotrexate or pyrimethamine is reversed by giving the reduced folate, folinic acid (5-formyl THF).

Vitamin B_{12} deficiency

In Western countries, severe deficiency is usually caused by (Addisonian) pernicious anaemia (Table 5.3). Less commonly, it may be caused by veganism in which the diet lacks B_{12} (usually in Hindu Indians), gastrectomy or small intestinal lesions. Mild degrees of B_{12} deficiency have been reported in the elderly and ascribed to poor diet and malab-sorption of food B_{12}. There is no syndrome of B_{12} deficiency as a result of increased utilization or loss of the vitamin. The deficiency takes at least 2 years to develop (i.e. the time needed for body stores to deplete at the rate of 1–2 μg/day) when there is severe malabsorption of B_{12} from the diet. Nitrous oxide, however, may rapidly inactivate body B_{12} (see p. 71).

Pernicious anaemia

This is caused by autoimmune attack on the gastric mucosa leading to atrophy of the stomach. The wall of the stomach becomes thin, with a plasma cell and lymphoid infiltrate of the lamina propria. Intestinal metaplasia may occur. There is achlorhydria and secretion of IF is absent or almost absent. Serum gastrin levels are raised. *Helicobater pylori* infection may initiate an autoimmune gastritis which presents in younger subjects as iron deficiency and in the elderly as pernicious anaemia.

More females than males are affected (1.6 : 1), with a peak occurrence at 60 years, and there may be associated autoimmune disease including the autoimmune polyendocrine syndrome (Table 5.4). The disease is found in all races but is most common in northern Europeans and tends to occur in families. There is also an increased incidence of carcinoma of the stomach (approximately 2–3% of all cases of pernicious anaemia).

Antibodies

Ninety per cent of patients show parietal cell antibody in the serum directed against gastric H^+/K^+-ATPase, and 50% type I or blocking antibody to IF which inhibits IF binding to B_{12}. Thirty-five per cent show a second (type II or precipitating) antibody to IF which inhibits its ileal binding site. IF antibodies are virtually specific for pernicious anaemia but occur in the serum of only half of patients, whereas the more common parietal cell antibody is less specific and occurs quite commonly in older subjects (e.g. 16% of normal women over 60 years).

Other causes of vitamin B_{12} deficiency

Congenital lack or abnormality of IF usually presents at approximately 2 years of age when stores of B_{12} that were derived from the mother *in utero* have been used up. There is also a form of autoimmune pernicious anaemia that presents in childhood. Specific malabsorption of B_{12} is brought about by genetic mutation of the IF–B_{12} receptor, cubilin or of amnionless which is involved in processing the IF–B_{12} complex. It usually presents in infancy or childhood and is associated with proteinuria in 90% of cases.

Lesser degrees of B_{12} deficiency occur resulting from inadequate intake of B_{12}, malabsorption of food B_{12}, especially in the elderly, atrophic gastritis (possibly triggered by *Helicobacter pylori*) without IF antibodies and other conditions listed in Table 5.3. Serum homocysteine and methylmalonic acid levels may be mildly raised and serum B_{12} levels subnormal but in these conditions megaloblastic anaemia or neuropathy rarely occur.

Table 5.4 Pernicious anaemia: associations.	
Female	Vitiligo
Blue eyes	Myxoedema
Early greying	Hashimoto's disease
Northern European	Thyrotoxicosis
Familial	Addison's disease
Blood group A	Hypoparathyroidism Hypogammaglobulinaemia Carcinoma of the stomach

Folate deficiency

This is most often a result of a poor dietary intake of folate alone or in combination with a condition of increased folate utilization or malabsorption (Table 5.5). Excess cell turnover of any sort, including pregnancy, is the main cause of an increased need for folate, because the folate molecule becomes degraded when DNA synthesis is increased. The mechanism by which anticonvulsants and barbiturates cause the deficiency is still controversial.

Table 5.5 Causes of folate deficiency.

Nutritional
Especially old age, institutions, poverty, famine, special diets, goat's milk anaemia, etc.

Malabsorption
Tropical sprue, gluten-induced enteropathy (adult or child). Possible contributory factor to folate deficiency in some patients with partial gastrectomy, extensive jejunal resection or Crohn's disease

Excess utilization

Physiological
Pregnancy and lactation, prematurity

Pathological
Haematological diseases: haemolytic anaemias, myelofibrosis
Malignant disease: carcinoma, lymphoma, myeloma
Inflammatory diseases: Crohn's disease, tuberculosis, rheumatoid arthritis, psoriasis, exfoliative dermatitis, malaria

Excess urinary folate loss
Active liver disease, congestive heart failure

Drugs
Anticonvulsants, sulfasalazine

Mixed
Liver disease, alcoholism, intensive care

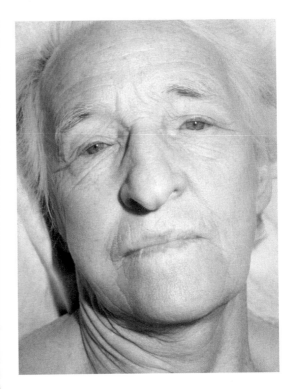

Figure 5.6 Megaloblastic anaemia: pallor and mild icterus in a patient with a haemoglobin count of 7.0 g/dL and a mean corpuscular volume of 132 fL.

Alcohol, sulfasalazine and other drugs may have multiple effects on folate metabolism.

Clinical features of megaloblastic anaemia

The onset is usually insidious with gradually progressive symptoms and signs of anaemia (see Chapter 2). The patient may be mildly jaundiced (lemon yellow tint) (Fig. 5.6) because of the excess breakdown of haemoglobin resulting from increased ineffective erythropoiesis in the bone marrow. Glossitis (a beefy-red sore tongue) (Fig. 5.7), angular stomatitis (Fig. 5.8) and mild symptoms of malab-

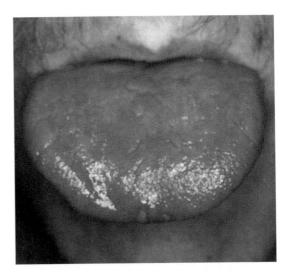

Figure 5.7 Megaloblastic anaemia: glossitis – the tongue is beefy-red and painful.

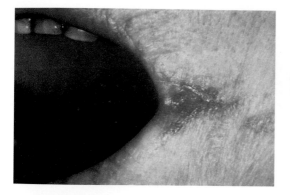

Figure 5.8 Megaloblastic anaemia: angular cheilosis (stomatitis).

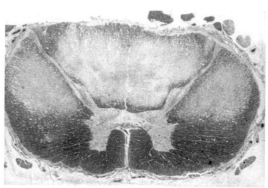

Figure 5.9 Cross-section of the spinal cord in a patient who died with subacute combined degeneration of the cord (Weigert–Pal stain). There is demyelination of the dorsal and dorsolateral columns.

Table 5.6 Effects of vitamin B_{12} or folate deficiency.

Megaloblastic anaemia

Macrocytosis of epithelial cell surfaces

Neuropathy (for vitamin B_{12} only)

Sterility

Rarely, reversible melanin skin pigmentation

Decreased osteoblast activity

Neural tube defects in the fetus are related to folate or B_{12} deficiency

Cardiovascular disease, e.g. stroke

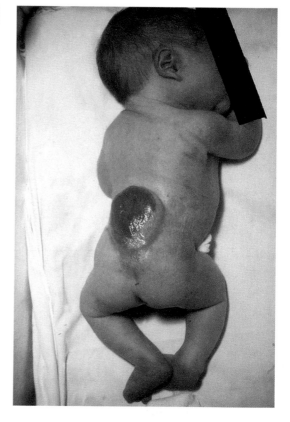

Figure 5.10 A baby with neural tube defect (spina bifida). (Courtesy of Professor C.J. Schorah.)

sorption with loss of weight may be present because of the epithelial abnormality. Purpura as a result of thrombocytopenia and widespread melanin pigmentation (the cause of which is unclear) are less frequent presenting features (Table 5.6). Many asymptomatic patients are diagnosed when a blood count that has been performed for another reason reveals macrocytosis.

Vitamin B_{12} neuropathy (subacute combined degeneration of the cord)

Severe B_{12} deficiency can cause a progressive neuropathy affecting the peripheral sensory nerves and posterior and lateral columns (Fig. 5.9). The neuropathy is symmetrical and affects the lower limbs more than the upper limbs. The patient notices tingling in the feet, difficulty in walking and may fall over in the dark. Rarely, optic atrophy or severe psychiatric symptoms are present. Anaemia may be severe, mild or even absent, but the blood film and bone marrow appearances are always abnormal.

The cause of the neuropathy is likely to be related to the accumulation of *S*-adenosyl homocysteine and reduced levels of *S*-adenosyl methionine in nervous tissue resulting in defective methylation of myelin and other substrates. The evidence that folate deficiency in the adult can cause a neuropathy is conflicting although there are some data suggesting it may cause psychiatric changes. Also that B_{12} and/or folate therapy may improve cognitive function and delay Alzheimer's disease in the elderly.

Neural tube defect

Folate or B_{12} deficiency in the mother predisposes to neural tube defect (NTD) (anencephaly, spina bifida or encephalocoele) in the fetus (Fig. 5.10). The lower the maternal serum or red cell folate or serum B_{12} levels (even when these are in the normal range), the higher the incidence of NTDs. Moreover, supplementation of the diet with folic acid at the time of conception and in early pregnancy reduces the incidence of NTD by 75%. The exact mechanism is uncertain but is thought to be related to build-up of homocysteine and *S*-adenosyl homocysteine in the fetus which may impair methylation of various proteins and lipids. A common polymorphism in the enzyme 5,10-methylene tetrahydrofolate reductase (5,10-MTHFR) (677C → T) (see p. 367) results in higher serum homocysteine and lower serum and red cell folate levels compared with controls. The incidence of the mutation is higher in the parents and fetus with NTD than in controls.

Other tissue abnormalities

Sterility is frequent in either sex with severe B_{12} or folate deficiency. Macrocytosis, excess apoptosis and other morphological abnormalities of cervical, buccal, bladder and other epithelia occur. Widespread reversible melanin pigmentation may

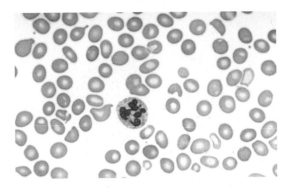

Figure 5.11 Megaloblastic anaemia: peripheral blood film showing oval macrocytes.

also occur. B_{12} deficiency is associated with reduced osteoblastic activity. The associations of folate deficiency with cardiovascular and malignant diseases are discussed on page 71.

Laboratory findings

The anaemia is macrocytic (MCV >98 fL and often as high as 120–140 fL in severe cases) and the macrocytes are typically oval in shape (Fig. 5.11). The reticulocyte count is low and the total white cell and platelet counts may be moderately reduced, especially in severely anaemic patients. A proportion of the neutrophils show hypersegmented nuclei (with six or more lobes). The bone marrow is usually hypercellular and the erythroblasts are large and show failure of nuclear maturation maintaining an open, fine, lacy primitive chromatin pattern but normal haemoglobinization (Fig. 5.12). Giant and abnormally shaped metamyelocytes are characteristic.

The serum unconjugated bilirubin and lactate dehydrogenase are raised as a result of marrow cell breakdown.

Diagnosis of vitamin B_{12} or folate deficiency

It is usual to assay serum B_{12} and folate (Table 5.7). The serum B_{12} is low in megaloblastic anaemia or neuropathy caused by B_{12} deficiency. The serum and red cell folate are both low in megaloblastic anaemia caused by folate deficiency. In B_{12} deficiency, the

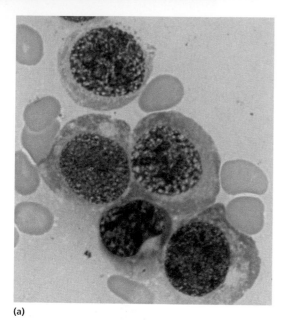 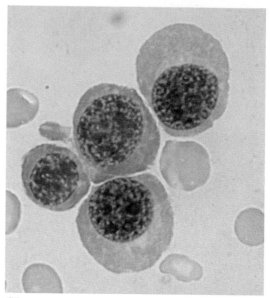

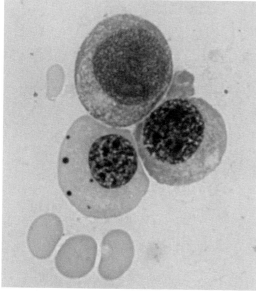 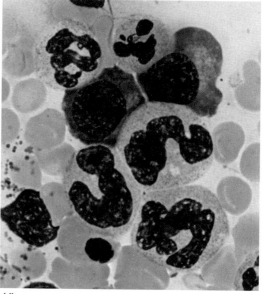

Figure 5.12 Megaloblastic changes in the bone marrow in a patient with severe megaloblastic anaemia. **(a–c)** Erythroblasts showing fine, open stippled (primitive) appearance of the nuclear chromatin even in late cells (pale cytoplasm with some haemoglobin formation). **(d)** Abnormal giant metamyelocytes and band forms.

Table 5.7 Laboratory tests for vitamin B_{12} and folate deficiency.

Test	Normal values*		Result in	
			Vitamin B_{12} deficiency	Folate deficiency
Serum vitamin B_{12}	160–925 ng/L	120–680 pmol/L	Low	Normal or borderline
Serum folate	3.0–15.0 μg/L	4–30 nmol/L	Normal or raised	Low
Red cell folate	160–640 μg/L	360–1460 nmol/L	Normal or low	Low

*Normal values differ slightly with different commercial kits.

serum folate tends to rise but the red cell folate falls. In the absence of B_{12} deficiency, however, the red cell folate is a more accurate guide of tissue folate status than the serum folate. Measurement of serum methylmalonic acid is a test for B_{12} deficiency and of homocysteine for folate or B_{12} deficiency. These are not specific, however, and it is difficult to establish normal levels in different age groups. These tests are not widely available.

Tests for cause of vitamin B_{12} or folate deficiency

For B_{12} deficiency, absorption tests using an oral dose of radioactive labelled cyanocobalamin were valuable in distinguishing malabsorption from an inadequate diet but are not now available.

Useful tests are listed in Table 5.8. These are mainly concerned with assessing gastric function and testing for antibodies to gastric antigens. In all cases of pernicious anaemia endoscopy studies should be performed to confirm the presence of gastric atrophy and exclude carcinoma of the stomach.

For folate deficiency, the dietary history is most important, although it is difficult to estimate folate intake accurately. Unsuspected gluten-induced enteropathy or other underlying conditions should also be considered (Table 5.5).

Treatment

Most cases only need therapy with the appropriate vitamin (Table 5.9). If large doses of folic acid (e.g. 5 mg/day) are given in B_{12} deficiency they cause a haematological response but may aggravate the neuropathy. They should therefore not be given alone unless B_{12} deficiency has been excluded. In severely anaemic patients who need treatment urgently it may be safer to initiate treatment with both vita-

Table 5.8 Tests for cause of vitamin B_{12} or folate deficiency.

Vitamin B_{12}	Folate
Diet history	Diet history
Serum gastrin	Tests for intestinal malabsorption
IF, parietal cell antibodies	Anti-transglutaminase and endomysial antibodies
Endoscopy	Duodenal biopsy Underlying disease

IF, intrinsic factor.

Table 5.9 Treatment of megaloblastic anaemia.

	Vitamin B_{12} deficiency	Folate deficiency
Compound	Hydroxocobalamin	Folic acid
Route	Intramuscular*	Oral
Dose	1000 µg	5 mg
Initial dose	6 × 1000 µg over 2–3 weeks	Daily for 4 months
Maintenance	1000 µg every 3 months	Depends on underlying disease; life-long therapy may be needed in chronic inherited haemolytic anaemias, myelofibrosis, renal dialysis
Prophylactic	Total gastrectomy Ileal resection	Pregnancy, severe haemolytic anaemias, dialysis, prematurity

*Some authors have recommended daily oral or sublingual therapy of vitamin B_{12} deficiency.

mins after blood has been taken for B_{12} and folate estimation and a bone marrow test has been performed. In the elderly, the presence of heart failure should be corrected with diuretics. Blood transfusion should be avoided if possible as it may cause circulatory overload.

Response to therapy

The patient feels better after 24–48 hours of correct vitamin therapy with increased appetite and well-being. The haemoglobin should rise by 2–3 g/dL each fortnight. The white cell and platelet counts become normal in 7–10 days (Fig. 5.13) and the marrow is normoblastic in about 48 hours,

although giant metamyelocytes persist for up to 12 days.

The peripheral neuropathy may partly improve but spinal cord damage is irreversible. The shorter the history of neurological symptoms, the greater the chance of recovery.

Prophylactic therapy

Vitamin B_{12} is given for life to patients who have total gastrectomy or ileal resection. Folic acid is given in pregnancy at a recommended dosage of 400 µg/day and all women of child-bearing age are recommended to have an intake of at least 400 µg/day (by increased intake of folate-rich or

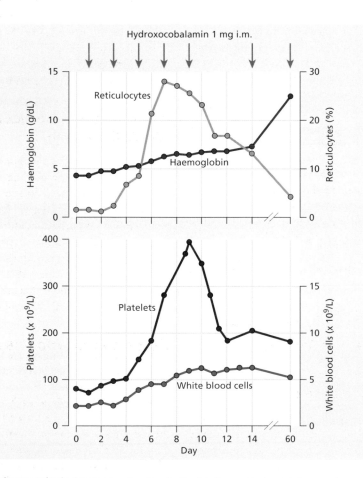

Figure 5.13 Typical haematological response to vitamin B_{12} (hydroxocobalamin) therapy in pernicious anaemia.

folate-supplemented foods or as folic acid) to prevent a first occurrence of an NTD in the fetus. Folic acid is also given to patients undergoing chronic dialysis and with severe haemolytic anaemias and primary myelofibrosis, and to premature babies. Food fortification with folic acid (e.g. in flour) is currently recommended in the UK to reduce the incidence of NTDs and is already practised in over 40 countries including North America.

Other megaloblastic anaemias

See Table 5.1.

Abnormalities of vitamin B_{12} or folate metabolism

These include congenital deficiencies of enzymes concerned in B_{12} or folate metabolism or of the serum transport protein for B_{12}, TC. Nitrous oxide (N_2O) anaesthesia causes rapid inactivation of body B_{12} by oxidizing the reduced cobalt atom of methyl B_{12}. Megaloblastic marrow changes occur with several days of N_2O administration and can cause pancytopenia. Chronic exposure (as in dentists and anaesthetists) has been associated with neurological damage resembling B_{12} deficiency neuropathy. Antifolate drugs, particularly those which inhibit DHF reductase (e.g. methotrexate and pyrimethamine) may also cause megaloblastic change. Trimethoprim, which inhibits bacterial DHF reductase, has only a slight action against the human enzyme and causes megaloblastic change only in patients already B_{12} or folate deficient.

Systemic diseases associated with folate or vitamin B_{12} deficiency

Cardiovascular diseases

Raised serum homocysteine levels are associated with an increased incidence of myocardial infarct, peripheral and cerebral vascular disease and venous thrombosis (see Chapter 27). Raised serum homocysteine levels are associated with low serum and red cell folate and low serum B_{12} or vitamin B_6 levels. Although folate deficiency (and in some studies, the presence of the polymorphism in the 5,10-MTHFR gene) has been associated with an increased incidence of cardiovascular disease, recent large randomized studies have not shown a reduction in the rate of myocardial infarction by the use of prophylactic folic acid but a reduction in incidence of stroke of about 15% has been found on meta-analysis.

Malignant diseases

Various associations have been found between folate status or polymorphisms in folate metabolizing enzymes and malignant diseases such as colon or breast cancer and acute lymphoblastic leukaemia in childhood. In most but not all, reduced folate status has been associated with an increased risk of malignancy. Large-scale studies of prophylactic folic acid undertaken for cardiovascular disease, have generally not shown in any difference in cancer incidence between those taking folic acid and controls.

Defects of DNA synthesis not related to vitamin B_{12} or folate

Congenital deficiency of one or other enzyme concerned in purine or pyrimidine synthesis can cause megaloblastic anaemia identical in appearance to that caused by a deficiency of B_{12} or folate. The best known is orotic aciduria. Therapy with drugs that inhibit purine or pyrimidine synthesis (such as hydroxyurea, cytosine arabinoside, 6-mercaptopurine and zidovudine (AZT)) and some forms of acute myeloid leukaemia or myelodysplasia also cause megaloblastic anaemia.

Other macrocytic anaemias

There are many non-megaloblastic causes of macrocytic anaemia (Table 5.10). The exact mechanisms creating large red cells in each of these conditions is not clear although increased lipid deposition on the red cell membrane or alterations of erythroblast maturation time in the marrow may be implicated. Alcohol is the most frequent cause of a raised MCV in the absence of anaemia. Reticulocytes are bigger

Table 5.10 Causes of macrocytosis other than megaloblastic anaemia.

Alcohol
Liver disease
Myxoedema
Myelodysplastic syndromes
Cytotoxic drugs
Aplastic anaemia
Pregnancy
Smoking
Reticulocytosis
Myeloma and paraproteinaemia
Neonatal

than mature red cells and so haemolytic anaemia is an important cause of macrocytic anaemia. The other underlying conditions listed in Table 5.10 are usually easily diagnosed provided that they are considered and the appropriate investigations to exclude B_{12} or folate deficiency are carried out.

Differential diagnosis of macrocytic anaemias

The clinical history and physical examination may suggest B_{12} or folate deficiency as the cause. Diet, drugs, alcohol intake, family history, history suggestive of malabsorption, presence of autoimmune diseases or other associations with pernicious anaemia (Table 5.4), previous gastrointestinal disease or operations are all important. The presence of jaundice, glossitis or a neuropathy are also valuable indications of megaloblastic anaemia.

The laboratory features of particular importance are the shape of macrocytes (oval in megaloblastic anaemia), the presence of hypersegmented neutrophils and of leucopenia and thrombocytopenia in megaloblastic anaemia and the bone marrow appearance. Assay of serum B_{12} and folate is essential. Exclusion of alcoholism (particularly if the patient is not anaemic), liver and thyroid function tests, and bone marrow examination for myelodysplasia, aplasia or myeloma are important in the investigation of macrocytosis not caused by B_{12} or folate deficiency.

SUMMARY

- Macrocytic anaemias show an increased size of circulating red cells (MCV > 98 fl). Causes include vitamin B_{12} (B_{12}, cobalamin) or folate deficiency, alcohol, liver disease, hypothyroidism, myelodysplasia, paraproteinaemia, cytotoxic drugs, aplastic anaemia, pregnancy and the neonatal period.
- B_{12} or folate deficiency cause megaloblastic anaemia, in which the bone marrow erythroblasts have a typical abnormal appearance.
- B_{12} deficiency is usually caused by B_{12} malabsorption brought about by pernicious anaemia in which there is autoimmune gastritis, resulting in severe deficiency of intrinsic factor, a glycoprotein made in the stomach which facilitates B_{12} absorption by the ileum.
- Other gastrointestinal diseases as well as a vegan diet may cause B_{12} deficiency.
- Folate deficiency may be caused by a poor diet, malabsorption (e.g. gluten-induced enteropathy) or excess cell turnover (e.g. pregnancy, haemolytic anaemias, malignancy).
- Treatment of B_{12} deficiency is usually with injections of hydroxocobalamin and of folate deficiency with oral folic (pteroylglutamic) acid.
- Rare causes of megaloblastic anaemia include inborn errors of B_{12} or folate transport or metabolism, and defects of DNA synthesis not related to B_{12} or folate.

Now visit www.wiley.com/go/essentialhaematology to test yourself on this chapter.

CHAPTER 6
Haemolytic anaemias

Key topics

Essential Haematology, 6th Edition. © A. V. Hoffbrand and P. A. H. Moss. Published 2011 by Blackwell Publishing Ltd.

Normal red cell destruction

Red cell destruction normally occurs after a mean lifespan of 120 days when the cells are removed extravascularly by the macrophages of the reticulo-endothelial (RE) system, especially in the marrow but also in the liver and spleen. As the cells have no nucleus, red cell metabolism gradually deteriorates as enzymes are degraded and not replaced and the cells become non-viable. The breakdown of haem from red cells liberates iron for recirculation via plasma transferrin mainly to marrow erythroblasts, and protoporphyrin which is broken down to bilirubin. Bilirubin circulates to the liver where it is conjugated to glucuronides which are excreted into the duodenum via bile and converted to sterco-bilinogen and stercobilin (excreted in faeces) (Fig. 6.1). Stercobilinogen and stercobilin are partly reabsorbed and excreted in urine as urobilinogen and urobilin. Globin chains are broken down to amino acids which are reutilized for general protein synthesis in the body.

Haptoglobins are proteins present in normal plasma capable of binding haemoglobin. The haemoglobin–haptoglobin complex is removed from plasma by the RE system. Intravascular haemolysis (breakdown of red cells within blood vessels) plays little or no part in normal red cell destruction.

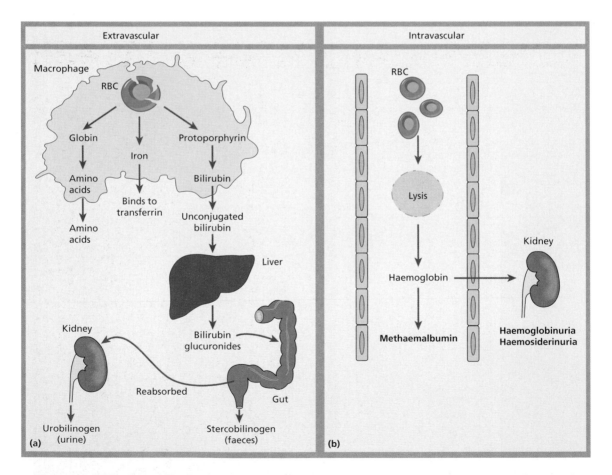

Figure 6.1 (a) Normal red blood cell (RBC) breakdown. This takes place extravascularly in the macrophages of the reticuloendothelial system. **(b)** Intravascular haemolysis occurs in some pathological disorders.

Introduction to haemolytic anaemias

Haemolytic anaemias are defined as those anaemias that result from an increase in the rate of red cell destruction. Because of erythropoietic hyperplasia and anatomical extension of bone marrow, red cell destruction may be increased several-fold before the patient becomes anaemic – compensated haemolytic disease. The normal adult marrow, after full expansion, is able to produce red cells at 6–8 times the normal rate provided this is 'effective'. Therefore, haemolytic anaemia may not be seen until the red cell lifespan is less than 30 days. It leads to a marked reticulocytosis, particularly in the more anaemic cases.

Classification

Table 6.1 is a simplified classification of the haemolytic anaemias. Hereditary haemolytic anaemias are the result of 'intrinsic' red cell defects whereas acquired haemolytic anaemias are usually the result of an 'extracorpuscular' or 'environmental' change. Paroxysmal nocturnal haemoglobinuria (PNH) is the exception because although it is an acquired disorder, the PNH red cells have an intrinsic defect.

Clinical features

The patient may show pallor of the mucous membranes, mild fluctuating jaundice and splenomegaly. There is no bilirubin in urine but this may turn dark

Table 6.1 Classification of haemolytic anaemias.

Hereditary	Acquired
Membrane Hereditary spherocytosis, hereditary elliptocytosis	**Immune** *Autoimmune* Warm antibody type Cold antibody type
Metabolism G6PD deficiency, pyruvate kinase deficiency	*Alloimmune* Haemolytic transfusion reactions Haemolytic disease of the newborn Allografts, especially stem cell transplantation
Haemoglobin Genetic abnormalities (Hb S, Hb C, unstable); see Chapter 7	*Drug associated*
	Red cell fragmentation syndromes See Table 6.6
	March haemoglobinuria
	Infections Malaria, clostridia
	Chemical and physical agents Especially drugs, industrial/domestic substances, burns
	Secondary Liver and renal disease
	Paroxysmal nocturnal haemoglobinuria

G6PD, glucose-6-phosphate dehydrogenase; Hb, haemoglobin.

on standing because of excess urobilinogen. Pigment (bilirubin) gallstones may complicate the condition (Fig. 6.2) and some patients (particularly with sickle cell disease) develop ulcers around the ankle. Aplastic crises may occur, usually precipitated by infection with parvovirus which 'switches off' erythropoiesis, and are characterized by a sudden increase in anaemia and drop in reticulocyte count (see Fig. 22.4).

Rarely, folate deficiency may cause an aplastic crisis in which the bone marrow is megaloblastic.

Laboratory findings

The laboratory findings are conveniently divided into three groups.

1 Features of increased red cell breakdown:
  (a) Serum bilirubin raised, unconjugated and bound to albumin;
  (b) Urine urobilinogen increased;
  (c) Serum haptoglobins absent because the haptoglobins become saturated with haemoglobin and the complex is removed by RE cells.
2 Features of increased red cell production:
  (a) Reticulocytosis;

  (b) Bone marrow erythroid hyperplasia; the normal marrow myeloid : erythroid ratio of 2 : 1 to 12 : 1 is reduced to 1 : 1 or reversed.
3 Damaged red cells:
  (a) Morphology (e.g. microspherocytes, elliptocytes, fragments);
  (b) Osmotic fragility, autohaemolysis, etc.;
  (c) Specific enzyme, protein or DNA tests.

Intravascular and extravascular haemolysis

There are two mechanisms whereby red cells are destroyed in haemolytic anaemia. There may be excessive removal of red cells by macrophages of the RE system (extravascular haemolysis) or they may be broken down directly in the circulation (intravascular haemolysis) (Table 6.2; Fig. 6.1). Whichever mechanism dominates will depend on the pathology involved. In intravascular haemolysis, free haemoglobin is released which rapidly saturates plasma haptoglobins and the excess free haemoglobin is filtered by the glomerulus. If the rate of haemolysis saturates the renal tubular reabsorptive capacity, free haemoglobin enters urine (Fig. 6.3a) and, as iron is released, the renal tubules become loaded with haemosiderin. Methaemalbumin is

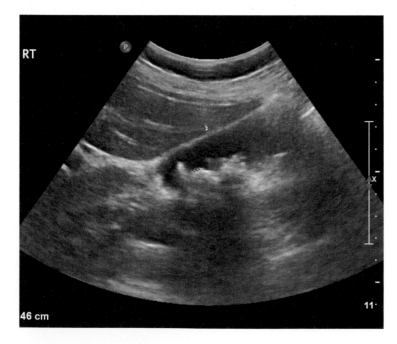

Figure 6.2 Ultrasound of multiple small pigment gallstones typical of those associated with hereditary spherocytosis. (Courtesy of Dr P. Wylie.)

Table 6.2 Causes of intravascular haemolysis.

Mismatched blood transfusion (usually ABO)

G6PD deficiency with oxidant stress

Red cell fragmentation syndromes

Some autoimmune haemolytic anaemias

Some drug- and infection-induced haemolytic anaemias

Paroxysmal nocturnal haemoglobinuria

March haemoglobinuria

Unstable haemoglobin

G6PD, glucose-6-phosphate dehydrogenase.

also formed from the process of intravascular haemolysis.

The main laboratory features of intravascular haemolysis are:

1 Haemoglobinaemia and haemoglobinuria;
2 Haemosiderinuria (iron storage protein in the spun deposit of urine (Fig. 6.3b));
3 Methaemalbuminaemia (detected spectrophotometrically by Schumm's test).

Hereditary haemolytic anaemias

Membrane defects

Hereditary spherocytosis

Hereditary spherocytosis (HS) is the most common hereditary haemolytic anaemia in northern Europeans.

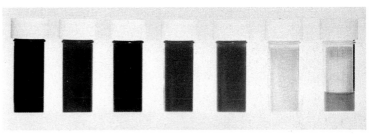

(a)

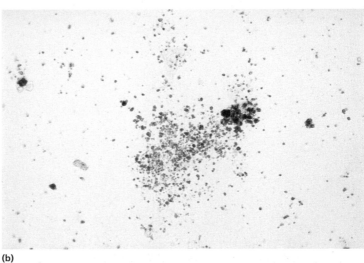

Figure 6.3 (a) Progressive urine samples in an acute episode of intravascular haemolysis showing haemoglobinuria of decreasing severity. **(b)** Prussian blue-positive deposits of haemosiderin in a urine spun deposit (Perls' stain).

(b)

Pathogenesis

HS is usually caused by defects in the proteins involved in the vertical interactions between the membrane skeleton and the lipid bilayer of the red cell (Table 6.3; see Fig. 2.12). The loss of membrane may be caused by the release of parts of the lipid bilayer that are not supported by the skeleton. In HS, the marrow produces red cells of normal biconcave shape but these lose membrane and become increasingly spherical (loss of surface area relative to volume) as they circulate through the spleen and the rest of the RE system. Ultimately, the spherocytes are unable to pass through the splenic microcirculation where they die prematurely.

Table 6.3 Molecular basis of hereditary spherocytosis and elliptocytosis.

Hereditary spherocytosis
Ankyrin deficiency or abnormalities
α- or β-spectrin deficiency or abnormalities
Band 3 abnormalities
Pallidin (protein 4.2) abnormalities

Hereditary elliptocytosis
α- or β-spectrin mutants leading to defective
  spectrin dimer formation
α- or β-spectrin mutants leading to defective
  spectrin–ankyrin associations
Protein 4.1 deficiency or abnormality

South-East Asian ovalocytosis (band 3 deletion)

Clinical features

The inheritance is autosomal dominant with variable expression; rarely it may be autosomal recessive. The anaemia can present at any age from infancy to old age. Jaundice is typically fluctuating and is particularly marked if the haemolytic anaemia is associated with Gilbert's disease (a defect of hepatic conjugation of bilirubin); splenomegaly occurs in most patients. Pigment gallstones are frequent (Fig. 6.2); aplastic crises, usually precipitated by parvovirus infection, may cause a sudden increase in severity of anaemia (see Fig. 22.5).

Haematological findings

Anaemia is usual but not invariable; its severity tends to be similar in members of the same family. Reticulocytes are usually 5–20%. The blood film shows microspherocytes (Fig. 6.4a) that are densely staining with smaller diameters than normal red cells.

Investigation and treatment

A rapid fluorescent flow analysis of eosin-maleimide bound to red cells is used as a test for HS and membrane band 3 protein deficiency (Fig. 6.5). This has replaced the classic osmotic fragility test which showed the HS red cells to be excessively fragile in dilute saline solution. The identification of the exact molecular defect is not needed for management. The direct antiglobulin (Coombs) test is

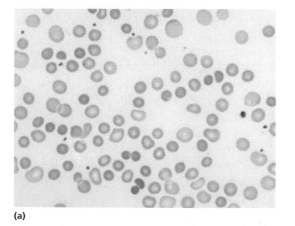
(a)

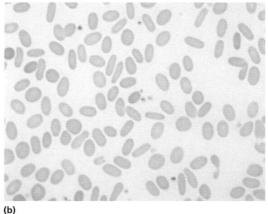
(b)

Figure 6.4 (a) Blood film in hereditary spherocytosis. The spherocytes are deeply staining and of small diameter. Larger polychromatic cells are reticulocytes (confirmed by supravital staining). **(b)** Blood film in hereditary elliptocytosis.

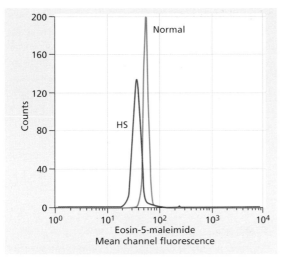

Figure 6.5 Eosin-5-maleimide staining in hereditary spherocytosis (HS) showing reduced mean channel fluorescence due to membrane band 3 protein deficiency. (Courtesy of Mr G. Ellis.)

normal, excluding an autoimmune cause of spherocytosis and haemolysis.

The principal form of treatment is splenectomy, preferably laparoscopic, although this should not be performed unless clinically indicated because of symptomatic anaemia, gallstones, leg ulcers or growth retardation. This is because of the risk of post-splenectomy sepsis, particularly in early childhood (see p. 148). There is also evidence for late vascular complications. Cholecystectomy should be performed with splenectomy if symptomatic gallstones are present. Splenectomy should always produce a rise in the haemoglobin level to normal, even though microspherocytes formed in the rest of the RE system will remain.

Hereditary elliptocytosis

This has similar clinical and laboratory features to HS except for the appearance of the blood film (Fig. 6.4b), but it is usually a clinically milder disorder. It is usually discovered by chance on a blood film and there may be no evidence of haemolysis. Occasional patients require splenectomy. The basic defect is a failure of spectrin heterodimers to self-associate into heterotetramers. A number of genetic mutations affecting horizontal interactions have been detected (Table 6.3). Patients with homozygous or doubly heterozygous elliptocytosis present with

a severe haemolytic anaemia with microspherocytes, poikilocytes and splenomegaly (hereditary pyropoikilocytosis).

South-East Asian ovalocytosis

This is common in Melanesia, Malaysia, Indonesia and the Philippines and is caused by a nine amino acid deletion at the junction of the cytoplasmic and transmembrane domains of the band 3 protein. The cells are rigid and resist invasion by malarial parasites. Most cases are not anaemic and are asymptomatic.

Defective red cell metabolism

Glucose-6-phosphate dehydrogenase deficiency

Glucose-6-phosphate dehydrogenase (G6PD) functions to reduce nicotinamide adenine dinucleotide phosphate (NADP). It is the only source of NADPH that is needed for the production of reduced glutathione. Deficiency of G6PD renders the red cell susceptible to oxidant stress (Fig. 6.6).

Epidemiology

There is a wide variety of normal genetic variants of the enzyme G6PD, the most common being type B (Western) and type A in Africans. In addition, more than 400 variants caused by point mutations or deletions of the enzyme G6PD have been characterized that show less activity than normal and worldwide over 400 million people are G6PD deficient in enzyme activity (Fig. 6.7).

The inheritance is sex-linked, affecting males, and carried by females who show approximately half the normal red cell G6PD values. The female heterozygotes have an advantage of resistance to *Falciparum* malaria. The main races affected are in West Africa, the Mediterranean, the Middle East and South-East Asia. The degree of deficiency varies, often being mild (10–15% of normal activity) in black Africans, more severe in Orientals and most severe in Mediterraneans. Severe deficiency occurs occasionally in white people.

Clinical features

G6PD deficiency is usually asymptomatic. Although G6PD is present in all cells, the main syndromes that occur are as follow:

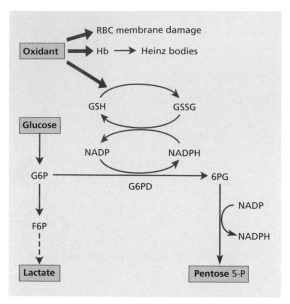

Figure 6.6 Haemoglobin and red blood cell (RBC) membranes are usually protected from oxidant stress by reduced glutathione (GSH). In G6PD deficiency, NADPH and GSH synthesis is impaired. F6P, fructose-6-phosphate; G6P, glucose-6-phosphate; G6PD, glucose-6-phosphate dehydrogenase; GSSG, glutathione (oxidized form); NADP, nicotinamide adenine dinucleotide phosphate.

1 Acute haemolytic anaemia in response to oxidant stress, e.g. drugs, fava beans or infections (Table 6.4). The acute haemolytic anaemia is caused by rapidly developing intravascular haemolysis with haemoglobinuria (Fig. 6.3a). The anaemia may be self-limiting as new young red cells are made with near normal enzyme levels.
2 Neonatal jaundice.
3 Rarely, a congenital non-spherocytic haemolytic anaemia.

These syndromes may result from different types of severe enzyme deficiency.

Diagnosis

Between crises the blood count is normal. The enzyme deficiency is detected by one of a number of screening tests or by direct enzyme assay on red cells. During a crisis the blood film may show contracted and fragmented cells, 'bite' cells and 'blister' cells (Fig. 6.8) which have had Heinz bodies removed by the spleen. Heinz bodies (oxidized, denatured haemoglobin) may be seen in the reticulocyte preparation, particularly if the spleen is absent. There are also features of intravascular haemolysis. Because of the higher enzyme level in

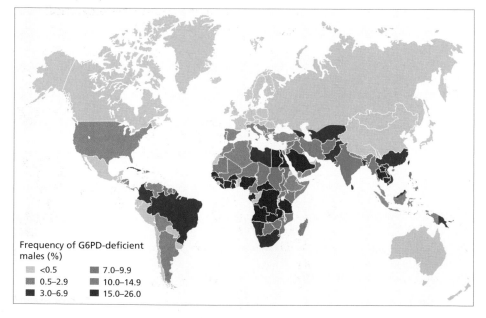

Figure 6.7 Global distribution of *G6PD* gene variants causing G6PD deficiency. Shaded areas indicate the prevalence of G6PD deficiency. (From Luzzatto L. & Notaro R. (2001) *Science* **293**: 442, with permission.)

Table 6.4 Agents that may cause haemolytic anaemia in glucose-6-phosphate dehydrogenase (G6PD) deficiency.

Infections and other acute illnesses (e.g. diabetic ketoacidosis)

Drugs

Antimalarials (e.g. primaquine, pamaquine, chloroquine, Fansidar®, Maloprim®)

Sulphonamides and sulphones (e.g. co-trimoxazole, sulfanilamide, dapsone, Salazopyrin®)

Other antibacterial agents (e.g. nitrofurans, chloramphenicol)

Analgesics (e.g. aspirin), moderate doses are safe

Antihelminths (e.g. β-naphthol, stibophen)

Miscellaneous (e.g. vitamin K analogues, naphthalene (mothballs), probenecid)

Fava beans (possibly other vegetables)

NB. Many common drugs have been reported to precipitate haemolysis in G6PD deficiency in some patients (e.g. aspirin, quinine and penicillin) but not at conventional dosage.

young red cells, red cell enzyme assay may give a 'false' normal level in the phase of acute haemolysis with a reticulocyte response. Subsequent assay after the acute phase reveals the low G6PD level when the red cell population is of normal age distribution.

Treatment

The offending drug is stopped, any underlying infection is treated, a high urine output is maintained and blood transfusion undertaken where necessary for severe anaemia. G6PD-deficient babies are prone to neonatal jaundice and in severe cases phototherapy and exchange transfusion may be needed. The jaundice is usually not caused by excess haemolysis but by deficiency of G6PD affecting neonatal liver function.

Glutathione deficiency and other syndromes

Other defects in the pentose phosphate pathway leading to similar syndromes to G6PD deficiency have been described – particularly glutathione deficiency.

Glycolytic (Embden–Meyerhof) pathway defects

These are all uncommon and lead to a congenital non-spherocytic haemolytic anaemia. In some there

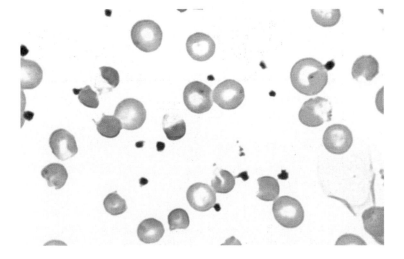

Figure 6.8 Blood film in G6PD deficiency with acute haemolysis after an oxidant stress. Some of the cells show loss of cytoplasm with separation of remaining haemoglobin from the cell membrane ('blister' cells). There are also numerous contracted and deeply staining cells. Supravital staining (as for reticulocytes) showed the presence of Heinz bodies (see Fig. 2.17).

are defects of other systems (e.g. a myopathy). The most frequently encountered is pyruvate kinase deficiency.

Pyruvate kinase deficiency

This is inherited as an autosomal recessive, the affected patients being homozygous or doubly heterozygous. Over 100 different mutations have been described. The red cells become rigid as a result of reduced adenosine triphosphate (ATP) formation. The severity of the anaemia varies widely (haemoglobin 4–10 g/dL) and causes relatively mild symptoms because of a shift to the right in the oxygen (O_2) dissociation curve caused by a rise in intracellular 2,3-diphosphoglycerate (2,3-DPG). Clinically, jaundice is usual and gallstones frequent. Frontal bossing may be present. The blood film shows poikilocytosis and distorted 'prickle' cells, particularly post-splenectomy. Direct enzyme assay is needed to make the diagnosis. Splenectomy may alleviate the anaemia but does not cure it and is indicated in those patients who need frequent transfusions.

Hereditary disorders of haemoglobin synthesis

Several of these cause clinical haemolysis. They are discussed in Chapter 7.

Acquired haemolytic anaemias

Immune haemolytic anaemias

Autoimmune haemolytic anaemias

Autoimmune haemolytic anaemias (AIHAs) are caused by antibody production by the body against its own red cells. They are characterized by a positive direct antiglobulin test (DAT) also known as the Coombs' test (see Fig. 29.5) and divided into 'warm' and 'cold' types (Table 6.5) according to whether the antibody reacts more strongly with red cells at 37°C or 4°C.

Warm autoimmune haemolytic anaemias

The red cells are coated with immunoglobulin (Ig), usually immunoglobulin G (IgG) alone or with

---

Table 6.5 Immune haemolytic anaemias: classification.

Warm type	Cold type
Autoimmune	
Idiopathic	*Idiopathic*
Secondary	*Secondary*
SLE, other 'autoimmune' diseases	Infections – *Mycoplasma* pneumonia, infectious mononucleosis
CLL, lymphomas	Lymphoma
Drugs (e.g. methyldopa)	Paroxysmal cold haemoglobinuria (rare, sometimes associated with infections, e.g. syphilis)
Alloimmune	
Induced by red cell antigens	
Haemolytic transfusion reactions	
Haemolytic disease of the newborn	
Post stem cell grafts	
Drug induced	
Drug–red cell membrane complex	
Immune complex	

CLL, chronic lymphocytic leukaemia; SLE, systemic lupus erythematosus.

complement, and are therefore taken up by RE macrophages which have receptors for the Ig Fc fragment. Part of the coated membrane is lost so the cell becomes progressively more spherical to maintain the same volume and is ultimately prematurely destroyed, predominantly in the spleen. When the cells are coated with IgG and complement (C3d, the degraded fragment of C3) or complement alone, red cell destruction occurs more generally in the RE system.

Clinical features

The disease may occur at any age, in either sex, and presents as a haemolytic anaemia of varying severity. The spleen is often enlarged. The disease tends to remit and relapse. It may occur alone or in association with other diseases (Table 6.5). When associated with idiopathic thrombocytopenic purpura (ITP), which is a similar condition affecting platelets (see p. 334), it is known as Evans' syndrome. When secondary to systemic lupus erythematosus the cells typically are coated with immunoglobulin and complement.

Laboratory findings

The haematological and biochemical findings are typical of an extravascular haemolytic anaemia with spherocytosis prominent in the peripheral blood (Fig. 6.9a). The DAT is positive as a result of IgG, IgG and complement or IgA on the cells and, in some cases, the autoantibody shows specificity within the Rh system. The antibodies both on the cell surface and free in serum are best detected at 37°C.

Treatment

1 Remove the underlying cause (e.g. methyldopa).
2 Corticosteroids. Prednisolone is the usual first-line treatment; 60 mg/day is a typical starting dose in adults and should then be tapered down. Those with predominantly IgG on red cells do best whereas those with complement often respond poorly, both to corticosteroids and splenectomy.
3 Splenectomy may be of value in those who fail to respond well or fail to maintain a satisfactory haemoglobin level on an acceptably small steroid dosage.

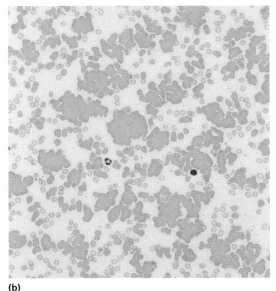

(a) (b)

Figure 6.9 **(a)** Blood film in warm autoimmune haemolytic anaemia. Numerous microspherocytes are present and larger polychromatic cells (reticulocytes). **(b)** Blood film in cold autoimmune haemolytic anaemia. Marked red cell agglutination is present in films made at room temperature. The background is caused by the raised plasma protein concentration.

4 Immunosuppression may be tried if steroids and/ or splenectomy have failed. This may be with drugs or monoclonal antibodies. Azathioprine, cyclophosphamide, chlorambucil, ciclosporin and mycophenolate mofetil have been tried.

5 Monoclonal antibodies. Anti-CD20 (rituximab) has produced prolonged remissions in a proportion of cases and anti-CD52 (Campath-1H) has been tried successfully in a few cases.

6 High-dose immunoglobulin has been used but with less success than in ITP (see p. 336).

7 It may be necessary to treat the underlying disease, e.g. chronic lymphocytic leukaemia or lymphoma.

8 Folic acid is given in severe cases.

9 Blood transfusion may be needed if anaemia is severe and causing symptoms. The blood should be the least incompatible and if the specificity of the autoantibody is known, donor blood is chosen that lacks the relevant antigen(s). The patients also readily make alloantibodies against donor red cells.

Cold autoimmune haemolytic anaemias

In these syndromes the autoantibody, whether monoclonal (as in the idiopathic cold haemagglutinin syndrome or associated with lymphoproliferative disorders) or polyclonal (as following infection, e.g. infectious mononucleosis or *Mycoplasma* pneumonia) attaches to red cells mainly in the peripheral circulation where the blood temperature is cooled (Table 6.5). The antibody is usually IgM and binds to red cells best at 4°C. IgM antibodies are highly efficient at fixing complement and both intravascular and extravascular haemolysis can occur. Complement alone is usually detected on the red cells, the antibody having eluted off the cells in warmer parts of the circulation. Interestingly, in nearly all these cold AIHA syndromes the antibody is directed against the 'I' antigen on the red cell surface. In infectious mononucleosis it is anti-i.

Clinical features

The patient may have a chronic haemolytic anaemia aggravated by the cold and often associated with intravascular haemolysis. Mild jaundice and splenomegaly may be present. The patient may develop acrocyanosis (purplish skin discoloration) at the tip of the nose, ears, fingers and toes caused by the agglutination of red cells in small vessels.

Laboratory findings are similar to those of warm AIHA except that spherocytosis is less marked, red cells agglutinate in the cold (Fig. 6.9b) and the DAT reveals complement (C3d) only on the red cell surface. The serum shows a high titre of "cold" autoantibodies to red cells.

Treatment consists of keeping the patient warm and treating the underlying cause, if present. Alkylating agents such as chlorambucil or purine nucleoside analogues (e.g. fludarabine) may be helpful in the chronic varieties. Both anti-CD20 (rituximab) and anti-CD52 (Campath-1H) have been used. Rituximab is particularly effective when there is an associated B-lymphoproliferative disease. Splenectomy does not usually help unless massive splenomegaly is present. Steroids are not helpful. Underlying lymphoma should be excluded in 'idiopathic' cases.

Paroxysmal cold haemoglobinuria is a rare syndrome of acute intravascular haemolysis after exposure to the cold. It is caused by the Donath–Landsteiner antibody, an IgG antibody with specificity for the P blood group antigens, which binds to red cells in the cold but causes lysis with complement in warm conditions. Viral infections and syphilis are predisposing causes and the condition is usually self-limiting.

Alloimmune haemolytic anaemias

In these anaemias, antibody produced by one individual reacts with red cells of another. Two important situations are transfusion of ABO-incompatible blood and Rh disease of the newborn which are considered in Chapters 29 and 30. The increased use of allogeneic transplantation for renal, hepatic, cardiac and bone marrow diseases has led to the recognition of alloimmune haemolytic anaemia resulting from the production of red cell antibodies in the recipient by donor lymphocytes transferred in the allograft.

Drug-induced immune haemolytic anaemias

Drugs can cause immune haemolytic anaemias via three mechanisms (Fig. 6.10):

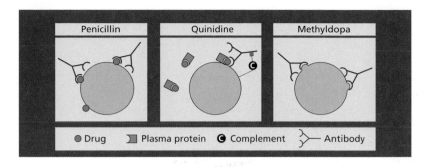

Figure 6.10 Three different mechanisms of drug-induced immune haemolytic anaemia. In each case the coated (opsonized) cells are destroyed in the reticuloendothelial system.

1 Antibody directed against a drug–red cell membrane complex (e.g. penicillin, ampicillin). This only occurs with massive doses of the antibiotic.
2 Deposition of complement via a drug–protein (antigen)–antibody complex onto the red cell surface (e.g. quinidine, rifampicin); or
3 A true autoimmune haemolytic anaemia in which the role of the drug is unclear (e.g. methyldopa).

In each case, the haemolytic anaemia gradually disappears when the drug is discontinued.

Red cell fragmentation syndromes

These arise through physical damage to red cells either on abnormal surfaces (e.g. artificial heart valves or arterial grafts), arteriovenous malformations or as a microangiopathic haemolytic anaemia. This is caused by red cells passing through abnormal small vessels. The latter may be caused by deposition of fibrin strands often associated with disseminated intravascular coagulation (DIC) or platelet adherence as in thrombotic thrombocytopenic purpura (TTP) (see p. 337) or vasculitis (e.g. polyarteritis nodosa; Table 6.6). The peripheral blood contains many deeply staining, red cell fragments (Fig. 6.11). When DIC underlies the haemolysis, clotting abnormalities (see p. 335) and a low platelet count are also present. TTP is discussed in detail on page 337.

March haemoglobinuria

This is caused by damage to red cells between the small bones of the feet, usually during prolonged marching or running. The blood film does not show fragments.

Infections

Infections can cause haemolysis in a variety of ways. They may precipitate an acute haemolytic crisis in G6PD deficiency or cause microangiopathic haemolytic anaemia (e.g. with meningococcal or

Table 6.6 Red cell fragmentation syndromes.	
Cardiac haemolysis	Prosthetic heart valves
	Patches, grafts
	Perivalvular leaks
Arteriovenous malformations	
Microangiopathic	TTP-HUS
	Disseminated intravascular coagulation
	Malignant disease
	Vasculitis (e.g. polyarteritis nodosa)
	Malignant hypertension
	Pre-eclampsia/HELLP
	Renal vascular disorders/ HELLP syndrome
	Ciclosporin
	Homograft rejection

HELLP, haemolysis with elevated liver function tests and low platelets; HUS, haemolytic uraemic syndrome; TTP, thrombotic thrombocytopenic purpura.

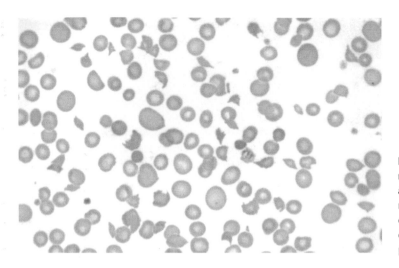

Figure 6.11 Blood film in microangiopathic haemolytic anaemia (in this patient, Gram-negative septicaemia). Numerous contracted and deeply staining cells and cell fragments are present.

pneumococcal septicaemia). Malaria causes haemolysis by extravascular destruction of parasitized red cells as well as by direct intravascular lysis. Blackwater fever is an acute intravascular haemolysis accompanied by acute renal failure caused by *Falciparum* malaria. *Clostridium perfringens* septicaemia can cause intravascular haemolysis with marked microspherocytosis.

Chemical and physical agents

Certain drugs (e.g. dapsone and Salazopyrin®) in high doses cause oxidative intravascular haemolysis with Heinz body formation in normal subjects. In Wilson's disease an acute haemolytic anaemia can occur as a result of high levels of copper in the blood. Chemical poisoning (e.g. with lead, chlorate or arsine) can cause severe haemolysis. Severe burns damage red cells causing acanthocytosis or spherocytosis.

Secondary haemolytic anaemias

In many systemic disorders red cell survival is shortened. This may contribute to anaemia (see Chapter 28).

Paroxysmal nocturnal haemoglobinuria

PNH is a rare acquired clonal disorder of marrow stem cells in which there is deficient synthesis of the

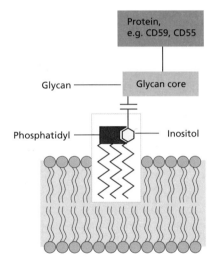

Figure 6.12 Schematic representation of the phosphatidylinositol glycan which anchors many different proteins to the cell membrane (e.g. CD59).

glycosylphosphatidylinositol (GPI) anchor, a structure that attaches several surface proteins to the cell membrane. It results from acquired mutations in the X chromosome gene coding for phosphatidylinositol glycan protein class A (PIG-A) which is essential for the formation of the GPI anchor. The net result is that GPI-linked proteins (such as CD55 and CD59) are absent from the cell surface of all the cells derived from the abnormal stem cell (Fig. 6.12). The lack of surface molecules decay-activating factor (DAF, CD55) and membrane inhibitor of reactive lysis (MIRL, CD59) render red cells sensitive to lysis by complement and the result is chronic intravascular haemolysis. Haemosiderinuria is a constant feature and can give rise to iron deficiency which may exacerbate the anaemia. CD55 and CD59 are also present on white cells and platelets. The other main clinical problem seen in PNH is thrombosis and patients may develop recurrent thromboses of large veins including portal and hepatic veins, as well as intermittent abdominal pain brought about by thrombosis of mesenteric veins.

PNH is almost invariably associated with some form of bone marrow hypoplasia, often frank aplastic anaemia. It appears that the PNH clone may expand as a result of a selective pressure, possibly immunologically mediated, against cells that have normal GPI-linked membrane proteins.

PNH is diagnosed by flow cytometry which shows loss of expression of the GPI-linked proteins, CD55 and CD59. Alternatively, a test for loss of the GPI anchor on WBC (FLAER) may be used.

Eculizumab, a humanized antibody against complement C5, inhibits the activation of terminal components of complement and reduces haemolysis and transfusion requirements. Iron therapy is used for iron deficiency and long-term anticoagulation with warfarin may be needed. Immunosuppression can be useful and allogeneic stem cell transplantation is a definitive treatment. The disease occasionally remits and the median survival is approximately 10 years.

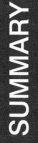

SUMMARY

- Haemolytic anaemia is caused by shortening of the red cell life. The red cells may break down in the reticuloendothelial system (extravascular) or in the circulation (intravascular).
- Haemolytic anaemia may be caused by inherited red cell defects, which are usually intrinsic to the red cell, or to acquired causes, which are usually caused by an abnormality of the red cell environment.
- Features of extravascular haemolysis include jaundice, gallstones and splenomegaly with raised reticulocytes, unconjugated bilirubin and absent haptoglobins. In intravascular haemolysis (e.g. caused by ABO mismatched blood transfusion), there is haemoglobinaemia, methaemalbuminaemia, haemoglobinuria and haemosiderinuria.
- Genetic defects include those of the red cell membrane (e.g. hereditary spherocytosis), enzyme deficiencies (e.g. glucose-6-phosphate dehydrogenase or pyruvate kinase deficiency) or haemoglobin defects (e.g. sickle cell anaemia).
- Acquired causes of haemolytic anaemia include warm or cold, auto- or allo-antibodies to red cells, red cell fragmentation syndromes, infections, toxins and paroxysmal nocturnal haemoglobinuria.

Now visit www.wiley.com/go/essentialhaematology to test yourself on this chapter.

CHAPTER 7
Genetic disorders of haemoglobin

Key topics

This chapter deals with inherited diseases caused by reduced or abnormal synthesis of globin. Mutations in the globin genes are the most prevalent monogenic disorders worldwide and affect approximately 7% of the world's population. The synthesis of normal haemoglobin in the fetus and adult is described first.

Haemoglobin synthesis

Normal adult blood contains three types of haemo-globin (see Table 2.2). The major component is haemoglobin A with the molecular structure $\alpha_2\beta_2$. The minor haemoglobins contain γ (fetal Hb or Hb F) or δ (Hb A_2) globin chains instead of β chains. In the embryo and fetus, Gower 1, Portland, Gower 2 and fetal Hb dominate at different stages (Fig. 7.1). The genes for the globin chains occur in two clusters: ε, γ, δ and β on chromosome 11 and ζ and α on chromosome 16. Two types of γ chain occur, G_γ and A_γ, which differ by a glycine or alanine amino acid at position 136 in the polypeptide

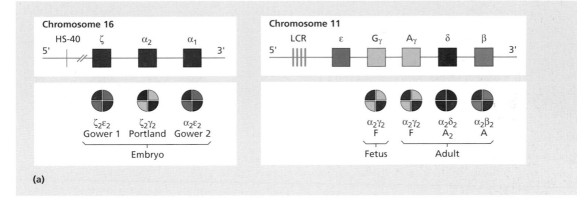

(a)

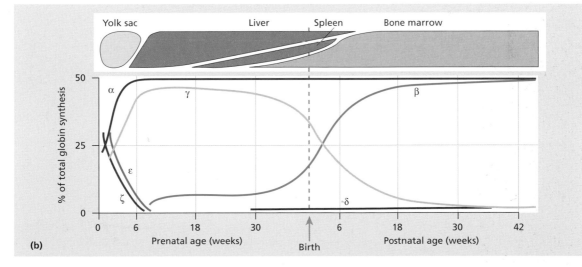

(b)

Figure 7.1 (a) The globin gene clusters on chromosomes 16 and 11. In embryonic, fetal and adult life different genes are activated or suppressed. The different globin chains are synthesized independently and then combine with each other to produce the different haemoglobins. The γ gene may have two sequences, which code for either a glutamic acid or alanine residue at position 136 (G_γ or A_γ, respectively). LCR, locus control region, HS-40, see text. **(b)** Synthesis of individual globin chains in prenatal and postnatal life.

chain. The α-chain gene is duplicated and both α genes (α₁ and α₂) on each chromosome are active (Fig. 7.1).

Molecular aspects

All the globin genes have three exons (coding regions) and two introns (non-coding regions whose DNA is not represented in the finished protein). The initial RNA is transcribed from both introns and exons, and from this transcript the RNA derived from introns is removed by a process known as splicing (Fig. 7.2). The introns always begin with a G-T dinucleotide and end with an A-G dinucleotide. The splicing machinery recognizes these sequences as well as neighbouring conserved sequences. The RNA in the nucleus is also 'capped' by addition of a structure at the 5′ end which contains a seven methyl-guanosine group. The cap structure may be important for attachment of the mRNA to ribosomes. The newly formed mRNA is also polyadenylated at the 3′ end (Fig. 7.2). This stabilizes it. Thalassaemia may arise from mutations or deletions of any of these sequences.

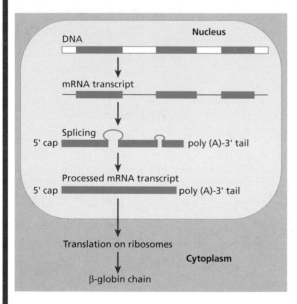

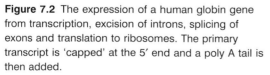

Figure 7.2 The expression of a human globin gene from transcription, excision of introns, splicing of exons and translation to ribosomes. The primary transcript is 'capped' at the 5′ end and a poly A tail is then added.

A number of other conserved sequences are important in globin synthesis and mutations at these sites may also give rise to thalassaemia. These sequences influence gene transcription, ensure its fidelity, specify sites for the initiation and termination of translation, and ensure the stability of newly synthesized mRNA. Promoters are found 5′ of the gene, either close to the initiation site or more distally. They are the sites where RNA polymerases bind and catalyse gene transcription (see Fig. 1.9). Enhancers occur either 5′ or 3′ to the gene (Fig. 7.2). Enhancers are important in the tissue-specific regulation of globin gene expression and in regulation of the synthesis of the various globin chains during fetal and postnatal life. The locus control region (LCR) is a genetic regulatory element, situated a long way upstream of the β-globin cluster, that controls the genetic activity of each domain, probably by physically interacting with the promoter region and opening up the chromatin to allow transcription factors to bind. The α-globin gene cluster also contains an LCR-like region termed HS40. GATA-1, FOG and NF-E2 transcription factors, expressed mainly in erythroid precursors, are important in determining the expression of globin genes in erythroid cells.

Globin mRNA enters the cytoplasm and attaches to ribosomes (translation) where the synthesis of globin chains takes place. This occurs by attachment of transfer RNAs, each with its individual amino acid, by codon–anticodon base pairing to an appropriate position on the mRNA template.

Switch from fetal to adult haemoglobin

The globin genes are arranged on chromosomes 11 and 16 in the order in which they are expressed (Fig. 7.1). Certain embryonic haemoglobins are usually only expressed in yolk sac erythroblasts. The β-globin gene is expressed at a low level in early fetal life, but the main switch to adult haemoglobin occurs 3–6 months after birth when synthesis of the γ chain is largely replaced by the β chain. *BCL11A* is a transcriptional regulator of the switch and of the silencing of δ chain synthesis in the adult. The methylation state of the gene (expressed genes tend to be hypomethylated, non-expressed hypermethylated), the state of the chromosome packaging and various enhancer sequences all play a part in determining whether a particular gene will be transcribed.

Haemoglobin abnormalities

These result from the following:

1 Synthesis of an abnormal haemoglobin.
2 Reduced rate of synthesis of normal α- or β-globin chains (the α- and β-thalassaemias).

Table 7.1 shows some of the first group of syndromes that arise from synthesis of an α or β chain with an amino acid substitution. In many cases, however, the abnormality is completely silent. The clinically most important abnormality is sickle cell anaemia. Haemoglobin (Hb) C, D and E are also common and, like Hb S, are substitutions in the β chain. Unstable haemoglobins are rare and cause a chronic haemolytic anaemia of varying severity with intravascular haemolysis (see Table 6.2). Abnormal haemoglobins may also cause (familial) polycythaemia (see Chapter 15) or congenital methaemoglobinaemia (see Chapter 2).

The genetic defects of haemoglobin are the most common genetic disorders worldwide. They occur in tropical and subtropical areas (Fig. 7.3) and most

appear to have been selected because the carrier state affords some protection against malaria.

Thalassaemias

These are a heterogeneous group of genetic disorders that result from a reduced rate of synthesis of α or β chains. β-Thalassaemia is more common in the Mediterranean region while α-thalassaemia is more common in the Far East.

Table 7.1 The clinical syndromes produced by haemoglobin abnormalities.

Syndrome	Abnormality
Haemolysis	Crystalline haemoglobins (Hb S, C, D, E, etc.) Unstable haemoglobin
Thalassaemia	α or β resulting from reduced globin chain synthesis
Familial polycythaemia	Altered oxygen affinity
Methaemoglobinaemia	Failure of reduction (Hb Ms)

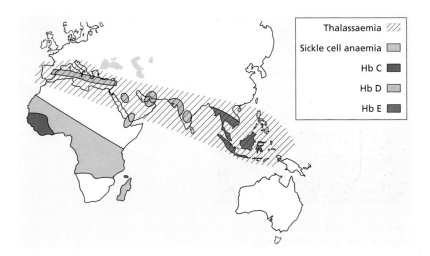

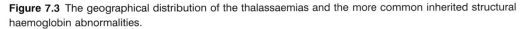

Figure 7.3 The geographical distribution of the thalassaemias and the more common inherited structural haemoglobin abnormalities.

α-Thalassaemia syndromes

These are usually caused by gene deletions and are listed in Table 7.2. As there are normally four copies of the α-globin gene, the clinical severity can be classified according to the number of genes that are missing or inactive. Loss of all four genes completely suppresses α-chain synthesis (Fig. 7.4) and because the α chain is essential in fetal as well as in adult haemoglobin this is incompatible with life and leads to death *in utero* (hydrops fetalis; Fig. 7.5). Three α gene deletions leads to a moderately severe (haemoglobin 7–11 g/dL) microcytic, hypochromic anaemia (Fig. 7.6) with splenomegaly. This is known as Hb H disease because haemoglobin H (β_4) can be detected in red cells of these patients by electrophoresis or in reticulocyte preparations (Fig. 7.6). In fetal life, Hb Barts (γ_4) occurs.

The α-thalassaemia traits are caused by loss of one or two genes and are usually not associated with anaemia, although the mean corpuscular volume (MCV) and mean corpuscular haemoglobin (MCH) are low and the red cell count is over 5.5×10^{12}/L. Haemoglobin electrophoresis is normal and DNA analysis is needed to be certain of the diagnosis. Uncommon non-deletional forms of α-thalassaemia are caused by point mutations producing dysfunction of the genes or rarely by mutations affecting termination of translation which give rise to an elongated but unstable chain (e.g. Hb Constant Spring). Two rare forms of α-thalassaemia are associated with mental retardation. They are caused by mutation in a gene on chromosome 16 (ATR-16) or on chromosome X (ATR-X) which control the transcription of the α globin and other genes.

β-Thalassaemia syndromes

β-Thalassaemia major

This condition occurs on average in one in four offspring if both parents are carriers of the β-thalassaemia trait. Either no β chain (β^0) or small amounts (β^+) are synthesized. Excess α chains precipitate in erythroblasts and in mature red cells causing the severe ineffective erythropoiesis and haemolysis that are typical of this disease. The

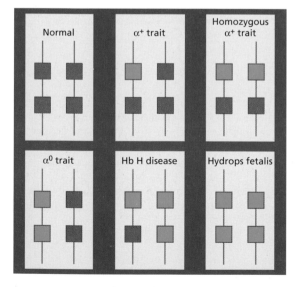

Figure 7.4 The genetics of α-thalassaemia. Each α gene may be deleted or (less frequently) dysfunctional. The orange boxes represent normal genes, and the blue boxes represent gene deletions or dysfunctional genes.

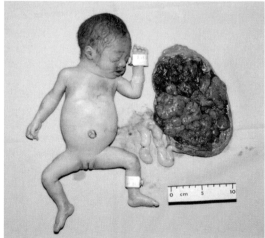

Figure 7.5 α-Thalassaemia: hydrops fetalis, the result of deletion of all four α-globin genes (homozygous α^0-thalassaemia). The main haemoglobin present is Hb Barts (γ_4). The condition is incompatible with life beyond the fetal stage. (Courtesy of Professor D. Todd)

Table 7.2 Classification of thalassaemia.

Clinical

Hydrops fetalis
Four gene deletion α-thalassaemia

Thalassaemia major
Transfusion dependent, homozygous
β^0-thalassaemia or other combinations
of β-thalassaemia trait

Thalassaemia intermedia
See Table 6.5

Thalassaemia minor
β^0-Thalassaemia trait
β^+-Thalassaemia trait
Hereditary persistence of fetal haemoglobin
δβ-Thalassaemia trait
α^0-Thalassaemia trait
α^+-Thalassaemia trait

Genetic

Type	Haplotype	Heterozygous thalassaemia trait (minor)*	Homozygous
α-Thalassaemias[†]			
α^0	$--/$	MCV, MCH low	Hydrops fetalis
α^+	$-\alpha/$	MCV, MCH minimally reduced	As heterozygous α^0-thalassaemia
β-Thalassaemias			
β^0		MCV, MCH low (Hb $A_2 > 3.5\%$)	Thalassaemia major (Hb F 98%, Hb A_2 2%)
β^+		MCV, MCH low (Hb $A_2 > 3.5\%$)	Thalassaemia major or intermedia (Hb F 70–80%, Hb A 10–20%, Hb A_2 variable)
δβ-Thalassaemia and hereditary persistence of fetal haemoglobin		MCV, MCH low (Hb F 5–20%, Hb A_2 normal)	Thalassaemia intermedia (Hb F 100%)
Hb Lepore		MCV, MCH low (Hb A 80–90%, Hb Lepore 10%, Hb A_2 reduced)	Thalassaemia major or intermedia (Hb F 80%, Hb Lepore 10–20%, Hb A, Hb A_2 absent)

MCH, mean corpuscular haemoglobin; MCV, mean corpuscular volume.
*Occasionally heterozygous β-thalassaemia is dominant (associated with the clinical picture of thalassaemia intermedia). There are several explanations.
[†]Compound heterozygote $\alpha^0\alpha^+$ ($--/-\alpha$) is haemoglobin H disease.

greater the α-chain excess, the more severe the anaemia. Production of γ chains helps to 'mop up' excess α chains and to ameliorate the condition. Over 400 different genetic defects have now been detected (Figs 7.7 and 7.8).

Unlike α-thalassaemia, the majority of genetic lesions are point mutations rather than gene dele-tions. These mutations may be within the gene complex itself or in promoter or enhancer regions. Certain mutations are particularly frequent in some communities (Fig. 7.7) and this may simplify ante-natal diagnosis aimed at detecting the mutations in fetal DNA. Thalassaemia major is often a result of inheritance of two different mutations, each

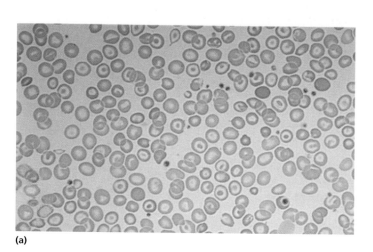

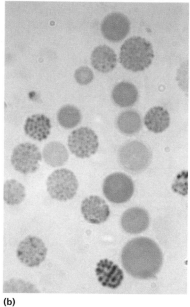

(a)

(b)

Figure 7.6 **(a)** α-Thalassaemia: haemoglobin H disease (three α-globin gene deletion). The blood film shows marked hypochromic microcytic cells with target cells and poikilocytosis. **(b)** α-Thalassaemia: haemoglobin H disease. Supravital staining with brilliant cresyl blue reveals multiple fine, deeply stained deposits ('golf ball' cells) caused by precipitation of aggregates of β-globin chains. Hb H can also be detected as a fast-moving band on haemoglobin electrophoresis (Fig. 7.12).

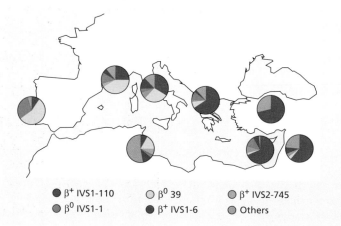

Figure 7.7 Distribution of different mutations of β-thalassaemia major in the Mediterranean area. IVSI, IVS2 intervening sequences; 1, 6, 39, 110, 745 are mutations of corresponding codons. (Courtesy of Professor A. Cao.)

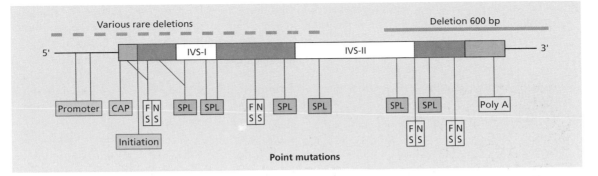

Figure 7.8 Examples of mutations that produce β-thalassaemia. These include single base changes, small deletions and insertions of one or two bases affecting introns, exons or the flanking regions of the β-globin gene. FS, 'frameshifts': deletion of nucleotide(s) that places the reading frame out of phase downstream of the lesion; NS, 'non-sense': premature chain termination as a result of a new translational stop codon (e.g. UAA); SPL, 'splicing': inactivation of splicing or new splice sites generated (aberrant splicing) in exons or introns; promoter, CAP, initiation: reduction of transcription or translation as a result of lesion in promoter, CAP or initiation regions; Poly A, mutations on the poly A addition signal resulting in failure of poly A addition and an unstable mRNA.

affecting β-globin synthesis (compound heterozygotes). In some cases, deletion of the β gene, δ and β genes or even δ, β and γ genes occurs. In others, unequal crossing-over has produced δβ fusion genes (so-called Lepore syndrome named after the first family in which this was diagnosed) (see p. 99).

Clinical features

1 Severe anaemia becomes apparent at 3–6 months after birth when the switch from γ- to β-chain production should take place.
2 Enlargement of the liver and spleen occurs as a result of excessive red cell destruction, extramedullary haemopoiesis and later because of iron overload. The large spleen increases blood requirements by increasing red cell destruction and pooling, and by causing expansion of the plasma volume.
3 Expansion of bones caused by intense marrow hyperplasia leads to a thalassaemic facies (Fig. 7.9) and to thinning of the cortex of many bones with a tendency to fractures and bossing of the skull with a 'hair-on-end' appearance on X-ray (Fig. 7.10).
4 Thalassaemia major is the disease that most frequently underlies transfusional iron overload. This is because regular transfusions are usually

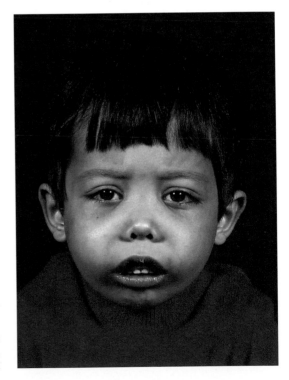

Figure 7.9 The facial appearance of a child with β-thalassaemia major. The skull is bossed with prominent frontal and parietal bones; the maxilla is enlarged.

commenced in the first year of life and unless the disease is cured by stem cell transplantantion, are continued for life. Also iron absorption is increased because of low serum hepcidin levels because of release of GDF 15 and TWSG1 from early red cell precursors which are increased because of ineffective erythropoisis. The tests for iron overload, clinical features (cardiac, hepatic and endocrine) and chelation therapy are discussed in Chapter 4.

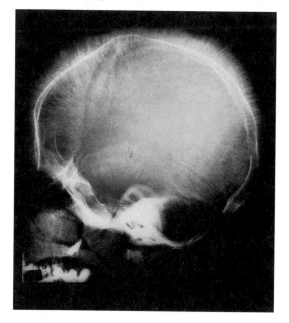

Figure 7.10 The skull X-ray in β-thalassaemia major. There is a 'hair-on-end' appearance as a result of expansion of the bone marrow into cortical bone.

5 Infections can occur for a variety of reasons. In infancy, without adequate transfusion, the anaemic child is prone to bacterial infections. Pneumococcal, *Haemophilus* and meningococcal infections are likely if splenectomy has been carried out and prophylactic penicillin is not taken. *Yersinia enterocolitica* occurs, particularly in iron-loaded patients being treated with deferoxamine; it may cause severe gastroenteritis. Iron overload also predisposes to baterial infections, e.g. *Klebsiella* and fungal infections. Transfusion of viruses by blood transfusion may occur.

Liver disease in thalassaemia is most frequently a result of hepatitis C but hepatitis B is also common where the virus is endemic. Human immunodeficiency virus (HIV) has been transmitted to some patients by blood transfusion. As a result of better iron chelation therapy reducing substantially death from cardiac iron overload, infections now account for an increasing proportion of deaths in thalassaemia major in the UK.

6 Osteoporosis may occur in well-transfused patients. It is more common in diabetic patients with endocrine abnormalities and with marrow expansion resulting from ineffective erythopoiesis.

Laboratory diagnosis

1 There is a severe hypochromic microcytic anaemia, raised reticulocyte percentage with normoblasts, target cells and basophilic stippling in the blood film (Fig. 7.11).

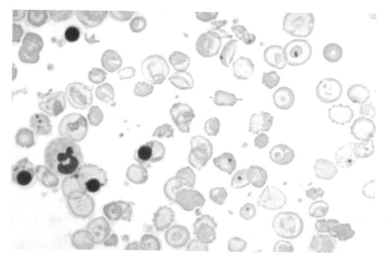

Figure 7.11 Blood film in β-thalassaemia major postsplenectomy. There are hypochromic cells, target cells and many nucleated red cells (normoblasts). Howell–Jolly bodies are seen in same red cells.

2 High performance liquid chromatography (HPLC) is now usually used as first-line method to diagnose haemoglobin disorders (Fig. 7.12b). HPLC or haemoglobin electrophoresis reveals absence or almost complete absence of Hb A, with almost all the circulating haemoglobin being Hb F. The Hb A₂ percentage is normal, low or slightly raised (Fig. 7.12a). DNA analysis is used to identify the defect on each allele.

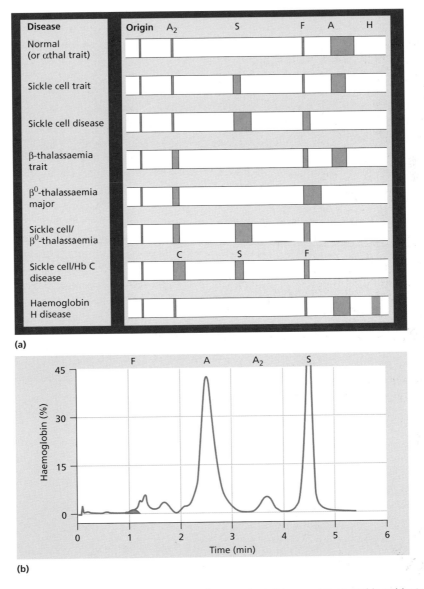

Figure 7.12 (a) Haemoglobin electrophoretic patterns in normal adult human blood and in subjects with sickle cell (Hb S) trait or disease, β-thalassaemia trait, β-thalassaemia major, Hb S/β-thalassaemia or Hb S/Hb C disease and Hb H disease. **(b)** High performance liquid chromatography. The different haemoglobins elute at different times from the column and their concentrations are read automatically. In this example, the patient is a carrier of sickle cell disease.

Treatment

1 Regular blood transfusions are needed to maintain the haemoglobin over 10 g/dL at all times. This usually requires 2–3 units every 4–6 weeks. Blood, filtered to remove white cells, gives the fewest reactions. The patients should be genotyped at the start of the transfusion programme in case red cell antibodies against transfused red cells develop.

2 Regular folic acid (e.g. 5 mg/day) is given if the diet is poor.

3 Iron chelation therapy (see Chapter 4).

4 Splenectomy may be needed to reduce blood requirements. This should be delayed until the patient is over 6 years old because of the high risk of dangerous infections post-splenectomy. The vaccinations and antibiotics to be given are described in Chapter 10.

5 Endocrine therapy is given either as replacement because of end-organ failure or to stimulate the pituitary if puberty is delayed. Diabetic patients will require insulin therapy. Patients with osteoporosis may need additional therapy with increased calcium and vitamin D in their diet, together with a bisphosphonate and appropriate endocrine therapy.

6 Immunization against hepatitis B should be carried out in all non-immune patients. Treatment for transfusion-transmitted hepatitis C with α-interferon, ribavirin and newer antivirals is needed if viral genomes are detected in plasma.

7 Allogeneic stem cell transplantation offers the prospect of permanent cure. The success rate (long-term thalassaemia major-free survival) is over 80–90% in well-chelated younger patients without liver fibrosis or hepatomegaly. A human leucocyte antigen (HLA) matching sibling (or rarely other family member or matching unrelated donor) acts as donor. Failure is mainly a result of recurrence of thalassaemia, death (e.g. from infection) or severe chronic graft-versus-host disease.

β-Thalassaemia trait (minor)

This is a common, usually symptomless, abnormality characterized like α-thalassaemia trait by a hypochromic microcytic blood picture (MCV and MCH very low) but high red cell count ($>5.5 \times 10^{12}$/L) and mild anaemia (haemoglobin 10–12 g/dL). It is usually more severe than α-thalassaemia trait. A raised Hb A_2 (>3.5%) confirms the diagnosis. One of the most important indications for making the diagnosis is that it allows the possibility of prenatal counselling to patients with a partner who also has a significant haemoglobin disorder. If both carry β-thalassaemia trait there is a 25% risk of having a child with thalassaemia major.

Thalassaemia intermedia

Cases of thalassaemia of moderate severity (haemoglobin 7.0–10.0 g/dL) who do not need regular transfusions are called thalassaemia intermedia (Table 7.3). This is a *clinical* syndrome which may be caused by a variety of genetic defects: homozygous β-thalassaemia with production of more Hb F than usual, e.g. from mutations of the *BCL11A* gene or with mild defects in β-chain synthesis, by β-thalassaemia trait alone of unusual severity ('dominant' β-thalassaemia) or β-thalassaemia trait in association with mild globin abnormalities such as Hb Lepore. The coexistence of α-thalassaemia trait improves the haemoglobin level in homozygous β-thalassaemia by reducing the degree of chain imbalance and thus of α-chain precipitation and

Table 7.3 Thalassaemia intermedia.

Homozygous β-thalassaemia
Homozygous mild β⁺-thalassaemia
Coinheritance of α-thalassaemia
Enhanced ability to make fetal haemoglobin
  (γ-chain production)

Heterozygous β-thalassaemia
Coinheritance of additional α-globin genes
  (αααα/αα or αααα/αααα)
Dominant β-thalassaemia trait

*δβ-Thalassaemia and hereditary persistence of
  fetal haemoglobin*
Homozygous δβ-thalassaemia
Heterozygous δβ-thalassaemia/β-thalassaemia
Homozygous Hb Lepore (some cases)

Haemoglobin H disease

ineffective erythropoiesis. Conversely, patients with β-thalassaemia trait who also have excess (five or six) α genes tend to be more anaemic than usual. The patient with thalassaemia intermedia may show bone deformity, enlarged liver and spleen, extramedullary erythropoiesis (Fig. 7.13) and features of iron overload caused by increased iron absorption. Iron chelation with oral drugs or (gentle) venesections may be needed to treat this. Hb H disease (three-gene deletion α-thalassaemia) is a type of thalassaemia intermedia without iron overload or extramedullary haemopoiesis.

δβ-Thalassaemia

This involves failure of production of both β and δ chains. Fetal haemoglobin production is increased to 5–20% in the heterozygous state which resembles thalassaemia minor haematologically. In the homozygous state only Hb F is present and haematologically the picture is of thalassaemia intermedia. Haemoglobin F gives up oxygen to tissues less well than haemoglobin A.

Haemoglobin Lepore

This is an abnormal haemoglobin caused by unequal crossing-over of the β and δ genes to produce a polypeptide chain consisting of the δ chain at its amino end and β chain at its carboxyl end. The δβ-fusion chain is synthesized inefficiently and normal δ- and β-chain production is abolished. The homozygotes show thalassaemia intermedia and the heterozygotes thalassaemia trait.

Hereditary persistence of fetal haemoglobin

These are a heterogeneous group of genetic conditions caused by deletions or cross-overs affecting the production of β and γ chains or, in non-deletion forms, by point mutations upstream from the γ-globin genes or in the *BCL11A* gene (see p. 90).

Association of β-thalassaemia trait with other genetic disorders of haemoglobin

The combination of β-thalassaemia trait with Hb E trait usually causes a transfusion-dependent thalassaemia major syndrome, but some cases are intermediate. β-Thalassaemia trait with Hb S trait produces the clinical picture of sickle cell anaemia rather than of thalassaemia (see p. 104). β-Thalassaemia trait with Hb D trait causes a hypochromic microcytic anaemia of varying severity.

Sickle cell anaemia

Sickle cell disease is a group of haemoglobin disorders resulting from the inheritance of the sickle β-

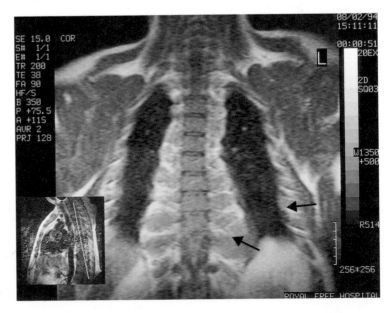

Figure 7.13 β-Thalassaemia intermedia: magnetic resonance imaging (MRI) scan showing masses of extramedullary haemopoietic tissue arising from the ribs (arrowed) and in the paravertebral region (arrowed) without encroachment of the spinal cord.

Normal β-chain	Amino acid	pro	glu	glu
	Base composition	CCT	G(A)G	GAG
Sickle β-chain	Base composition	CCT	G(T)G	GAG
	Amino acid	pro	val	glu

Figure 7.14 Molecular pathology of sickle cell anaemia. There is a single base change in the DNA coding for the amino acid in the sixth position in the β-globin chain (adenine is replaced by thymine). This leads to an amino acid change from glutamic acid to valine. A, adenine; C, cytosine; G, guanine; glu, glutamic acid; pro, proline; T, thymine; val, valine.

globin gene. Homozygous sickle cell anaemia (Hb SS) is the most common severe syndrome while the doubly heterozygote conditions of Hb SC and Hb Sβthal also cause sickling disease. Hb S (Hb $\alpha_2\beta_2^S$) is insoluble and forms crystals when exposed to low oxygen tension. Deoxygenated sickle haemoglobin polymerizes into long fibres, each consisting of seven intertwined double strands with cross-linking. The red cells sickle and may block different areas of the microcirculation or large vessels causing infarcts of various organs. The sickle β-globin abnormality is caused by substitution of valine for glutamic acid in position 6 in the β chain (Fig. 7.14). The carrier state is very widespread and is found in up to one in four West Africans, maintained at this level because of the protection against malaria that is afforded by the carrier state.

Homozygous disease

Clinical features

Clinical features are of a severe haemolytic anaemia punctuated by crises. The symptoms of anaemia are often mild in relation to the severity of the anaemia because Hb S gives up oxygen (O_2) to tissues relatively easily compared with Hb A, its O_2 dissociation curve being shifted to the right (see Fig. 2.9). The clinical expression of Hb SS is very variable, some patients having an almost normal life free of crises but others develop severe crises even as infants and may die in early childhood or as young adults. Crises may be vaso-occlusive, visceral, aplastic or haemolytic.

Vaso-occlusive crises

These are the most frequent and are precipitated by such factors as infection, acidosis, dehydration or deoxygenation (e.g. altitude, operations, obstetric delivery, stasis of the circulation, exposure to cold, violent exercise). Infarcts causing severe pain occur in the bones (hips, shoulders and vertebrae are commonly affected) (Fig. 7.15). The 'hand–foot' syndrome (painful dactylitis caused by infarcts of the small bones) is frequently the first presentation of the disease and may lead to digits of varying lengths (Fig. 7.16). Soft tissues affected include the lungs and the spleen. The most serious vaso-occlusive crisis is of the brain (a stroke occurs in 7% of all patients) or spinal cord. Transcranial Doppler ultrasonography detects abnormal blood flow indicative of arterial stenosis. This predicts for strokes in children. These can be largely prevented by regular blood transfusions in these cases.

Visceral sequestration crises

These are caused by sickling within organs and pooling of blood, often with a severe exacerbation of anaemia. The acute sickle chest syndrome is a feared complication and the most common cause of death after puberty. Patients present with dyspnoea, falling arterial P_{O_2}, chest pain and pulmonary infiltrates on chest X-ray. Treatment is with analgesia, oxygen, exchange transfusion and ventilatory support if necessary. Hepatic and girdle sequestration crises and splenic sequestration may lead to severe illness requiring exchange transfusions. Splenic sequestration is typically seen in infants and presents with an enlarging spleen, falling haemoglobin and abdominal pain. Treatment is with transfusion and patients must be monitored at regular intervals as progression may be rapid. Attacks tend to be recurrent and splenectomy is often needed.

Aplastic crises

These occur as a result of infection with parvovirus or from folate deficiency and are characterized by a sudden fall in haemoglobin, usually requiring transfusion. They are characterized by a fall in reticulocytes as well as haemoglobin (see Fig. 22.5).

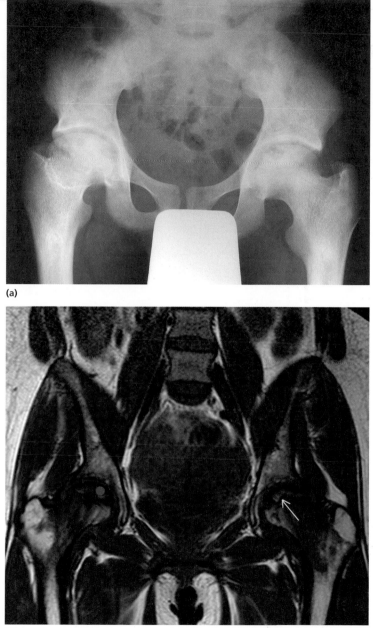

(a)

(b)

Figure 7.15 Sickle cell anaemia. **(a)** Radiograph of the pelvis of a young man of West Indian origin which shows avascular necrosis with flattening of the femoral heads, more marked on the right hip, coarsening of the bone architecture and cystic areas in the right femoral neck caused by previous infarcts. **(b)** Coronal hip MRI image revealing established osteonecrosis of femoral heads bilaterally (yellow arrow) with crescentric sclerotic margin (blue dot) as a consequence of sickle cell. (Courtesy of Dr A. Malhotra.)

Haemolytic crises

These are characterized by an increased rate of haemolysis with a fall in haemoglobin but rise in reticulocytes and usually accompany a painful crisis.

Other clinical features

Ulcers of the lower legs are common, as a result of vascular stasis and local ischaemia (Fig. 7.17). The spleen is enlarged in infancy and early childhood but later is often reduced in size as a result of infarcts

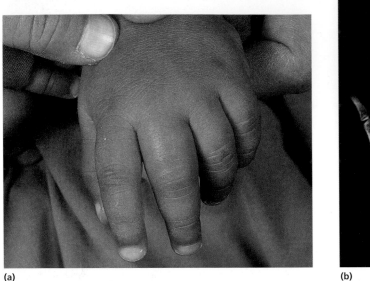

(a)

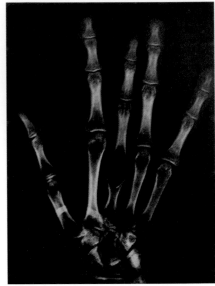

(b)

Figure 7.16 Sickle cell anaemia: **(a)** painful swollen fingers (dactylitis) in a child; and **(b)** the hand of an 18-year-old Nigerian boy with the 'hand–foot' syndrome. There is marked shortening of the right middle finger because of dactylitis in childhood affecting the growth of the epiphysis.

(autosplenectomy). Pulmonary hypertension detected by Doppler echocardiography and an increased tricuspid regurgitant velocity is common and increases the risk of death. A proliferative retinopathy and priapism are other clinical complications.

Chronic damage to the liver may occur through microinfarcts. Pigment (bilirubin) gallstones are frequent. The kidneys are vulnerable to infarctions of the medulla with papillary necrosis. Failure to concentrate urine aggravates the tendency to dehydration and crisis, and nocturnal enuresis is common. Osteomyelitis may also occur, usually from *Salmonella* spp. (Fig. 7.18).

Laboratory findings

1 The haemoglobin is usually 6–9 g/dL – low in comparison to symptoms of anaemia.
2 Sickle cells and target cells occur in the blood (Fig. 7.19). Features of splenic atrophy (e.g. Howell–Jolly bodies) may also be present.
3 Screening tests for sickling are positive when the blood is deoxygenated (e.g. with dithionate and $Na_2 HPO_4$).

4 HPLC or haemoglobin electrophoresis (Fig. 7.12): in Hb SS, no Hb A is detected. The amount of Hb F is variable and is usually 5–15%, larger amounts are normally associated with a milder disorder.

Treatment

1 Prophylactic – avoid those factors known to precipitate crises, especially dehydration, anoxia, infections, stasis of the circulation and cooling of the skin surface.
2 Folic acid (e.g. 5 mg once weekly).
3 Good general nutrition and hygiene.
4 Pneumococcal, *Haemophilus* and meningococcal vaccination and regular oral penicillin are effective at reducing the infection rate with these organisms. Oral penicillin should start at diagnosis and continue at least until puberty. Hepatitis B vaccination is also given as transfusions may be needed.
5 Crises – treat by rest, warmth, rehydration by oral fluids and/or intravenous normal saline (3 L in 24 hours) and antibiotics if infection

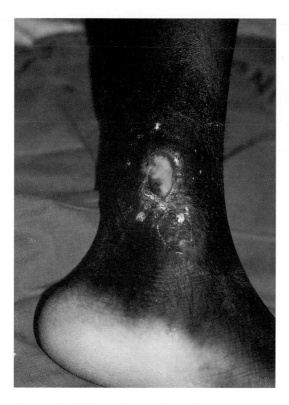

Figure 7.17 Sickle cell anaemia: medial aspect of the ankle of a 15-year-old Nigerian boy showing necrosis and ulceration.

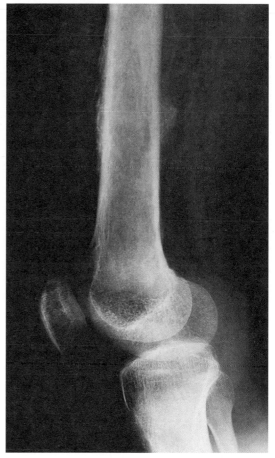

Figure 7.18 *Salmonella* osteomyelitis: lateral radiograph of the lower femur and knee. The periosteum is irregularly raised in the lower third of the femur.

is present. Analgesia at the appropriate level should be given. Suitable drugs are paracetamol, a non-steroidal anti-inflammatory agent and opiates (e.g. continuous subcutaneous diamorphine). Blood transfusion is given only if there is very severe anaemia with symptoms. Exchange transfusion may be needed particularly if there is neurological damage, a visceral sequestration crisis or repeated painful crises. This is aimed at achieving an Hb S percentage of less than 30 in severe cases and after a stroke is continued for at least 2 years.

6 Particular care is needed in pregnancy and anaesthesia. There is debate as to whether patients need transfusions with normal blood to reduce Hb S levels during pregnancy or before delivery or for minor operations. Careful anaesthetic and recovery techniques must be used to avoid hypoxaemia or acidosis. Routine transfusions throughout pregnancy are given to those with a poor obstetric history or a history of frequent crises.

7 Transfusions – these are also sometimes given repeatedly as prophylaxis to patients having frequent crises or who have had major organ damage (e.g. of the brain) or show abnormal transcranial Doppler studies. The aim is to suppress Hb S production over a period of several months or even years. Iron overload, which may need iron chelation therapy, and alloimmunization against donated blood are common problems.

8 Hydroxycarbamide (hydroxyurea) (15.0–20.0 mg/kg) can increase Hb F levels and has been shown to improve the clinical course of

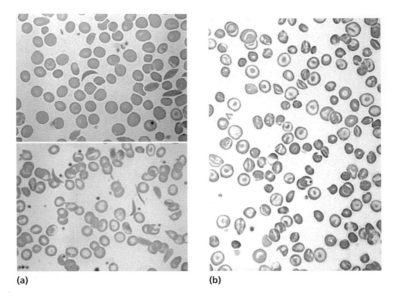

(a)   (b)

Figure 7.19 (a) Sickle cell anaemia: peripheral blood films showing deeply staining sickle cells, target cells and polychromasia. **(b)** Homozygous Hb C disease: peripheral blood film showing many target cells, deeply staining rhomboidal and spherocytic cells.

some children or adults who are having three or more painful crises each year. It should not be used during pregnancy.

9 Stem cell transplantation can cure the disease and many patients have now been successfully treated. The mortality rate is less than 10%. Transplantation is only indicated in the severest of cases whose quality of life or life expectancy are substantially impaired.

10 Research into other drugs (e.g. butyrates) to enhance Hb F synthesis or to increase the solubility of Hb S is taking place.

Sickle cell trait

This is a benign condition with no anaemia and normal appearance of red cells in a blood film. Haematuria is the most common symptom and is thought to be caused by minor infarcts of the renal papillae. Hb S varies from 25 to 45% of the total haemoglobin (Fig. 7.12). Care must be taken with anaesthesia, pregnancy and at high altitudes.

Combination of haemoglobin S with other genetic defects of haemoglobin

The most common of these are Hb S/β-thalassaemia, and sickle cell/C disease. In Hb S/β-thalassaemia, the MCV and MCH are lower than in homozygous Hb SS. The clinical picture is of sickle cell anaemia; splenomegaly is usual. Patients with Hb SC disease have a particular tendency to thrombosis and pulmonary embolism, especially in pregnancy. In general, when compared with Hb SS disease, they have a higher incidence of retinal abnormalities, milder anaemia, splenomegaly and generally a longer life expectancy. Diagnosis is made by haemoglobin electrophoresis, particularly with family studies.

Haemoglobin C disease

This genetic defect of haemoglobin is frequent in West Africa and is caused by substitution of lysine for glutamic acid in the β-globin chain at the same point as the substitution in Hb S. Hb C tends to form rhomboidal crystals and in the homozygous state there is a mild haemolytic anaemia with marked target cell formation, cells with rhomboidal shape and microspherocytes (Fig. 7.19b). The spleen is enlarged. The carriers show a few target cells only.

Haemoglobin D disease

This is a group of variants all with the same electrophoretic mobility. Heterozygotes show no haematological abnormality while homozygotes have a mild haemolytic anaemia.

Haemoglobin E disease

This is the most common haemoglobin variant in South-East Asia. In the homozygous state, there is a mild microcytic hypochromic anaemia. Haemoglobin E/β^0-thalassaemia, however, resembles homozygous β^0-thalassaemia both clinically and haematologically.

Prenatal diagnosis of genetic haemoglobin disorders

It is important to give genetic counselling to couples at risk of having a child with a major haemoglobin defect. If a pregnant woman is found to have a haemoglobin abnormality, her partner should be tested to determine whether he also carries a defect. When both partners show an abnormality and there is a risk of a serious defect in the offspring, particularly β-thalassaemia major, it is important to offer antenatal diagnosis. Several techniques are available, the choice depending on the stage of pregnancy and the potential nature of the defect.

DNA diagnosis

The majority of samples are obtained by chorionic villus biopsy although amniotic fluid cells are sometimes used. Techniques to sample maternal blood for fetal cells or fetal DNA are being developed. The DNA is then analysed using one of the following methods.

Polymerase chain reaction (PCR) is the most commonly used technique (Fig. 7.20) and may be performed by using primer pairs that only amplify individual alleles ('allele-specific priming') (Fig. 7.21) or by using consensus primers that amplify all the alleles followed by restriction digestion to detect a particular allele. This is best illustrated by Hb S in which the enzyme DdeI detects the A-T change (Fig. 7.22).

Gap-PCR analysis is useful for detecting gene deletions in α-thalassaemia (Fig. 7.23), for $\delta\beta$-thalassaemia and Hb Lepore. Small deletions and point mutations are diagnosed by cycle-sequencing of PCR product using fluorescent labels and analysis of the fragments on a capillary-based automatic sequencer. This approach is useful for rare and unknown mutations, for confirming prenatal diagnosis of β-thalassaemia and sickle cell disorders by other PCR methods, and for the rare non-deletion α^+-thalassaemia mutations that result in severe Hb H hydrops fetalis syndrome.

Pre-implantation genetic diagnosis which avoids the need for pregnancy termination involves per-

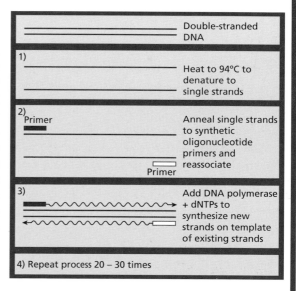

Figure 7.20 Polymerase chain reaction (PCR). The primers hybridize to DNA on either side of the piece of DNA to be analysed. Repeated cycles of denaturation, association with the primers, incubation with a DNA polymerase and deoxyribonucleotides (dNTPs) results in amplification of the DNA over a million times within a few hours.

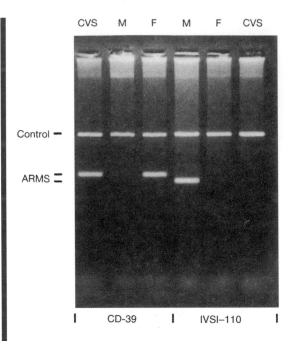

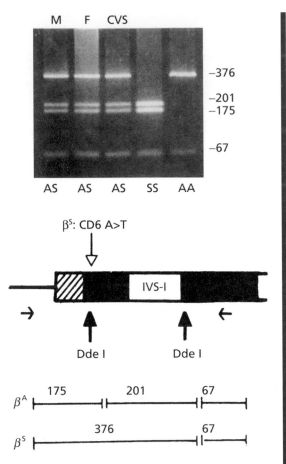

Figure 7.21 The rapid prenatal diagnosis of β-thalassaemia by amplification refractory mutation system (ARMS). The father has the common Mediterranean codon 39 (CD39) mutation, the mother the IVS1–110 G→A mutation. The fetus is hetero-zygous for the CD39 mutation. CVS, fetal DNA from chorionic villus sampling; F, father; M, mother. (Courtesy of Dr J. Old and Professor D.J. Weatherall.)

Figure 7.22 Sickle cell anaemia: antenatal diagnosis by DdeI-PCR analysis. The DNA is amplified by two primers that span the sickle cell gene mutation site and produces a product of 473 base pairs (bp) in size. The product is digested with the restriction enzyme DdeI and the resulting fragments analysed by agarose gel electrophoresis. The replacement of an adenine base in the normal β-globin gene by thymine results in Hb S and removes a normal restriction site for DdeI, producing a larger 376 bp fragment than the normal 175 and 201 bp fragments in the digested amplified product. In this case, the chorionic villus sample (CVS) DNA shows both the normal fragments and the larger sickle cell product and so is AS. The gel shows DNA from the mother (M), father (F), fetal DNA from a CVS, a normal DNA control (AA) and a homozygous sickle cell DNA control (SS). (Courtesy of Dr J. Old.)

forming conventional *in vitro* fertilization, followed by removing one or two cells from the blastomeres on day 3. PCR is used to detect thalassaemia muta-tions so that unaffected blastomeres can be selected for implantation. HLA typing can also be used to select an HLA matching blastomere matching a previous thalassaemia major child. Ethical consid-erations are important in deciding to use these applications.

Fetal blood sampling

Fetal blood sampling may be performed in mid-second trimester and allows DNA study and protein synthesis studies.

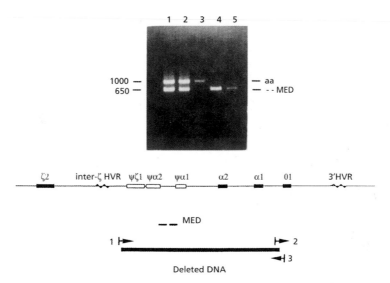

Figure 7.23 α^0-Thalassaemia: antenatal diagnosis by gap-PCR analysis. The common α^0-thalassaemia deletion mutations are diagnosed using primers which bind to flanking sequences on either side of the deletion break-point. For the −MED deletion, the primer pair (1 & 2) produce an amplified product of 650 base pairs (bp) in size. The primers are too far apart to amplify the normal DNA sequence, so a third primer (3) is included that is complementary to the deleted sequence near one of the breakpoints. This produces a normal fragment of 1000 bp. The gel electrophoresis photograph shows the mother's DNA (lane 1, heterozygous), father's DNA (lane 2, heterozygous), CVS DNA (lane 3, normal) and two homozygous control DNAs (lanes 4 & 5). (Courtesy of Dr. J. Old.)

SUMMARY

- Genetic disorders of haemoglobin fall into two main groups:
  1 The thalassaemias in which synthesis of the α or β globin chain is reduced.
  2 Structural disorders in which an abnormal haemoglobin is produced.
- The α- or β-thalassaemias occur clinically as minor forms with microcytic hypochromic red cells and a raised red cell count with or without anaemia. Total absence of function of all four α globin genes causes hydrops fetalis.
- Total absence of function of both β globin genes causes β-thalassaemia major, a transfusion-dependent anaemia associated with iron overload. Thalassaemia intermedia is a clinical term for a group of disorders showing mild to moderate anaemia and is usually caused by variants of β-thalassaemia.
- The most frequent structural defect of haemoglobin is the sickle mutation in the β-globin chain causing, in the homozygous form, a severe haemolytic anaemia, associated with vaso-occlusive crises. These may be painful affecting bone or affect soft tissues (e.g. chest, spleen or central nervous system). Crises may also be haemolytic or aplastic.
- Antenatal diagnosis using PCR technology to amplify chorionic villous DNA is used to detect severe genetic defects of haemoglobin production, with termination of the pregnancy if appropriate.

Now visit www.wiley.com/go/essentialhaematology to test yourself on this chapter.

CHAPTER 8

The white cells 1: granulocytes, monocytes and their benign disorders

Key topics

Essential Haematology, 6th Edition. © A. V. Hoffbrand and P. A. H. Moss. Published 2011 by Blackwell Publishing Ltd.

The white blood cells (leucocytes) may be divided into two broad groups: the phagocytes and the immunocytes. Granulocytes, which include three types of cell – neutrophils (polymorphs), eosinophils and basophils – together with monocytes comprise the phagocytes. Their normal development and function, and benign disorders are dealt with in this chapter. Only mature phagocytic cells and lymphocytes are found in normal peripheral blood (Table 8.1; Fig. 8.1). The lymphocytes, their

Adults	Blood count	Children	Blood count
Table 8.1 White cells: normal blood counts.			
Total leucocytes	$4.00–11.0 \times 10^9$/L*	*Total leucocytes*	
Neutrophils	$2.5–7.5 \times 10^9$/L*	Neonates	$10.0–25.0 \times 10^9$/L
Eosinophils	$0.04–0.4 \times 10^9$/L	1 year	$6.0–18.0 \times 10^9$/L
Monocytes	$0.2–0.8 \times 10^9$/L	4–7 years	$6.0–15.0 \times 10^9$/L
Basophils	$0.01–0.1 \times 10^9$/L	8–12 years	$4.5–13.5 \times 10^9$/L
Lymphocytes	$1.5–3.5 \times 10^9$/L		

*Normal black and Middle Eastern subjects may have lower counts. In normal pregnancy the upper limits are: total leucocytes 14.5×10^9/L, neutrophils 11×10^9/L.

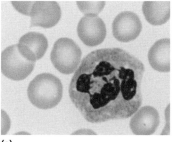
(a)

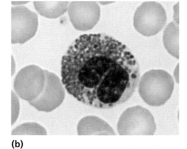
(b)

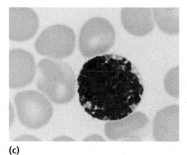
(c)

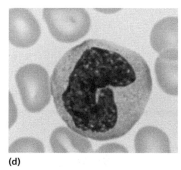
(d)

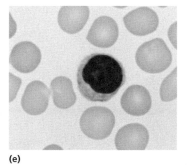
(e)

Figure 8.1 White blood cells (leucocytes): **(a)** neutrophil (polymorph); **(b)** eosinophil; **(c)** basophil; **(d)** monocyte; **(e)** lymphocyte.

precursor cells and plasma cells, which make up the immunocyte population, are considered in Chapter 9.

The function of phagocytes and immunocytes in protecting the body against infection is closely connected with two soluble protein systems of the body: immunoglobulins and complement. These proteins, which may also be involved in blood cell destruction in a number of diseases, are discussed together with the lymphocytes in Chapter 9.

Granulocytes

Neutrophil (polymorph)

This cell has a characteristic dense nucleus consisting of between two and five lobes, and a pale cytoplasm with an irregular outline containing many fine pink–blue (azurophilic) or grey–blue granules (Fig. 8.1a). The granules are divided into primary, which appear at the promyelocyte stage, and secondary (specific) which appear at the myelocyte

stage and predominate in the mature neutrophil (Fig 8.7). Both types of granule are lysosomal in origin (Fig. 8.7). The lifespan of neutrophils in the blood is only 6–10 hours.

Neutrophil precursors

These do not normally appear in normal peripheral blood but are present in the marrow (Fig. 8.2). The earliest recognizable precursor is the myeloblast, a cell of variable size that has a large nucleus with fine chromatin and usually two to five nucleoli (see Fig. 13.4). The cytoplasm is basophilic and no cytoplasmic granules are present. The normal bone marrow contains up to 5% of myeloblasts. Myeloblasts give rise by cell division to promyelocytes which are slightly larger cells and have developed primary granules in the cytoplasm. These cells then divide and differentiate to myelocytes which have specific or secondary granules. The nuclear chromatin is now more condensed and nucleoli are not visible. Separate myelocytes of the neutrophil, eosinophil

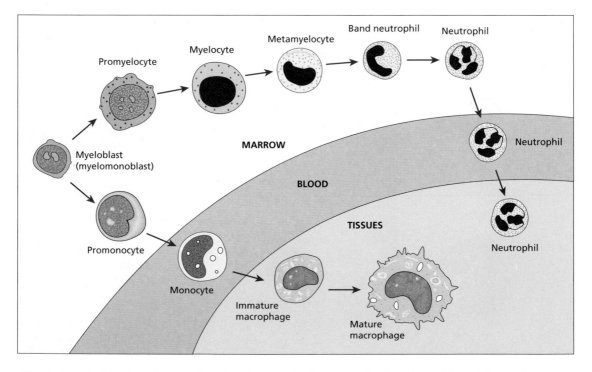

Figure 8.2 The formation of the neutrophil and monocyte phagocytes. Eosinophils and basophils are also formed in the marrow in a process similar to that for neutrophils.

and basophil series can be indentified. The myelo-cytes give rise by cell division and differentiation to metamyelocytes, non-dividing cells, which have an indented or horseshoe-shaped nucleus and a cyto-plasm filled with primary and secondary granules. Neutrophil forms between the metamyelocyte and fully mature neutrophil are termed 'band', 'stab' or 'juvenile'. These cells may occur in normal periph-eral blood. They do not contain the clear, fine fila-mentous connections between nuclear lobes that is seen in mature neutrophils.

Monocytes

These are usually larger than other peripheral blood leucocytes and possess a large central oval or indented nucleus with clumped chromatin (Fig. 8.1d). The abundant cytoplasm stains blue and con-tains many fine vacuoles, giving a ground-glass appearance. Cytoplasmic granules are also often present. The monocyte precursors in the marrow (monoblasts and promonocytes) are difficult to dis-tinguish from myeloblasts and monocytes.

Eosinophils

These cells are similar to neutrophils, except that the cytoplasmic granules are coarser and more deeply red staining and there are rarely more than three nuclear lobes (Fig. 8.1b). Eosinophil myelocytes can be recognized but earlier stages are indistinguishable from neutrophil precursors. The blood transit time for eosinophils is longer than for neutrophils. They enter inflammatory exudates and have a special role in allergic responses, defence against parasites and removal of fibrin formed during inflammation.

Basophils

These are only occasionally seen in normal periph-eral blood. They have many dark cytoplasmic gran-ules which overlie the nucleus and contain heparin and histamine (Fig. 8.1c). In the tissues they become mast cells. They have immunoglobulin E (IgE) attachment sites and their degranulation is associ-ated with histamine release.

Granulopoiesis

The blood granulocytes and monocytes are formed in the bone marrow from a common precursor cell (see Fig. 1.2). In the granulopoietic series progeni-tor cells, myeloblasts, promyelocytes and myelo-cytes form a proliferative or mitotic pool of cells while the metamyelocytes, band and segmented granulocytes make up a post-mitotic maturation compartment (Fig. 8.3). Large numbers of band and segmented neutrophils are held in the marrow

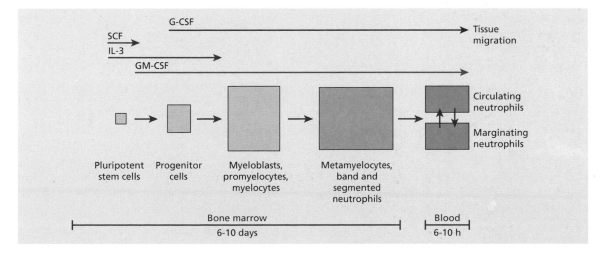

Figure 8.3 Neutrophil kinetics. CSF, colony-stimulating factor; G, granulocyte; IL, interleukin; M, monocyte; SCF, stem cell factor.

as a 'reserve pool' or storage compartment. The bone marrow normally contains more myeloid cells than erythroid cells in the ratio of 2:1 to 12:1, the largest proportion being neutrophils and metamyelocytes. In the stable or normal state, the bone marrow storage compartment contains 10–15 times the number of granulocytes found in the peripheral blood.

Following their release from the bone marrow, granulocytes spend only 6–10 hours in the circulation before moving into the tissues where they perform their phagocytic function. In the bloodstream there are two pools usually of about equal size: the circulating pool (included in the blood count) and the marginating pool (not included in the blood count). They spend on average 4–5 days in the tissues before they are destroyed during defensive action or as the result of senescence.

Control of granulopoiesis: myeloid growth factors

The granulocyte series arises from bone marrow progenitor cells which are increasingly specialized. Many growth factors are involved in this maturation process including interleukin-1 (IL-1), IL-3, IL-5 (for eosinophils), IL-6, IL-11, granulocyte–macrophage colony-stimulating factor (GM-CSF), granulocyte CSF (G-CSF) and monocyte CSF (M-CSF) (see Fig. 1.7). The growth factors stimulate proliferation and differentiation and also affect the function of the mature cells on which they act (e.g. phagocytosis, superoxide generation and cytotoxicity in the case of neutrophils; phagocytosis, cytotoxicity and production of other cytokines by monocytes) (Fig. 1.6).

Increased granulocyte and monocyte production in response to an infection is induced by increased production of growth factors from stromal cells and T lymphocytes, stimulated by endotoxin, IL-1 or tumour necrosis factor (TNF) (Fig. 8.4).

Clinical applications of G-CSF

Clinical administration of G-CSF intravenously or subcutaneously produces a rise in circulating neutrophils. G-CSF is used in clinical practice. Short-acting G-CSF is given daily. A longer acting

pegylated (PEG) G-CSF can be given once in 7–14 days. Some of the indications are as follows:

* *Post-chemotherapy, radiotherapy or stem cell transplantation* In these situations, G-CSF accelerates granulocytic recovery and shortens the period of neutropenia (Fig. 8.5). This may translate into a reduction of length of time in hospital, antibiotic usage and frequency of infection but periods of extreme neutropenia after intensive chemotherapy cannot be prevented.
* *Acute myeloid leukaemia* As in other haematological malignancies treated with intensive chemotherapy G-CSF has been used to reduce infections, hospital stay and antibiotic usage. There is no evidence that G-CSF injections can precipitate relapse of the disease.
* *Myelodysplasia* G-CSF has been given alone or in conjunction with erythropoietin in an attempt to improve bone marrow function (without accelerating leukaemic transformation).
* *Lymphomas* G-CSF is given to reduce infection, delay in giving chemotherapy and hospitalization after chemotherapy. A single injection of pegylated G-CSF immediately after chemotherapy is often used.
* *Severe neutropenia* Both congenital and acquired neutropenia, including cyclical and drug-induced neutropenia, have been found to respond well to G-CSF.
* *Severe infection* G-CSF has been used as an adjuvant to antimicrobial therapy.
* *Peripheral blood stem cell harvesting* G-CSF is used to increase the number of circulating multipotent progenitors, improving the harvest of sufficient peripheral blood stem cells for transplantation.

Monocytes

Monocytes spend only a short time in the marrow and, after circulating for 20–40 hours, leave the blood to enter the tissues where they mature and carry out their principal functions. Their extravascular lifespan after their transformation to macrophages (histiocytes) may be as long as several months or even years. They may assume specific functions in different tissues (e.g. skin, gut, liver) (Fig. 8.6). One particularly important lineage is that of

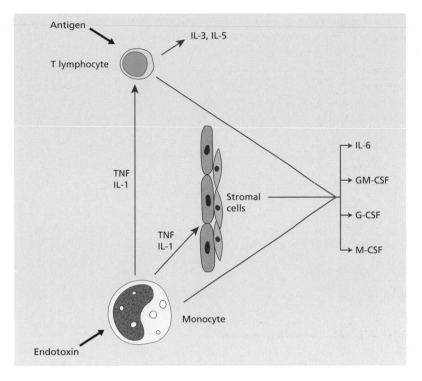

Figure 8.4 Regulation of haemopoiesis; pathways of stimulation of leucopoiesis by endotoxin, for example from infection. It is likely that endothelial and fibroblast cells release basal quantities of granulocyte–macrophage colony-stimulating factor (GM-CSF) and granulocyte colony-stimulating factor (G-CSF) in the normal resting state and that this is enhanced substantially by tumour necrosis factor (TNF) and interleukin-1 (IL-1) from monocytes.

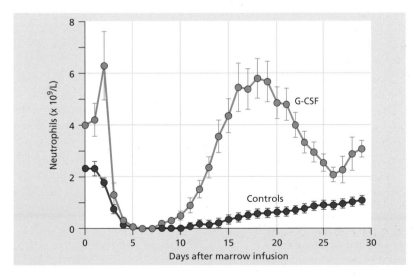

Figure 8.5 Typical effect of granulocyte colony-stimulating factor (G-CSF) on recovery of neutrophils following autologous bone marrow transplantation.

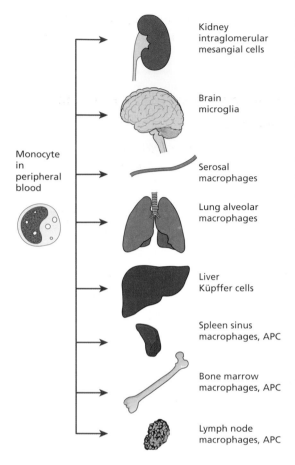

Monocyte
in
peripheral
blood

Kidney
intraglomerular
mesangial cells

Brain
microglia

Serosal
macrophages

Lung alveolar
macrophages

Liver
Küpffer cells

Spleen sinus
macrophages, APC

Bone marrow
macrophages, APC

Lymph node
macrophages, APC

Figure 8.6 Reticuloendothelial system: distribution of macrophages. APC, antigen presenting cells.

dendritic cells which are involved in antigen presentation to T cells (see Chapter 9). GM-CSF and M-CSF are involved in their production and activation.

Disorders of neutrophil and monocyte function

The normal function of neutrophils and monocytes may be divided into three phases.

Chemotaxis (cell mobilization and migration)

The phagocyte is attracted to bacteria or the site of inflammation by chemotactic substances released from damaged tissues or by complement components and also by the interaction of leucocyte adhesion molecules with ligands on the damaged tissues. The leucocyte adhesion molecules also mediate recruitment, migration and interaction with other immune cells. They are also variously expressed on endothelial cells and platelets (see Chapter 1).

Phagocytosis

The foreign material (e.g. bacteria, fungi) or dead or damaged cells of the host are phagocytosed (Fig. 8.7). Recognition of a foreign particle is aided by opsonization with immunoglobulin or complement because both neutrophils and monocytes have Fc and C3b receptors (see Chapter 9). Opsonization of normal body cells (e.g. red cells or platelets) also makes them liable to destruction by macrophages of the reticuloendothelial system, as in autoimmune haemolysis, idiopathic (autoimmune) thrombocytopenic purpura or many of the drug-induced cytopenias.

Macrophages have a central role in antigen presentation: processing and presenting foreign antigens on human leucocyte antigen (HLA) molecules to the immune system. They also secrete a large number of growth factors and chemokines that regulate inflammation and immune responses.

Chemokines are chemotactic cytokines of which there are two main classes: CXC (α) chemokines, small (8–10 000 MW) pro-inflammatory cytokines which mainly act on neutrophils, and CC (β) chemokines such as macrophage inflammatory protein-1α (MIP-1α) and RANTES, which act on monocytes, basophils, eosinophils and natural killer (NK) cells. Chemokines may be produced constitutively and control lymphocyte traffic under physiological conditions; inflammatory chemokines are induced or up-regulated by inflammatory stimuli. They bind to and activate cells via chemokine receptors and play an important part in recruiting appropriate cells to the sites of inflammation.

Killing and digestion

This occurs by oxygen-dependent and oxygen-independent pathways. In the oxygen-dependent reactions, superoxide (O_2^-), hydrogen peroxide

(H_2O_2) and other activated oxygen (O_2) species, are generated from O_2 and reduced nicotinamide adenine dinucleotide phosphate (NADPH). In neutrophils, H_2O_2 reacts with myeloperoxidase and intracellular halide to kill bacteria; activated oxygen may also be involved. The non-oxidative microbicidal mechanisms involve microbicidal proteins. These may act alone (e.g. cathepsin G) or in conjunction with H_2O_2 (e.g. lysozyme, elastase). They may also act with a fall in pH within phagocytic vacuoles into which lysosomal enzymes are released. An additional iron binding protein, lactoferrin, is present in neutrophil granules and is bacteriostatic by depriving bacteria of iron and generating free radicals (Fig. 8.7). Finally, nitric oxide (NO) generated through NO synthase from L-arginine is another mechanism by which phagocytes kill microbes.

Defects of phagocytic cell function

Chemotaxis

These defects occur in rare congenital abnormalities (e.g. 'lazy leucocyte' syndrome) and in more common acquired abnormalities either of the environment (e.g. corticosteroid therapy) or of the leucocytes themselves (e.g. in acute or chronic myeloid leukaemia, myelodysplasia and the myeloproliferative syndromes).

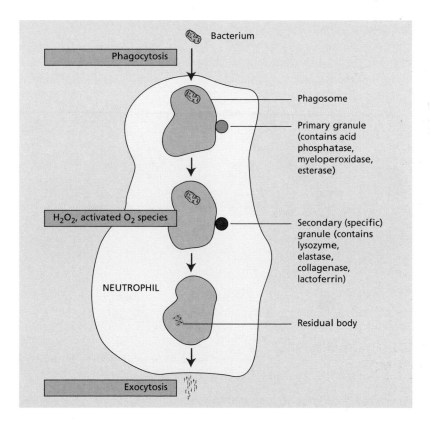

Figure 8.7 Phagocytosis and bacterial destruction. On entering the neutrophil, the bacterium is surrounded by an invaginated surface membrane and fuses with a primary lysosome to form a phagosome. Enzymes from the lysosome attack the bacterium. Secondary granules also fuse with the phagosomes, and new enzymes from these granules including lactoferrin attack the organism. Various types of activated oxygen, generated by glucose metabolism, also help to kill bacteria. Undigested residual bacterial products are excreted by exocytosis.

Phagocytosis

These defects usually arise because of a lack of opsonization which may be caused by congenital or acquired causes of hypogammaglobulinaemia or lack of complement components.

Killing

This abnormality is clearly illustrated by the rare X-linked or autosomal recessive chronic granulomatous disease that results from abnormal leucocyte oxidative metabolism. There is an abnormality affecting different elements of the respiratory burst oxidase or its activating mechanism. The patients have recurring infections, usually bacterial but sometimes fungal, which present in infancy or early childhood in most cases.

Other rare congenital abnormalities may also result in defects of bacterial killing (e.g. myeloperoxidase deficiency and the Chédiak–Higashi syndrome; see below). Acute or chronic myeloid leukaemia and myelodysplastic syndromes may also be associated with defective killing of ingested microorganisms.

Benign disorders

A number of the hereditary conditions may give rise to changes in granulocyte morphology (Fig. 8.8).

Pelger–Huët anomaly

In this uncommon condition bilobed neutrophils are found in the peripheral blood. Occasional unsegmented neutrophils are also seen. Inheritance is autosomal dominant.

May–Hegglin anomaly

In this rare condition the neutrophils contain basophilic inclusions of RNA (resembling Döhle bodies) in the cytoplasm. There is an associated

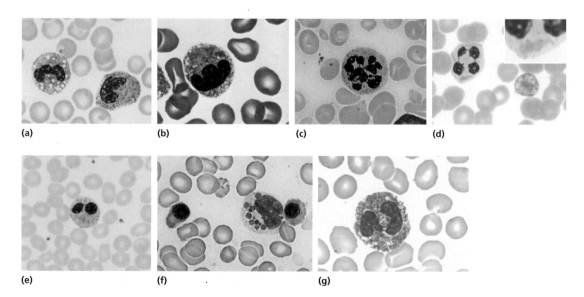

(a) (b) (c) (d)

(e) (f) (g)

Figure 8.8 Abnormal white blood cells. **(a)** Neutrophil leucocytosis: toxic changes shown by the presence of red–purple granules in the band form neutrophils. **(b)** Neutrophil leucocytosis: a Döhle body can be seen in the cytoplasm of the neutrophil. **(c)** Megaloblastic anaemia: hypersegmented oversized neutrophil in peripheral blood. **(d)** May–Hegglin anomaly: the neutrophils contain basophilic inclusions 2–5 μm in diameter; there is an associated mild thrombocytopenia with giant platelets. **(e)** Pelger–Huët anomaly: coarse clumping of the chromatin in *pince nez* configuration. **(f)** Chédiak–Higashi syndrome: bizarre giant granules in the cytoplasm of a monocyte. **(g)** Alder's anomaly: coarse violet granules in the cytoplasm of a neutrophil.

mild thrombocytopenia with giant platelets. Inheritance is autosomal dominant.

Other rare disorders

In contrast to these two relatively benign anomalies, other rare congenital leucocyte disorders may be associated with severe disease. The Chédiak–Higashi syndrome is inherited in an autosomal recessive manner, and there are giant granules in the neutrophils, eosinophils, monocytes and lymphocytes accompanied by neutropenia, thrombocytopenia and marked hepatosplenomegaly. Abnormal leucocyte granulation or vacuolation is also seen in patients with rare mucopolysaccharide disorders (e.g. Hurler's syndrome).

Common morphological abnormalities

Figure 8.8 also shows some of the more common abnormalities of neutrophil morphology that can be seen in peripheral blood. Hypersegmented forms occur in megaloblastic anaemia, Döhle bodies and toxic changes in infection. The 'drumstick' appears on the nucleus of a proportion of the neutrophils in normal females and is caused by the presence of two X chromosomes. Pelger cells are seen in the benign congenital abnormality but also in patients with acute myeloid leukaemia or myelodysplasia.

Causes of leucocytosis and monocytosis

Neutrophil leucocytosis

An increase in circulating neutrophils to levels greater than 7.5×10^9/L is one of the most frequently observed blood count changes. The causes of neutrophil leucocytosis are given in Table 8.2. Neutrophil leucocytosis is sometimes accompanied by fever as a result of the release of leucocyte pyrogens. Other characteristic features of reactive neutrophilia may include: (a) a 'shift to the left' in the peripheral blood differential white cell count (i.e. an increase in the number of band forms) and the

Table 8.2 Causes of neutrophil leucocytosis.

Bacterial infections (especially pyogenic bacterial, localized or generalized)
Inflammation and tissue necrosis (e.g. myositis, vasculitis, cardiac infarct, trauma)
Metabolic disorders (e.g. uraemia, eclampsia, acidosis, gout)
Neoplasms of all types (e.g. carcinoma, lymphoma, melanoma)
Acute haemorrhage or haemolysis
Drugs (e.g. corticosteroid therapy (inhibits margination): lithium, tetracycline)
Chronic myeloid leukaemia, myeloproliferative disease: polycythaemia vera, myelofibrosis, essential thrombocythaemia
Treatment with myeloid growth factors (e.g. G-CSF)
Rare inherited disorders
Asplenia

occasional presence of more primitive cells such as metamyelocytes and myelocytes; (b) the presence of cytoplasmic toxic granulation and Döhle bodies (Fig. 8.8a,b).

The leukaemoid reaction

The leukaemoid reaction is a reactive and excessive leucocytosis usually characterized by the presence of immature cells (e.g. myeloblasts, promyelocytes and myelocytes) in the peripheral blood. Occasionally, lymphocytic reactions occur. Associated disorders include severe or chronic infections, severe haemolysis or metastatic cancer. Leukaemoid reactions are often particularly marked in children. Granulocyte changes such as toxic granulation and Döhle bodies help to differentiate the leukaemoid reaction from chronic myeloid leukaemia.

Leucoerythroblastic reaction

This is characterized by the presence of erythroblast and granulocyte precursors in the blood (Fig 8.9). It is caused by metastatic infiltration of the marrow or certain benign or neoplastic blood disorders (Table 8.3).

Neutropenia

The lower limit of the normal neutrophil count is $2.5 \times 10^9/L$ except in black people and in the Middle East where $1.5 \times 10^9/L$ is normal (see below). When the absolute neutrophil level falls below $0.5 \times 10^9/L$ the patient is likely to have recurrent infections and when the count falls to less than $0.2 \times 10^9/L$ the risks are very serious, particularly if there is also a functional defect. Neutropenia may be selective or part of a general pancytopenia (Table 8.4).

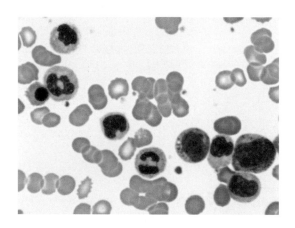

Figure 8.9 Leucoerythroblastic blood film. This shows an erythroblast, promyelocyte, myelocyte and metamyelocytes in a patient with metastatic breast carcinoma in the bone marrow. (Courtesy of Dr J.E. Pettit.)

Table 8.3 Causes of leucoerythroblastic blood film

Metastatic neoplasm in the marrow
Primary myelofibrosis
Acute and chronic myeloid leukaemia
Myeloma, lymphoma
Miliary tuberculosis
Severe megaloblastic anaemia
Severe haemolysis
Osteopetrosis

Table 8.4 Causes of neutropenia.

Selective neutropenia
Congenital
Kostmann's syndrome

Acquired
Drug-induced
 Anti-inflammatory drugs (phenylbutazone)
 Antibacterial drugs (chloramphenicol, co-trimoxazole, sulfasalazine, imipenem)
 Anticonvulsants (phenytoin, carbamazepine)
 Antithyroids (carbimazole)
 Hypoglycaemics (tolbutamide)
 Phenothiazines (chlorpromazine, thioridazine)
 Psychotropics and antidepressants (clozapine, mianserin, imipramine)
 Miscellaneous (gold, penicillamine, mepacrine, frusemide, deferiprone)

Benign (racial or familial)

Cyclical

Immune
Autoimmune
Systemic lupus erythematosus
Felty's syndrome
Hypersensitivity and anaphylaxis

Large granular lymphocytic leukaemia
(see p. 242)

Infections
Viral (e.g. hepatitis, influenza, HIV)
Fulminant bacterial infection (e.g. typhoid, miliary tuberculosis)

Part of general pancytopenia (see Table 22.1)
Bone marrow failure
Splenomegaly

HIV, human immunodeficiency virus.

Benign ethnic neutropenia

It has been known for many decades that black people often have a low neutrophil count. It is now clear that up to 98% of people of West African origin carry a polymorphism in the Duffy antigen chemokine receptor (DARC) gene which leads to loss of DARC expression on red cells. This has apparently been selected during evolution because the malaria parasite *Plasmodium vivax* uses DARC as a receptor to enter the red cell. DARC is a chemokine receptor and the loss of red cell DARC expression leads directly to the clinical state of benign ethnic neutropenia. The effect is to lower the median neutrophil count by around $0.5 \times 10^9/L$ in this population. There does not appear to be any significant clinical sequelae and the reduced blood cell count may result from an altered pattern of neutrophil margination. A similar effect is also seen in other populations, most notably in the Middle East.

Congenital neutropenia

Kostmann's syndrome is an autosomal recessive disease presenting in the first year of life with life-threatening infections. Most cases are caused by mutations of the gene coding for neutrophil elastase. G-CSF produces a clinical response although marrow fibrosis and acute myeloid leukaemia may supervene.

Drug-induced neutropenia

A large number of drugs have been implicated (Table 8.4) and may induce neutropenia either by direct toxicity or immune-mediated damage.

Cyclical neutropenia

This is a rare syndrome with 3- to 4-week periodicity. Severe but temporary neutropenia occurs. Monocytes tend to rise as the neutrophils fall. Mutation of the gene for neutrophil elastase underlies some cases.

Autoimmune neutropenia

In some cases of chronic neutropenia an autoimmune mechanism can be demonstrated. The antibody may be directed against one of the neutrophil-specific antigens (e.g. NA, NB).

Idiopathic benign neutropenia

An increase in the marginating fraction of blood neutrophils and a corresponding reduction in the circulating fraction is one cause of benign neutropenia. This may in some races be related to reduced DARC expression as discussed above. Many healthy Africans and other races, especially in the Middle East, have a low peripheral blood neutrophil count without excess margination. These subjects have no increased susceptibility to infection and the bone marrow appears normal although there is diminished neutrophil production.

Finally, the term chronic idiopathic neutropenia is used for unexplained acquired neutropenia (neutrophil count below normal for the ethnic group), without phasic variations or underlying disease. It is more common in females and thought to be brought about by immune cells causing inhibition of myelopoiesis in the bone marrow.

Clinical features

Severe neutropenia is particularly associated with infections of the mouth and throat. Painful and often intractable ulceration may occur at these sites (Fig. 8.10), on the skin or at the anus. Septicaemia rapidly supervenes. Organisms carried as commensals by healthy individuals, such as *Staphylococcus epidermidis* or Gram-negative organisms in the bowel, may become pathogens. Other features of infections associated with severe neutropenia are described on p. 169.

Diagnosis

Bone marrow examination is useful in determining the level of damage in granulopoiesis (i.e. whether there is reduction in early precursors or whether there is reduction only of circulating and marrow neutrophils with late precursors remaining in the marrow). Marrow aspiration and trephine biopsy may also provide evidence of leukaemia, myelodysplasia or other infiltration.

Management

The treatment of patients with acute severe neutropenia is described on p. 169. In many patients with drug-induced neutropenia spontaneous recovery occurs within 1–2 weeks after stopping the drug. Patients with chronic neutropenia have recurrent infections which are mainly bacterial in origin although fungal and viral infections (especially herpes) also occur. Early recognition and vigorous treatment with antibiotics, antifungal or antiviral agents, as appropriate, is essential. Prophylactic antibacterial agents (e.g. oral co-trimoxazole or ciprofloxacin and colistin) and antifungal agents (e.g. oral amphotericin and fluconazole or itraconazole) may be of value in reducing the incidence and severity of infections caused by severe neutropenia. The haemopoietic growth factor G-CSF may be used to stimulate neutrophil production and is effective in a variety of benign chronic neutropenic states. Corticosteroid therapy or splenectomy has been associated with good results in some patients with autoimmune neutropenia. Rituximab (anti-CD20) may also be effective. Conversely, corticosteroids impair neutrophil function and should not be used indiscriminately in patients with neutropenia.

Monocytosis

A rise in blood monocyte count above $0.8 \times 10^9/L$ is infrequent. The conditions listed in Table 8.5 may be responsible.

Eosinophilic leucocytosis (eosinophilia)

The causes of an increase in blood eosinophils (Fig. 8.11) above $0.4 \times 10^9/L$ are listed in Table 8.6.

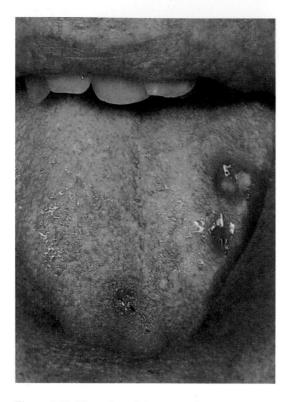

Figure 8.10 Ulceration of the tongue in severe neutropenia.

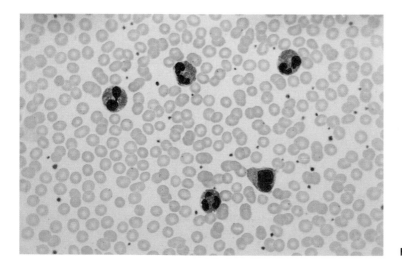

Figure 8.11 Eosinophilia.

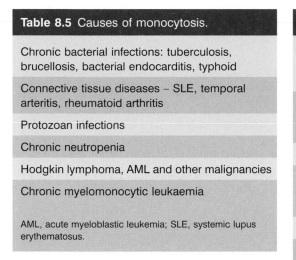

Table 8.5 Causes of monocytosis.

Chronic bacterial infections: tuberculosis, brucellosis, bacterial endocarditis, typhoid

Connective tissue diseases – SLE, temporal arteritis, rheumatoid arthritis

Protozoan infections

Chronic neutropenia

Hodgkin lymphoma, AML and other malignancies

Chronic myelomonocytic leukaemia

AML, acute myeloblastic leukemia; SLE, systemic lupus erythematosus.

Table 8.6 Causes of eosinophilia.

Allergic diseases, especially hypersensitivity of the atopic type (e.g. bronchial asthma, hay fever, urticaria and food sensitivity)

Parasitic diseases (e.g. amoebiasis, hookworm, ascariasis, tapeworm infestation, filariasis, schistosomiasis and trichinosis)

Recovery from acute infection

Certain skin diseases (e.g. psoriasis, pemphigus and dermatitis herpetiformis, urticaria and angioedema, atopic dermatitis)

Drug sensitivity

Polyarteritis nodosa, vasculitis, serum sickness

Graft-versus-host disease

Hodgkin lymphoma and some other tumours, especially clonal T-cell disorders

Metastatic malignancy with tumour necrosis

Hypereosinophilic syndrome

Chronic eosinophilic leukaemia

Myeloproliferative including systemic mastocytosis

Pulmonary syndromes
  Eosinophilic pneumonia, transient pulmonary infiltrates (Loeffler's syndrome), allergic granulomatosis (Churg–Strauss syndrome), tropical pulmonary eosinophilia

Eosinophilic leucocytosis is most frequently caused by allergic diseases, parasites, skin diseases or drugs. Sometimes no underlying cause is found, no clonal marker can be indicated and if the eosinophil count is elevated ($>1.5 \times 10^9$/L) for over 6 months and associated with tissue damage then the *hypereosinophilic syndrome* is diagnosed. The heart valves, central nervous system, skin and lungs may be affected and treatment is usually with steroids or cytotoxic drugs. In 25% of cases a clonal T-cell population is present. In other cases of chronic eosinophilia, often with similar clinical features, a clonal cytogenetic or molecular abnormality is present and the term chronic eosinophilic leukaemia is used (see p. 199).

Basophil leucocytosis (basophilia)

An increase in blood basophils above 0.1×10^9/L is uncommon. The usual cause is a myeloproliferative disorder such as chronic myeloid leukaemia or polycythaemia vera. Reactive basophil increases are sometimes seen in myxoedema, during smallpox or chickenpox infection and in ulcerative colitis.

Histiocytic and dendritic cell disorders

Histiocytes are myeloid-derived tissue macrophages (Table 8.7).

Dendritic cells

These are specialized antigen-presenting cells found mainly in the skin, lymph nodes, spleen and thymus. They comprise:

1 Myeloid-derived cells including Langerhans' cells which are present in skin and mucosa and are characterized by the presence of tennis racquet-shaped Birbeck granules in electron-microscopy sections in neutrophils, eosinophils, macrophages and lymphocytes; and

Table 8.7 Classification of the histiocytic and dendritic cell disorders.

Benign

Dendritic cell-related
Langerhans' cell histiocytosis
Solitary dendritic cell histiocytoma

Histiocyte-related
Haemophagocytic lymphohistiocytosis
  primary (familial)
  secondary – infection, drug, tumour
Sinus histiocytosis with massive
  lymphadenopathy (Rosai–Dorfman syndrome)

Malignant
Dendritic and histiocytic sarcomas (localized or
  disseminated)
AML, monocytic and myelomonocytic (see p.
  179)
Chronic myelomonocytic leukaemia (see p. 221)

AML, acute myeloid leukaemia.

2 A lymphocyte-derived subset. The primary role of dendritic cells is antigen presentation to T and B lymphocytes (see p. 133).

Langerhans' cell histiocytes

Langerhans' cell histiocytosis (LCH) includes diseases previously called *histiocytosis X, Letterer–Siwe disease, Hand–Schüller–Christian disease* and *eosinophilic granuloma*. The disease may be single organ or multisystem. There is a clonal proliferation of CD1a-positive cells. The multisystem disease affects children in the first 3 years of life with hepatosplenomegaly, lymphadenopathy and eczematous skin symptoms. Localized lesions may occur especially in the skull, ribs and long bones, the posterior pituitary causing diabetes insipidus, the central nervous system, gastrointestinal tract and lungs. The lesions include Langerhans' cells (characterized by the presence of tennis racquet-shaped Birbeck granules in electron-microscopy sections), eosinophils, lymphocytes, neutrophils and macrophages. The prognosis is better for localized disease but there is a 66% mortality in young children with multisystem disease who do not respond to chemotherapy.

Haemophagocytic lymphohistiocytosis (haemophagocytic syndrome)

This is a rare, recessively inherited or more frequently acquired disease, usually precipitated by a viral (especially Epstein–Barr or herpes viruses), bacterial or fungal infection or occuring in association with tumours. Often the patient is immunocompromised. Patients present with fever and pancytopenia, often with splenomegaly and liver dysfunction. There are increased numbers of histiocytes in the bone marrow which ingest red cells, white cells and platelets (Fig. 8.12). Clinical features are fever, pancytopenia and multiorgan dysfunction often with lymphadenopathy, hepatic and splenic enlargement, coagulopathy and CNS signs. Treatment is of the underlying infection, if known, with support care. T-cell activation is implicated in the aetiology. Chemotherapy with etoposide, corticosteroids, ciclosporin or rituximab (anti-CD20) may be tried. The condition is often fatal.

Sinus histiocytosis with massive lymphadenopathy

This is also known as the Rosai–Dorfman syndrome. There is painless, chronic cervical lymphadenopathy. There may be fever and weight loss. The histology is typical and the condition subsides over months or years.

Lysosomal storage diseases

Gaucher's, Tay–Sachs and Niemann–Pick diseases result from hereditary deficiency of enzymes required for glycolipid breakdown.

Gaucher's disease

Gaucher's disease is an uncommon autosomal recessive disorder characterized by an accumulation of glucosylceramide in the lysosomes of reticuloendothelial cells as a result of deficiency of glucocerebrosidase (Fig. 8.13. Three types occur: a chronic adult type (type I); an acute infantile neuronopathic

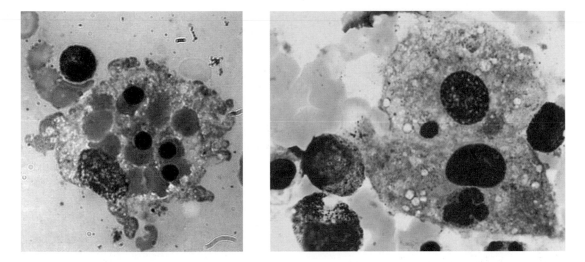

Figure 8.12 Haemophagocytic lymphohistiocytosis: bone marrow aspirates showing histiocytes that have ingested red cells, erythroblasts and neutrophils.

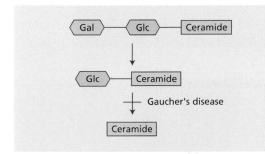

Figure 8.13 Gaucher's disease results from a deficiency of glucocerebrosidase. Gal, galactose; Glc, glucose.

type (type II); and a subacute neuronopathic type with onset in childhood or adolescence (type III). Type I is caused by a variety of mutations in the glucocerebrosidase gene, one type of which (a single base pair substitution in codon 444) is particularly common in Ashkenazi Jews and explains the high incidence of the disease in this group. In type I the outstanding physical sign is splenomegaly. Moderate liver enlargement and pingueculae (conjunctival deposits) are other characteristic findings. In many cases, bone deposits cause bone pain and pathologi-

cal fractures. Osteoporosis is also frequent. Expansion of the lower end of the femur may produce the 'Erlenmeyer flask deformity' (Fig. 8.14c).

The clinical manifestations are caused by the accumulation of glucocerebroside-laden macrophages in the spleen, liver and bone marrow (Fig. 8.14a,b). Gaucher cells are, however, not inert lipid storage containers but are metabolically active, secreting proteins that cause secondary pathology (e.g. pulmonary hypertension, alveolar fibrosis and cholesterol gallstones). Carriers of a Gaucher mutation also have an increased incidence and earlier onset of Parkinson's disease.

Gaucher's disease at all ages is commonly associated with marked anaemia, leucopenia and thrombocytopenia occurring singly or in combination. Polyclonal hypergammaglobulinaemia or monoclonal gammopathy are frequent with a risk of myeloma. Diagnosis is made by assay of white cell glucocerebrosidase and DNA analysis. Lysosomal enyzmes, chitotriosidase and acid phosphatase are raised and useful in monitoring therapy. Pulmonary activation regulated cytokine (PARC), angiotensin-converting enzyme (ACE), macrophage inflammation factor protein (MIP-1β) and ferritin are also elevated.

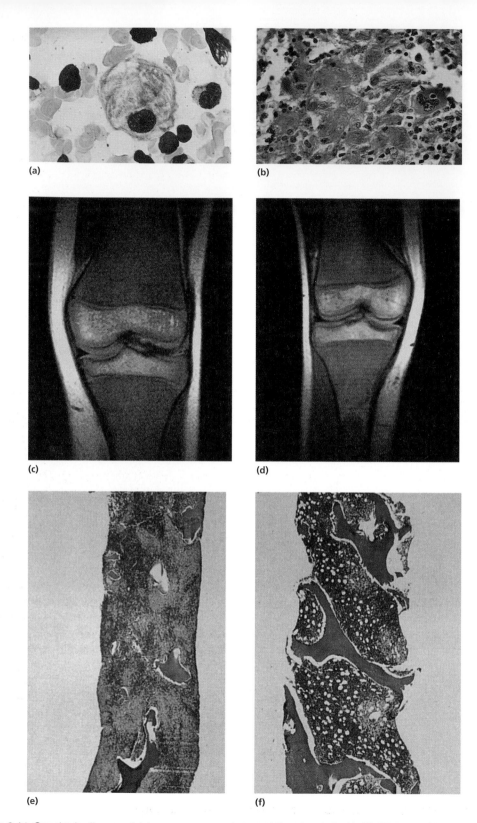

Figure 8.14 Gaucher's disease: **(a)** bone marrow aspirate – a Gaucher cell with 'fibrillar' cytoplasmic pattern; **(b)** spleen histology – pale clusters of Gaucher cells in the reticuloendothelial cord; **(c)** magnetic resonance imaging (MRI) scan of the left knee of a patient before treatment showing Erlenmeyer flask deformity with expansion of the marrow and thinning of the cortical bone; **(d)** following a year of glucocerebrosidase therapy with subsequent remodelling of bone; and bone marrow trephine biopsy before **(e)** and after **(f)** 2 years of glucocerebrosidase therapy.

Enzyme replacement therapy with glucocerebrosidase, imiglucerase (Cerezyme®), made by recombinant technology and given intravenously once every 2 weeks is very effective in treating the disease with shrinkage of spleen, rise in blood count and improved bone structure (Fig. 8.14d,f). Two new recombinant enzymes, velaglucerase and taliglucerase, are now available. An oral drug, miglustat, is useful in mild forms. It reduces the amount of substrate being produced in lysosomes and may be used in combination with the intravenous enzyme.

Newer preparations are becoming available. The use of imiglucerase has virtually eliminated the need for splenectomy but it cannot reverse established osteonecrosis, bone deformation, hepatic, splenic or marrow fibrosis. Stem cell transplantation has been carried out successfully in severely affected patients, usually with type II or III disease.

Niemann–Pick disease

Niemann–Pick disease shows certain clinical and pathological similarities to Gaucher's disease. It is caused by a sphingomyelinase deficiency. The majority of patients are infants who die in the first few years of life although occasional patients survive to adult life. Massive hepatosplenomegaly occurs and there is usually lung and nervous system involvement with retarded physical and mental development. A 'cherry-red' spot is commonly seen in the retina of affected infants. Pancytopenia is a regular feature and in marrow aspirates 'foam cells' of similar size to Gaucher cells are seen. Chemical analysis of the tissues reveals that the disorder is caused by an accumulation of sphingomyelin and cholesterol.

SUMMARY

- Granulocytes include neutrophils (polymorphs), eosinophils and basophils. They are made in the bone marrow under the control of a variety of growth factors and have a short lifespan in the blood stream before entering tissues.
- Phagocytes (neutrophils and monocytes) are the body's main defence against bacterial infection. Neutrophil leucocytosis occurs in bacterial infection and in other types of inflammation. Neutropenia, if severe, predisposes to infections. It may be caused by bone marrow failure, chemotherapy or radiotherapy drugs, immune mechanisms or occur congenitally.
- Eosinophilia is most frequently caused by allergic diseases, including skin diseases, parasitic infections or drugs. It can be caused by a clonal increase in eosinophils termed chronic eosinophilic leukaemia or an idiopathic condition, often associated with tissue damage.

- Defects of function of neutrophils and monocytes may affect their chemotaxis, phagocytosis or killing.
- Histiocytes are tissue macrophages derived from circulation monocytes. They may form clonal diseases called Langerhans' cell histiocytosis which affect single or multiple organs.
- The haemophagocytic syndrome involves destruction of red cells, granulocytes and platelets by tissue macrophages.
- Lysosomal storage diseases are caused by inherited defects in the enzymes responsible for breakdown of glycolipids. Gaucher's disease is caused by glucocerebrosidase deficiency and is associated with accumulation of glycolipids in the reticuloendothelial system with splenomegaly, pancytopenia and bone lesions causing the main clinical manifestations.

Now visit www.wiley.com/go/essentialhaematology to test yourself on this chapter.

CHAPTER 9
The white cells 2: lymphocytes and their benign disorders

Key topics

Essential Haematology, 6th Edition. © A. V. Hoffbrand and P. A. H. Moss. Published 2011 by Blackwell Publishing Ltd.

Lymphocytes are the immunologically competent cells that assist the phagocytes in defence of the body against infection and other foreign invasion (Fig. 9.1). Two unique features characteristic of the immune system are the ability to generate **antigenic specificity** and the phenomenon of **immunological memory**. A complete description of the functions of lymphocytes is beyond the scope of this book, but information essential to an understanding of the diseases of the lymphoid system, and of the role of lymphocytes in haematological diseases, is included here.

Lymphocytes

In postnatal life, the bone marrow and thymus are the **primary lymphoid organs** in which lymphocytes develop (Fig. 9.2). The **secondary lymphoid organs** in which specific immune responses are generated are the lymph nodes, spleen and lymphoid tissues of the alimentary and respiratory tracts.

B and T lymphocytes

The immune response depends upon two types of lymphocytes, B and T cells (Table 9.1), which derive from the haemopoietic stem cell. B cells mature in the bone marrow and circulate in the peripheral blood until they undergo recognition of antigen. The B-cell receptor is membrane-bound immunoglobulin and after activation this is secreted as free soluble immunoglobulin. At this point they mature into memory B cells or plasma cells. The latter home to the bone marrow and have a characteristic morphology with an eccentric round nucleus with a 'clock-face' chromatin pattern and strongly basophilic cytoplasm (Fig. 9.1d).

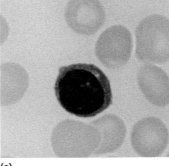
(a)

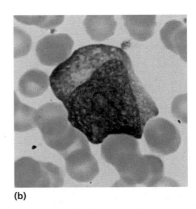
(b)

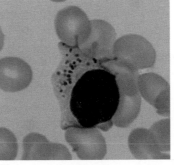
(c)

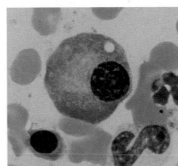
(d)

Figure 9.1 Lymphocytes: **(a)** small lymphocyte; **(b)** activated lymphocyte; **(c)** large granular lymphocyte; **(d)** plasma cell.

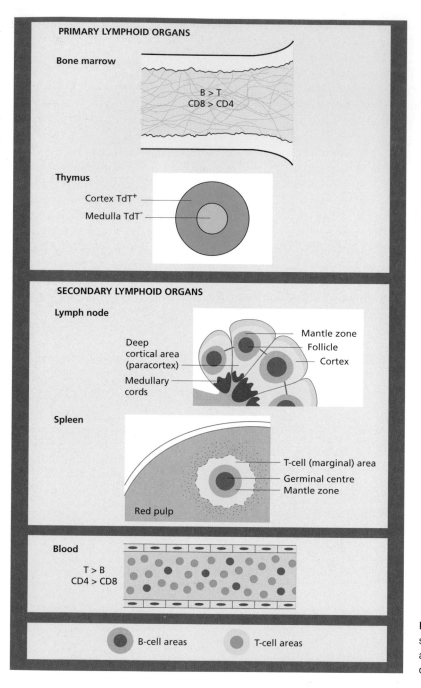

Figure 9.2 Primary and secondary lymphoid organs and blood. TdT, terminal deoxynucleotidyl.

Table 9.1 Functional aspects of T and B cells.

	T cells	B cells
Origin	Thymus	Bone marrow
Tissue distribution	Parafollicular areas of cortex in nodes, periarteriolar in spleen	Germinal centres of lymph nodes, spleen, gut, respiratory tract; also subcapsular and medullary cords of lymph nodes
Blood	80% of lymphocytes; CD4 > CD8	20% of lymphocytes
Membrane receptor	TCR for antigen	BCR (= immunoglobulin) for antigen
Function	CD8$^+$: CMI against intracellular organisms CD4$^+$: T-cell help for antibody production and generation of CMI	Humoral immunity by generation of antibodies
Characteristic surface markers	CD1 CD2 CD3 CD4 or 8 CD5 CD6 CD7 HLA class I HLA class II when activated	CD19 CD20 CD22 CD9 (pre B cells) CD10 (precursor B cells) CD79 a and b HLA class I and II
Genes rearranged	TCR α, β, γ, δ	IgH, Igκ, Igλ

BCR, B cell receptor; C, complement; CMI, cell-mediated immunity; HLA, human leucocyte antigen; Ig, immunoglobulin; TCR, T-cell receptor.

T cells develop from cells that have migrated to the thymus where they differentiate into mature T cells during passage from the cortex to the medulla. During this process, self-reactive T cells are deleted (negative selection) whereas T cells with some specificity for host human leucocyte antigen (HLA) molecules are selected (positive selection). The mature helper cells express CD4 and cytotoxic cells express CD8 (Table 9.1). The cells also express one of two T-cell antigen receptor heterodimers, $\alpha\beta$ (>90%) or $\gamma\delta$ (<10%), and recognize antigen only when it is presented at a cell surface (see below).

Natural killer cells

Natural killer (NK) cells are cytotoxic CD8$^+$ cells that lack the T-cell receptor (TCR). They are large cells with cytoplasmic granules and typically express surface molecules CD16 (Fc receptor), CD56 and CD57. NK cells are designed to kill target cells that have a low level of expression of HLA class I molecules such as may occur during viral infection or on a malignant cell. NK cells do this by displaying a number of receptors for HLA molecules on their surface. When HLA is expressed on the target cell these deliver an inhibitory signal into the NK cell.

When HLA molecules are absent on the target cell this inhibitory signal is lost and the NK cell can then kill its target. In addition, NK cells display antibody-dependent cell-mediated cytotoxicity (ADCC). In this, antibody binds to antigen on the surface of the target cell and then NK cells bind to the Fc portion of the bound antibody and kill the target cell.

Lymphocyte circulation

Lymphocytes in the peripheral blood migrate through *post-capillary venules* into the substance of the lymph nodes or into the spleen or bone marrow. T cells home to the perifollicular zones of the cortical areas of lymph nodes (paracortical areas) (Fig. 9.2) and to the periarteriolar sheaths surrounding the central arterioles of the spleen. B cells selectively accumulate in follicles of the lymph nodes and spleen. Lymphocytes return to the peripheral blood via the efferent lymphatic stream and the thoracic duct. CD4 helper cells predominate in normal peripheral blood and germinal centres, but in the marrow and gut the major T-cell subpopulation is CD8 positive.

Immunoglobulins

These are a group of proteins produced by plasma cells and B lymphocytes that bind to antigen. They are divided into five subclasses or *isotypes*: immunoglobulin G (IgG), IgA, IgM, IgD and IgE. IgG, the most common, contributes approximately 80%

of normal serum immunoglobulin and is further subdivided into four *subclasses*: IgG_1, IgG_2, IgG_3 and IgG_4. IgA is subdivided into two types.

IgM is usually produced first in response to antigen, IgG subsequently and for a more prolonged period. The same cell can switch from IgM to IgG, or to IgA or IgE synthesis. IgA is the main immunoglobulin in secretions, particularly of the gastrointestinal tract. IgD and IgE (involved in delayed hypersensitivity reactions) are minor fractions. Some important properties of the three main immunoglobulin subclasses are summarized in Table 9.2.

The immunoglobulins are all made up of the same basic structure (Fig. 9.3) consisting of two heavy chains which are called gamma (γ) in IgG, alpha (α) in IgA, mu (μ) in IgM, delta (δ) in IgD and epsilon (ε) in IgE, and two light chains – kappa (κ) or lambda (λ) – which are common to all five immunoglobulins. The heavy and light chains each have highly variable regions which give the immunoglobulin specificity, and constant regions in which there is virtual complete correspondence in amino acid sequence in all antibodies of a given isotype (e.g. IgA, IgG) or isotype subclass (e.g. IgG_1, IgG_2). IgG antibody can be broken into a constant Fc fragment and two highly variable Fab fragments. IgM molecules are much larger because they consist of five subunits.

The main role of immunoglobulins is defence of the body against foreign organisms. However, they also have a vital role in the pathogenesis of a number of haematological disorders. Secretion of a specific

Table 9.2 Some properties of the three main classes of immunoglobulin (Ig).

	IgG	IgA	IgM
Molecular weight	140 000	140 000	900 000
Normal serum level (g/L)	6.0–16.0	1.5–4.5	0.5–1.5
Present in	Serum and extracellular fluid	Serum and other body fluids (e.g. of bronchi and gut)	Serum only
Complement fixation	Usual	Yes (alternative pathway)	Usual and very efficient
Placental transfer	Yes	No	No
Heavy chain	(γ_{1-4})	α (α_1 or α_2)	μ

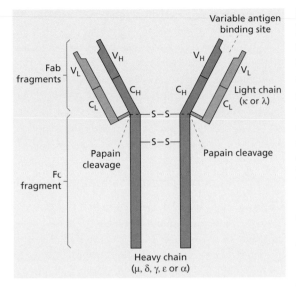

Figure 9.3 Basic structure of an immunoglobulin molecule. Each molecule is made up of two light (κ or λ) (blue areas) and two heavy (purple) chains, and each chain is made up of variable (V) and constant (C) portions, the V portions including the antigen-binding site. The heavy chain (μ, δ, γ, ε or α) varies according to the immunoglobulin class. IgA molecules form dimers, while IgM forms a ring of five molecules. Papain cleaves the molecules into an Fc fragment and two Fab fragments.

immunoglobulin from a monoclonal population of lymphocytes or plasma cells causes ***paraproteinaemia*** (see p. 273). Bence-Jones protein found in the urine in some cases of myeloma consists of a monoclonal secretion of light chains or light-chain fragments (either κ or λ). Immunoglobulins may bind to blood cells in a variety of immune disorders and cause their agglutination (e.g. in cold agglutinin disease; see p. 84) or destruction following direct complement lysis or after elimination by the reticuloendothelial system.

Antigen–receptor gene arrangements

Immunoglobulin gene rearrangements

The immunoglobulin heavy-chain and κ and λ light-chain genes occur on chromosomes 14, 2 and 22, respectively. In the germline state, the heavy-chain gene consists of separate segments for variable (V), diversity (D), joining (J) and constant (C) regions. Each of the V, D and J regions contain a number (*n*) of different ***gene segments*** (Fig. 9.4). In cells not committed to immunoglobulin synthesis these gene segments remain in their separate germ-

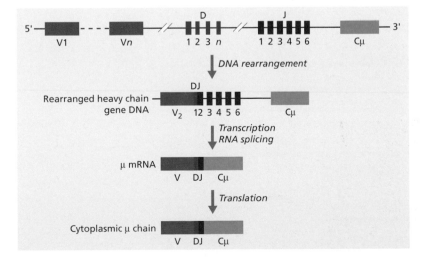

Figure 9.4 Rearrangement of a heavy-chain immunoglobulin gene. One of the V segments is brought into contact with a D, a J and a C (in this case Cμ) segment, forming an active transcriptional gene from which the corresponding mRNA is produced. The DJ rearrangement precedes VDJ joining. The class of immunoglobin depends on which of the nine constant regions (1μ, 1δ, 4γ, 2α, 1ε) is used.

line state. During early differentiation of B cells there is rearrangement of heavy-chain genes so that one of the V heavy-chain segments combines with one of the D segments, which has itself already combined with one of the J segments. Thus, they form a transcriptionally active gene for the heavy chain. The protein coding segments of the C region mRNA are joined to the V region after splicing out intervening RNA. The class of immunoglobulin that is secreted depends on which of the nine (4γ, 2α, 1μ, 1δ and 1ε) constant regions is used.

Diversity is introduced by the variability of which V segment joins with which D and with which J segment. In the arbitrary example shown in Fig. 9.4, V_2 joins with D_1 and J_2. Additional diversity is generated by the enzyme terminal deoxynucleotidyl transferase (TdT), which inserts a variable number of new bases into the DNA of the D region at the time of gene rearrangement. Similar rearrangements occur during generation of the light-chain gene (Fig. 9.5). Enzymes called ***recombinases*** are needed both in B and T cells to join up the adjacent pieces of DNA after excision of intervening sequences. These recognize certain heptamer- and nonamer-conserved sequences flanking the various gene segments. Mistakes in recombinase activity play an important part in the chromosome translocations of B- or T-cell malignancy.

The pattern of gene and protein expression that is seen during B cell development is valuable in determining the stage of B cell development and is useful in leukaemia diagnosis (Figs 9.5 and 9.6).

T-cell receptor gene rearrangements

The vast majority of T cells contain a TCR composed of a heterodimer of α and β chains. In a minority of T cells, the TCR is composed of γ and δ chains. The α, β, γ and δ genes of the TCRs each include V, D, J and C regions. During T-cell ontogeny, rearrangements of these gene segments occur in a similar fashion to those for immunoglobulin genes, thus creating T cells expressing a wide variety (10^8 or more) of TCR structures (Fig. 9.6). TdT is involved in creating additional diversity and the same recombinase enzymes used in B cells are involved in joining up TCR gene segments.

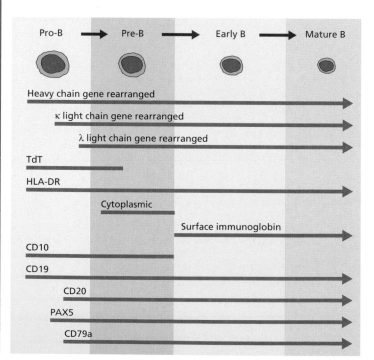

Figure 9.5 The sequence of immunoglobulin gene rearrangement, antigen and immunoglobulin expression during early B-cell development. Intracytoplasmic CD22 is a feature of very early B cells. HLA, human leucocyte antigen; TdT, terminal deoxynucleotidyl transferase.

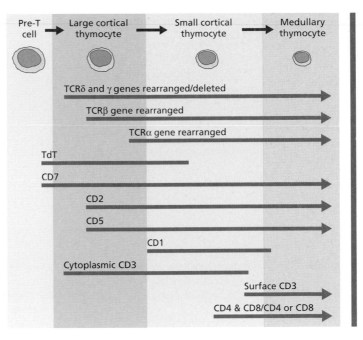

Figure 9.6 The sequence of events during early T-cell development. The earliest events appear to be the expression of surface CD7, intranuclear terminal deoxynucleotidyl transferase (TdT) and intracytoplasmic CD3 followed by T-cell receptor (TCR) gene rearrangement. Early medullary thymocytes may express both CD4 and CD8, but they then lose one or other of these structures.

Complement

This consists of a series of plasma proteins constituting an *amplification enzyme system* which is capable of lysis of bacteria (or of blood cells) or can 'opsonize' (coat) bacteria or cells so that they are phagocytosed. The complement sequence consists of nine major components – C1, C2, etc. – which are activated in turn (denoted thus C1) and form a cascade, resembling the coagulation sequence (Fig. 9.7). The most abundant and pivotal protein is C3, which is present in plasma at a level of approximately 1.2 g/L. The early (opsonizing) stages leading to coating of the cells with C3b can occur by two different pathways:

1 The *classic pathway* usually activated by IgG or IgM coating of cells; or
2 The *alternate pathway*, which is more rapid and activated by IgA, endotoxin (from Gram-negative bacteria) and other factors (Fig. 9.7).

Macrophages and neutrophils have C3b receptors and they phagocytose C3b-coated cells. C3b is degraded to C3d detected in the direct antiglobulin test using an anticomplement agent. If the complement sequence goes to completion (C9) there is generation of an active phospholipase that punches holes in the cell membrane (e.g. of the red cell or bacterium), causing direct lysis. The complement pathway also generates the biologically active fragments C3a and C5a which act directly on phagocytes to stimulate the respiratory burst (see p. 115). Both may trigger anaphylaxis by release of mediators from tissue mast cells and basophils which causes vasodilatation and increased permeability.

The immune response

One of the most striking features of the immune system is its capacity to produce a highly *specific* response. For both T and B cells this specificity is achieved by the presence of a particular receptor on the lymphocyte surface (Fig. 9.8). Naive (or virgin) B and T lymphocytes which leave the bone marrow and thymus are resting cells that are not in cell division. Specialized macrophages called dendritic cells (DCs; see p. 121) process antigens before presenting them to B and T lymphocytes – they are therefore known as *antigen-presenting cells* (APCs). The immune system contains many different lymphocytes. Each of these lymphocytes has a receptor that shows differences in structure from

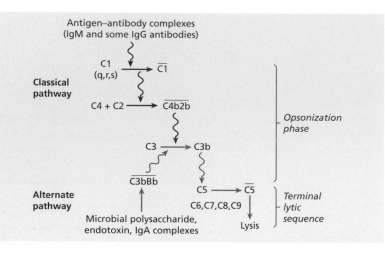

Figure 9.7 The complement (C) sequence. The activated factors are denoted by a bar over the number. Both pathways generate a C3 convertase. In the classic pathway, the convertase is the major (b) component of C4 and C2 (C4b2b). In the alternate pathway, it is the combination of C3b and the major fragment (b) of factor B (C3bBb).

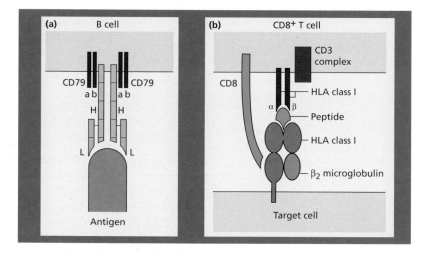

Figure 9.8 Antigen receptors on lymphocytes and their interaction with antigen. **(a)** The B-cell antigen receptor is membrane-bound immunoglobulin. Two heavy chains (H) are covalently bonded to two light chains (L). This antigen-binding unit is associated with the CD79 heterodimer which acts as a signal transduction unit. **(b)** The T-cell receptor consists of a number of components that together constitute the CD3 complex. Two antigen-binding chains (α, β) are associated with several proteins (γ, δ, ε, ζ) that mediate signal transduction. Antigen is recognized in the form of short peptides held on the surface of HLA molecules. CD8[+] T cells interact with peptide on a class I HLA molecule and the CD8 heterodimer interacts with the α_3 domain of the class I protein.

that of any other lymphocyte, and consequently will bind to only a restricted number of antigens. T and B cells undergo clonal expansion if they meet an APC that is presenting an antigen that can trigger their antigen receptor molecules. At this stage, lymphocytes may develop into effector cells (such as plasma cells or cytotoxic T cells) or memory cells.

DC precursors constitutively migrate at low levels from blood into tissues but their rate of migration is increased at the site of inflammation. Immature DCs are efficient at macropinocytosis which allows them to capture antigens from the environment. DCs can be matured by a variety of stimuli such as inflammatory cytokines – tumour necrosis factor-α (TNF-α) and interleukin-1 (IL-1) – and viral and bacterial products such as lipopolysaccharide (LPS) or double-stranded (ds) RNA. Mature DCs express high levels of co-stimulatory molecules and can efficiently present antigen to naïve antigen-specific T cells.

T cells are unable to bind antigen free in solution and require it to be presented on APCs in the form of peptides held on the surface of HLA molecules (Fig. 9.8b). T cells therefore recognize not only the antigen, but also 'self' HLA molecules and are known as **HLA-restricted**. The CD4 molecule on helper cells recognizes class II (HLA-DP, -DQ and -DR) molecules, whereas the CD8 molecule recognizes class I (HLA-A, -B and -C) molecules (see Fig. 23.5).

The antigen recognition site of the TCR is joined to several other subunits in the CD3 complex which together mediate signal transduction. During these structural interactions the cells release cytokines such as IL-1, -2, -4 and -10 which act to modify expansion of activated cells. Depending on their cytokine production, CD4+ T cells can be broadly subdivided into T helper type 1 (Th1) and Th2 cells. Th1 cells produce mainly IL-2, TNF-α and γ-interferon (IFN-γ), and are important in boosting cell-mediated immunity (and granuloma formation), whereas Th2 cells produce IL-4 and IL-10 and are mainly responsible for providing help for antibody production.

Antigen-specific immune responses are generated in **secondary lymphoid organs** and commence when antigen is carried into a lymph node (Fig. 9.9) on dendritic cells. B cells recognize antigen through their surface immunoglobulin and although most antibody responses require help from antigen-specific T cells, some antigens such as polysaccharides can lead to T-cell independent antibody production. T cells are screened for recognition of antigen and if a T cell makes an interaction it migrates into the follicle. In the follicle, germinal centres arise as a result of continuing response to antigenic stimulation (Fig. 9.10). These consist of follicular dendritic cells (FDCs), which are loaded with antigen, B cells and activated T cells which have migrated up from the T zone. Proliferating B cells move to the dark zone of the germinal centre as **centroblasts** where they undergo somatic mutation of their immunoglobulin variable-region genes. Their progeny are known as **centrocytes** and these must be selected by antigen on FDCs otherwise they will undergo apoptosis. If selected they become memory B cells or plasma cells (Fig. 9.10). Plasma cells migrate to the bone marrow and produce high affinity antibody. Although they contain intracellular immunoglobulin they do not express surface immunoglobulin.

Lymphocytosis

Lymphocytosis often occurs in infants and young children in response to infections that produce a neutrophil reaction in adults. Conditions particularly associated with lymphocytosis are listed in Table 9.3.

Glandular fever is a general term for a disease characterized by fever, sore throat, lymphadenopathy and atypical lymphocytes in the blood. It may be caused by primary infection with Epstein–Barr virus (EBV), cytomegalovirus (CMV), human immunodeficiency virus (HIV) or toxoplasma. EBV infection, otherwise known as infectious mononucleosis, is the most common cause.

Infectious mononucleosis

This is caused by primary infection with EBV and occurs only in a minority of infected individuals – in most cases infection is subclinical. The disease is characterized by a lymphocytosis caused by clonal expansions of T cells reacting against B lymphocytes infected with EBV. The disease is associated with a high titre of heterophile ('reacting with cells of

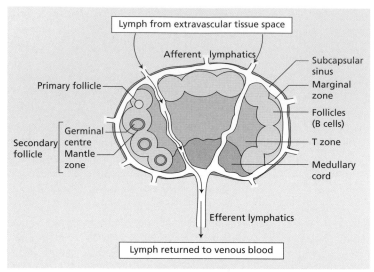

(a)

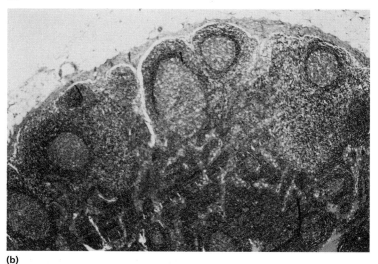

(b)

Figure 9.9 (a) Structure of a lymph node. **(b)** Lymph node showing germinal follicles surrounded by a darker mantle zone rim and lighter, more diffuse marginal and T-zone areas.

another species') antibody which reacts with sheep, horse or ox red cells.

Clinical features

The majority of patients are between the ages of 15 and 40 years. A prodromal period of a few days occurs with lethargy, malaise, headaches, stiff neck and a dry cough. In established disease the following features may be found:

1 Bilateral cervical lymphadenopathy is present in 75% of cases. Symmetrical generalized lymphadenopathy occurs in 50% of cases. The nodes are discrete and may be tender.
2 Over half of patients have a sore throat with inflamed oral and pharyngeal surfaces. Follicular tonsillitis is frequently seen.
3 Fever may be mild or severe.
4 A morbilliform rash, severe headache and eye signs (e.g. photophobia, conjunctivitis and peri-

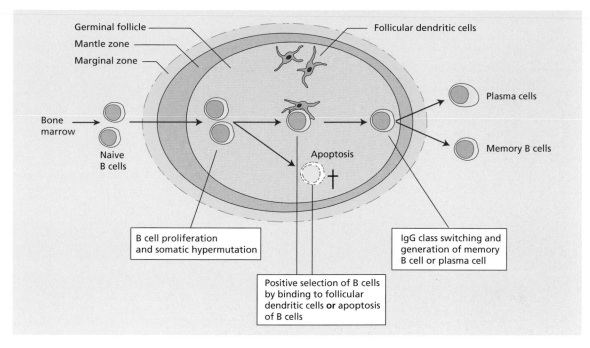

Figure 9.10 Generation of a germinal centre. B cells activated by antigen migrate from the T zone to the follicle where they undergo massive proliferation. Cells enter the dark zone as centroblasts and accumulate mutations in their immunoglobulin V genes. Cells then pass back into the light zone (Fig. 9.9) as centrocytes. Only those cells that can interact with antigen on follicular dendritic cells and receive signals from antigen-specific T cells (Fig. 9.8) are selected and migrate out as plasma cells and memory cells. Cells not selected die by apoptosis.

Table 9.3 Causes of lymphocytosis.

Infections
  Acute: infectious mononucleosis, rubella, pertussis, mumps, acute infectious lymphocytosis, infectious hepatitis, cytomegalovirus, HIV, herpes simplex or zoster
  Chronic: tuberculosis, toxoplasmosis, brucellosis, syphilis

Chronic lymphoid leukaemias (see Chapter 17)

Acute lymphoblastic leukaemia

Non-Hodgkin lymphoma (some)

Thyrotoxicosis

HIV, human immunodeficiency virus.

orbital oedema) are not uncommon. The rash may follow therapy with amoxicillin or ampicillin.

5 Palpable splenomegaly occurs in over half of patients and hepatomegaly in approximately 15%. Approximately 5% of patients are jaundiced.

6 Peripheral neuropathy, severe anaemia (caused by autoimmune haemolysis) or purpura (caused by thrombocytopenia) are less frequent complications.

Diagnosis

Pleomorphic atypical lymphocytosis

A moderate rise in white cell count (e.g. 10–$20 \times 10^9/L$) with an absolute lymphocytosis is usual, and some patients have even higher counts. Large numbers of atypical lymphocytes are seen in the peripheral blood film (Fig. 9.11). These T cells are

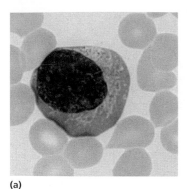
(a)

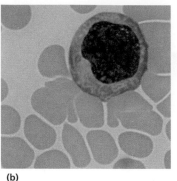
(b)

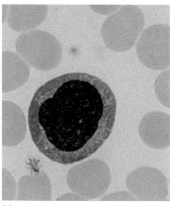
(c)

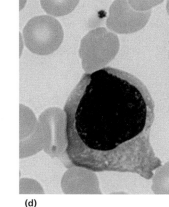
(d)

Figure 9.11 Infectious mononucleosis: representative 'reactive' T lymphocytes in the peripheral blood film of a 21-year-old man (see also Fig. 9.1b).

variable in appearance but most have nuclear and cytoplasmic features similar to those seen during reactive lymphocyte transformation. The greatest number of atypical lymphocytes are usually found between the seventh and tenth day of the illness.

Heterophile antibodies

Heterophile antibodies against sheep or horse red cells may be found in the serum at high titres. Modern slide screening tests, such as the *monospot test*, use formalinized horse red cells to test for the IgM antibodies that agglutinate the cells. Highest titres occur during the second and third week and the antibody persists in most patients for 6 weeks.

EBV antibody

If viral diagnostic facilities are available, a rise in the titre of IgM antibody against the EBV capsid antigen (VCA) may be demonstrated during the first 2–3 weeks. Specific IgG antibody to the EBV nuclear antigen (EBNA) and IgG VCA antibodies develop later and persist for life.

Haematological abnormalities

Haematological abnormalities other than the atypical lymphocytosis are frequent. Occasional patients develop an autoimmune haemolytic anaemia. The IgM autoantibody is typically of the 'cold' type and usually shows 'i' blood group specificity. Thrombocytopenia is frequent and an autoimmune thrombocytopenic purpura occurs in a smaller number of patients.

Differential diagnosis

The differential diagnosis of infectious mononucleosis includes cytomegalovirus, HIV or toxoplasmosis infection; acute leukaemia; influenza; rubella; bacterial tonsillitis; and infectious hepatitis.

Treatment

In the great majority of patients only symptomatic treatment is required. Corticosteroids are sometimes given to those with severe systemic symptoms. Patients characteristically develop an erythematous rash if given ampicillin therapy. Most patients recover fully 4–6 weeks after initial symptoms. However, convalescence may be slow and associated with severe malaise and lethargy.

Lymphopenia

Lymphopenia may occur in severe bone marrow failure, with corticosteroid and other immunosuppressive therapy, in Hodgkin lymphoma and with widespread irradiation. It also occurs during treatment with the monoclonal antibody alemtuzumab (anti-CD52) and in a variety of immunodeficiency syndromes, the most important of which is HIV infection (see p. 390).

Immunodeficiency

A large number of inherited or acquired defects in any of the components of the immune system can cause an impaired immune response with increased susceptibility to infection (Table 9.4). A primary lack of T cells (as in AIDS) leads not only to bacterial infections, but also to viral, protozoal, fungal and mycobacterial infections. In some cases, however, lack of specific subsets of T cells which control B-cell maturation may lead to a secondary lack of B-cell function, as in many cases of common variable immunodeficiency, which may develop in children or adults of either sex. In others, a primary defect of B cells or of APCs is present.

X-linked agammaglobulinaemia is caused by failure of B-cell development; pyogenic bacterial infections dominate the clinical course. Immunoglobulin replacement therapy can be given by monthly courses of intravenous immunoglobulin. Rare syndromes include aplasia of the thymus, severe combined (T and B) immunodeficiency as a result of adenosine deaminase deficiency and selective deficiencies of IgA or IgM. Acquired immune deficiency occurs with HIV infection and after

Table 9.4 Classification of immunodeficiencies.

Primary	
B cell (antibody deficiency)	X-linked agammaglobulinaemia, acquired common variable hypogammaglobulinaemia, selective IgA or IgG subclass deficiencies
T cell	Thymic aplasia (DiGeorge's syndrome), PNP deficiency
Mixed B and T cell	Severe combined immune deficiency (as a result of ADA deficiency or other causes); Bloom's syndrome; ataxia-telangiectasia; Wiskott–Aldrich syndrome
Secondary	
B cell (antibody deficiency)	Myeloma; nephrotic syndrome, protein-losing enteropathy, anti-CD20 (rituximab) therapy
T cell	AIDS; Hodgkin lymphoma, non-Hodgkin lymphoma; drugs: steroids, ciclosporin, azathioprine, fludarabine, etc.
T and B cell	Chronic lymphocytic leukaemia, post-stem cell transplantation, chemotherapy/radiotherapy, anti-CD52 (alemtuzumab)

ADA, adenosine deaminase; AIDS, acquired immune deficiency syndrome; Ig, immunoglobulin; PNP, purine nucleoside phosphorylase.

cytotoxic chemotherapy or radiotherapy and is particularly pronounced after stem cell transplantation where dysregulation of the immune system persists for 1 year or more and is responsible for a high incidence of serious viral infections (e.g. with cytomegalovirus or herpes zoster). Alemtuzemab (anti-CD52) causes a similar immunodeficiency. Immunodeficiency is also frequently associated with tumours of the lymphoid system including chronic lymphocytic leukaemia and myeloma.

Differential diagnosis of lymphadenopathy

The principal causes of lymphadenopathy are listed in Figure 9.12. The clinical history and examination give essential information. The age of the patient, length of history, associated symptoms of possible infectious or malignant disease, whether the nodes are painful or tender, consistency of the nodes and whether there is generalized or local lymphadenopathy are all important. The size of the liver and spleen are assessed. In the case of local node enlargement, inflammatory or malignant disease in the associated lymphatic drainage area are particularly considered.

Further investigations will depend on the initial clinical diagnosis but it is usual to include a full blood count, blood film and erythrocyte sedimentation rate (ESR). Chest X-ray, monospot test, cytomegalovirus and *Toxoplasma* titres, and anti-HIV and Mantoux tests are frequently needed. In many cases, it will be essential to make a histological diagnosis by node biopsy, usually trucut, in which a core of node is removed under radiological control. Fine needle aspirates give less material, destroy the architecture and so are less reliable in diagnosis.

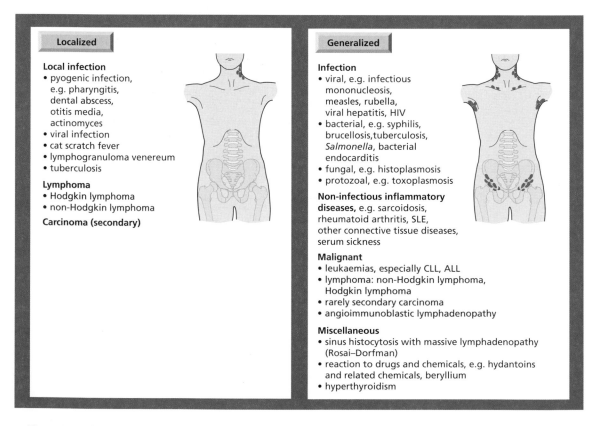

Localized

Local infection
• pyogenic infection, e.g. pharyngitis, dental abscess, otitis media, actinomyces
• viral infection
• cat scratch fever
• lymphogranuloma venereum
• tuberculosis

Lymphoma
• Hodgkin lymphoma
• non-Hodgkin lymphoma

Carcinoma (secondary)

Generalized

Infection
• viral, e.g. infectious mononucleosis, measles, rubella, viral hepatitis, HIV
• bacterial, e.g. syphilis, brucellosis, tuberculosis, *Salmonella*, bacterial endocarditis
• fungal, e.g. histoplasmosis
• protozoal, e.g. toxoplasmosis

Non-infectious inflammatory diseases, e.g. sarcoidosis, rheumatoid arthritis, SLE, other connective tissue diseases, serum sickness

Malignant
• leukaemias, especially CLL, ALL
• lymphoma: non-Hodgkin lymphoma, Hodgkin lymphoma
• rarely secondary carcinoma
• angioimmunoblastic lymphadenopathy

Miscellaneous
• sinus histocytosis with massive lymphadenopathy (Rosai–Dorfman)
• reaction to drugs and chemicals, e.g. hydantoins and related chemicals, beryllium
• hyperthyroidism

Figure 9.12 Causes of lymphadenopathy. ALL, acute lymphoblastic leukaemia; CLL, chronic lymphocytic leukaemia; SLE, systemic lupus erythematosus. Malignancies are listed in red.

Computed tomography (CT) scanning is valuable in determining the presence and extent of deep node enlargement. Subsequent investigations will depend on the diagnosis made and the patient's particular features. In some cases of deep node enlargement, where enlarged superficial nodes are not available for biopsy, bone marrow or liver biopsy, CT or ultrasound guided trucut deep node biopsy may be needed in an attempt to reach a histological diagnosis. Biopsy of the spleen is not performed as it may cause rupture requiring splenectomy.

SUMMARY

- Lymphocytes are immunologically competent white cells that are involved in antibody production (B cells) and with the body's defence against viral infection or other foreign invasion (T cells).
- They arise from haemopoietic stem cells in the marrow, T cells being subsequently processed in the thymus.
- B cells secrete gammaglobulin antibodies specific for individual antigens.
  T lymphocytes are further subdivided into helper (CD4+) and cytotoxic (CD8+) cells. They recognise peptides on HLA antigens. Natural killer cells are cytotoxic CD8+ cells that kill target cells with low expression of HLA molecules.
- The immune response occurs in the germinal centre of lymph nodes and involves B-cell and T-cell proliferation, somatic mutation, selection of cells by recognition of antigen on antigen-presenting cells and formation of plasma cells (which secrete immunoglobulin) or memory B cells.
- Immunoglobulins include five subclasses or isotypes, IgG, IgA, IgM, IgD and IgG, all made up of two heavy chains and two light chains (κ or λ).
- Complement is a cascade of plasma proteins that can either lyse cells or coat (opsonise) them so they are phagocytosed.
- Lymphocytosis is usually caused by acute or chronic infections or by lymphoid leukaemias or lymphomas.
- Lymphadenopathy may be localized (because of local infection or malignancy) or generalized because of infection, non-infectious inflammatory diseases, malignancy or drugs.

Now visit www.wiley.com/go/essentialhaematology to test yourself on this chapter.

CHAPTER 10
The spleen

Key topics

Essential Haematology, 6th Edition. © A. V. Hoffbrand and P. A. H. Moss. Published 2011 by Blackwell Publishing Ltd.

The spleen has an important and unique role in the function of the haemopoietic and immune systems. As well as being directly involved in many diseases of these systems, a number of important clinical features are associated with hypersplenic and hyposplenic states.

The anatomy and circulation of the spleen

The spleen lies under the left costal margin, has a normal weight of 150–250 g and a length of between 5 and 13 cm. It is normally not palpable but becomes palpable when the size is increased to over 14 cm.

Blood enters the spleen through the splenic artery which then divides into **trabecular arteries** which permeate the organ and give rise to **central arterioles** (Fig. 10.1). The majority of the arterioles end in **cords** which lack an endothelial lining and form an open blood system unique to the spleen with a loose reticular connective tissue network lined by fibroblasts and many macrophages. The blood re-enters the circulation by passing across the endothelium of venous **sinuses**. Blood then passes into the splenic vein and so back into the general circulation. The cords and sinuses form the **red pulp** which forms 75% of the spleen and has an essential role in monitoring the integrity of red blood cells (see below). A minority of the splenic vasculature is closed in which the arterial and venous systems are connected by capillaries with a continuous endothelial layer.

The central arterioles are surrounded by a core of lymphatic tissue known as *white pulp* which has an organization similar to lymph nodes (Fig. 10.1). The *periarteriolar lymphatic sheath* (PALS) lies directly around the arteriole and is equivalent to the T zone of the lymph node (see p. 128). B-cell follicles are found adjacent to the PALS and these are surrounded by the *marginal zone* and *perifollicular zone* which are rich in macrophages and dendritic cells. Lymphocytes migrate into white pulp from the sinuses of the red pulp or from vessels that end directly in the marginal and perifollicular zones.

There are both rapid (1–2 min) and slow (30–60 min) blood circulations through the spleen. The slow circulation becomes increasingly important in splenomegaly.

The functions of the spleen

The spleen is the largest filter of the blood in the body and several of its functions are derived from this.

Control of red cell integrity

The spleen has an essential role in the 'quality control' of red cells. Excess DNA, nuclear remnants

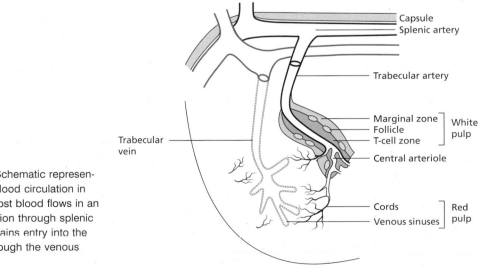

Figure 10.1 Schematic representation of the blood circulation in the spleen. Most blood flows in an 'open' circulation through splenic cords and regains entry into the circulation through the venous sinuses.

Capsule
Splenic artery
Trabecular artery
Marginal zone
Follicle — White pulp
T-cell zone
Central arteriole
Trabecular vein
Cords
Venous sinuses — Red pulp

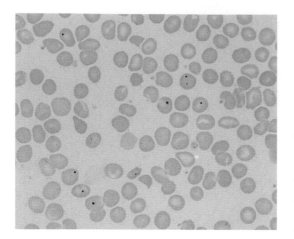

Figure 10.2 Splenic atrophy: peripheral blood film showing Howell–Jolly bodies, Pappenheimer bodies (siderotic granules; see p. 30) and misshapen cells.

(Howell–Jolly bodies) and siderotic granules are removed (Fig. 10.2). In the relatively hypoxic environment of the red pulp, and because of plasma skimming in the cords, the membrane flexibility of aged and abnormal red cells is impaired and they are retained within the sinus where they are ingested by macrophages.

Immune function

The lymphoid tissue in the spleen is in a unique position to respond to antigens filtered from the blood and entering the white pulp. Macrophages and dendritic cells in the marginal zone initiate an immune response and then present antigen to B and T cells to start adaptive immune responses. This arrangement is highly efficient at initiating immune responses to encapsulated bacteria and explains the susceptibility of hyposplenic patients to these organisms.

Extramedullary haemopoiesis

The spleen, like the liver, undergoes a transient period of haemopoiesis at around 3–7 months of fetal life but is not a site of erythropoiesis in the adult. However, haemopoiesis may be re-established in both organs as *extramedually haemopoiesis*, in disorders such as primary myelofibrosis or in chronic

severe haemolytic and megaloblastic anaemias. Extramedullary haemopoiesis may result either from reactivation of dormant stem cells within the spleen or homing of stem cells from the bone marrow to the spleen.

Imaging the spleen

Ultrasound is the most frequently used technique to image the spleen (Fig. 10.3). This can also detect whether or not blood flow in the splenic, portal and hepatic veins is normal, as well as liver size and consistency. Computed tomography (CT) is preferable for detecting structural detail and any associated lymphadenopathy (e.g. for lymphoma staging). Magnetic resonance imaging (MRI) also gives improved fine detail structure. Positron emission tomography (PET) is used particularly for initial staging and for detecting residual disease after treatment of lymphoma (Fig. 10.4).

Splenomegaly

Splenic size is increased in a wide range of conditions (Table 10.1). Splenomegaly is usually felt under the left costal margin but massive splenomegaly may be felt in the right iliac fossa (see Fig. 15.4). The spleen moves with respiration and a medial splenic notch may be palpable in some cases. In developed countries the most common causes of splenomegaly are infectious mononucleosis, haematological malignancy and portal hypertension, whereas malaria and schistosomiasis are more prevalent on a global scale (Table 10.1). Chronic myeloid leukaemia, primary myelofibrosis, lymphoma, Gaucher's disease, malaria, leishmaniasis and schistosomiasis are potential causes of *massive* splenomegaly.

Tropical splenomegaly syndrome

A syndrome of massive splenomegaly of uncertain aetiology has been found frequently in many malarious zones of the tropics including Uganda, Nigeria, New Guinea and the Congo. Smaller numbers of patients with this disorder are seen in southern Arabia, the Sudan and Zambia. Previously, such terms as 'big spleen disease', 'cryptogenic

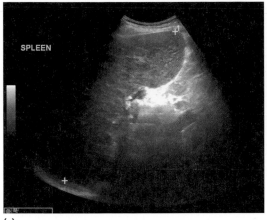

(a)

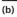

(b)

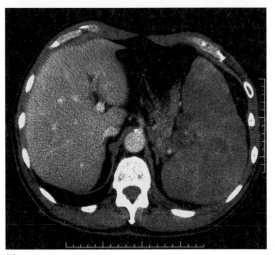

(c)

Figure 10.3 The spleen. **(a)** Ultrasound of spleen showing splenomegaly (15.3 cm). **(b)** Normal spleen (10 cm) on computed tomography (CT) scan. **(c)** CT scan: the spleen is enlarged and shows multiple low density areas. A diagnosis of diffuse large cell B lymphoma was made histologically after splenectomy. (Figs (a) and (b) courtesy of Dr T. Ogunremi.)

splenomegaly' and 'African macroglobulinaemia' have been used to describe this syndrome.

While it seems probable that malaria is the fundamental cause of tropical splenomegaly syndrome, this disease is not the result of active malarial infection as parasitaemia is usually scanty and malarial pigment is not found in biopsy material from the liver and spleen. The available evidence suggests that an abnormal host response to the continual presence of malarial antigen results in a reactive and relatively benign lymphoproliferative disorder that predominantly affects the liver and spleen.

Splenomegaly is usually gross and the liver is also enlarged. Portal hypertension may be a feature. The anaemia is often severe and the lowest haemoglobin levels are found in subjects with the largest spleens. While leucopenia is usual, some patients develop a marked lymphocytosis. The moderate degree of thrombocytopenia present does not often cause spontaneous bleeding. Serum immunoglobulin M (IgM) levels are high and fluorescent techniques reveal high titres of malarial antibody.

Although splenectomy corrects the pancytopenia, there is an increased risk of fulminant malarial infection. Trials of antimalarial prophylaxis have proved successful in the management of many affected patients, supporting the view that a con-

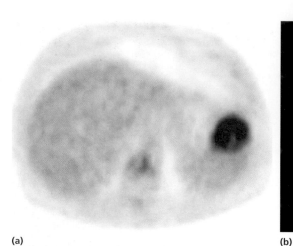

(a)

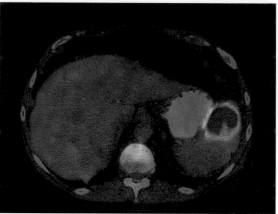

(b)

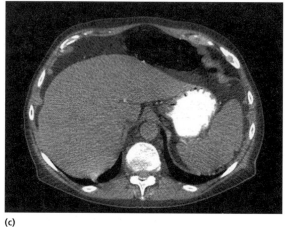

(c)

Figure 10.4 (a) Axial positron emission tomography (PET), **(b)** fused PET/CT and **(c)** CT images demonstrating a solitary focal area of [^{18}]FDG uptake on the PET image which is seen to localize to the spleen on the fused PET/CT image. (Courtesy of Dr V.S. Warbey and Professor G.J.R. Cook.)

tinuing presence of malarial antigen is needed for the perpetuation of the lymphoproliferation associated with this syndrome. Resistant cases have also been treated successfully with chemotherapy.

Hypersplenism

Normally, only approximately 5% (30–70 mL) of the total red cell mass is present in the spleen although up to half of the total marginating neutrophil pool and 30% of the platelet mass may be located there. As the spleen enlarges, the proportion of haemopoietic cells within the organ increases such that up to 40% of the red cell mass, and 90% of platelets (see Fig. 25.9), may be pooled in an enlarged spleen. ***Hypersplenism*** is a clinical syndrome that can be seen in any form of splenomegaly. It is characterized by:

- Enlargement of the spleen;
- Reduction of at least one cell line in the blood in the presence of normal bone marrow function.

Depending on the underlying cause, splenectomy may be indicated if the hypersplenism is symptomatic. It is followed by a rapid improvement in the peripheral blood count.

Hyposplenism

Functional hyposplenism is revealed by the blood film findings of Howell–Jolly bodies or

Table 10.1 Causes of splenomegaly.

Haematological
Chronic myeloid leukaemia*
Chronic lymphocytic leukaemia
Acute leukaemia
Lymphoma*
Primary myelofibrosis*
Polycythaemia vera
Hairy cell leukaemia
Thalassaemia major or intermedia*
Sickle cell anaemia (before splenic infarction)
Haemolytic anaemias
Megaloblastic anaemia

Portal hypertension
Cirrhosis
Hepatic, portal, splenic vein thrombosis

Storage diseases
Gaucher's disease*
Niemann–Pick disease
Histiocytosis X

Systemic diseases
Sarcoidosis
Amyloidosis
Collagen diseases – systemic lupus
  erythematosus, rheumatoid arthritis
Systemic mastocytosis

Infections
Acute: septicaemia, bacterial endocarditis,
  typhoid, infectious mononucleosis
Chronic: tuberculosis, brucellosis, syphilis,
  malaria, leishmaniasis,* schistosomiasis*

*Tropical**
Possibly caused by malaria

*Possible causes of massive (>20 cm) splenomegaly.

Table 10.2 Causes of hyposplenism and blood film features.

Causes	Blood film features
Splenectomy	*Red cells*
Sickle cell disease	Target cells
Essential	Acanthocytes
thrombocythaemia	Irregularly contracted
Adult gluten-induced	or crenated cells
enteropathy	Howell–Jolly bodies
Dermatitis	(DNA remnants)
herpetiformis	Siderotic (iron)
Rarely	granules
inflammatory bowel	(Pappenheimer
disease	bodies)
splenic arterial	
thrombosis	*White cells*
	± Mild lymphocytosis,
	monocytosis
	Platelets
	± Thrombocytosis

Table 10.3 Indications for splenectomy.

Splenic rupture

Chronic immune thrombocytopenia

Haemolytic anaemia (some cases), e.g.
hereditary spherocytosis, autoimmune
haemolytic anaemia, thalassaemia major or
intermedia

Chronic lymphocytic leukaemia and lymphomas

Primary myelofibrosis

Tropical splenomegaly

Pappenheimer bodies (siderotic granules on iron staining; Fig. 10.2). The most frequent cause is surgical removal of the spleen (e.g. after traumatic rupture) but hyposplenism can also occur in sickle cell anaemia, gluten-induced enteropathy, inflammatory bowel disease and splenic arterial thrombosis (Table 10.2).

Splenectomy

Surgical removal of the spleen may be indicated for treatment of haematological disorders as well as after splenic rupture or for splenic tumours or cysts (Table 10.3). Splenectomy can be performed by open abdominal laparotomy or by laparoscopic surgery.

The platelet count can often rise dramatically in the early postoperative period, reaching levels of up to 1000×10^9/L and peaking at 1–2 weeks. Thrombotic complications are seen in some patients and prophylactic aspirin or heparin are often required during this period. Long-term alterations in the peripheral blood cell count may also be seen, including a persistent thrombocytosis, lymphocytosis or monocytosis.

Prevention of infection in hyposplenic patients

Patients with hyposplenism are at lifelong increased risk of infection from a variety of organisms. This is seen particularly in children under the age of 5 years and those with sickle cell anaemia. The most characteristic susceptibility is to encapsulated bacteria such as *Streptococcus pneumoniae*, *Haemophilus influenzae* type B and *Neisseria meningitidis*. *Streptococcus pneumoniae* is a particular concern and can cause a rapid and fulminant disease. Malaria tends to be more severe in splenectomized individuals. Measures to reduce the risk of serious infection include the following:

1 The patient should be informed about the increased susceptibility to infection and advised to carry a card about their condition. They should be counselled about the increased risk of infection on foreign travel, including that from malaria and tick bites.
2 Prophylactic oral penicillin is recommended for life. Erythromycin may be prescribed for patients allergic to penicillin. A supply of tablets may also be given to the patient to take in the event of onset of fever before medical care is available.
3 Vaccination against pneumococcus, haemophilus, meningococcus and influenza infection is recommended (Table 10.4). All types of vaccine, including live vaccines, can be given safely to hyposplenic individuals although the immune response to vaccination may be impaired.

Table 10.4 Recommendations for vaccination of patients with hyposplenism.

Vaccine	Time of vaccination	Revaccination schedule	Comments
1 Pneumoccal polyvalent vaccine	If possible, at least 2 weeks prior to splenectomy	5 yearly	Assessment of antibody response may be useful
2 Combined *Haemophilus influenzae* type b conjugate and meningococcal C conjugate	Alternatively, 2 weeks post-splenectomy for all three vaccines	Not required Not required	Not required if previously vaccinated
3 Influenza	As soon as available for seasonal protection	Annual	Inactivated subunit vaccine

SUMMARY

- The normal adult spleen weighs 150–250 g and is 5–13 cm in diameter. It has a specialized circulation because the majority of arterioles end in 'cords' which lack an endothelial lining. The blood re-enters the circulation via venous sinuses. The cords and sinuses form the red pulp which monitors the integrity of red blood cells.

- The central arterioles are surrounded by lymphoid tissue called white pulp which is similar in structure to a lymph node.

- The spleen removes aged or abnormal red cells, and excess DNA and siderotic granules, from intact red cells. It also has a specialized immune function against capsulated bacteria, pneumococcus, haemophilus influenza and meningococcus to which splenectomized patients are immunized. Splenectomy is needed for splenic rupture and in some haematological diseases.

- Enlargement of the spleen (splenomegaly) occurs in many malignant and benign haematological diseases, in portal hypertension and with systemic diseases, including acute and chronic infections. Hyposplenism occurs in sickle cell anaemia, gluten-induced enteropathy and rarely in other diseases.

Now visit www.wiley.com/go/essentialhaematology to test yourself on this chapter.

CHAPTER 11

The aetiology and genetics of haematological malignancies

Key topics

Essential Haematology, 6th Edition. © A. V. Hoffbrand and P. A. H. Moss. Published 2011 by Blackwell Publishing Ltd.

The haemopoietic malignancies are clonal diseases that derive from a single cell in the marrow or peripheral lymphoid tissue that has undergone genetic alteration (Fig. 11.1). In this chapter we discuss the aetiology and genetic basis of haematological malignancy and subsequent chapters discuss the aetiology, diagnosis and management of the individual conditions.

The incidence of haematological neoplasms

Cancer is an increasingly important cause of morbidity and mortality with recent improvements in the prevention and treatment of cardiovascular disease. Nearly 40% of the population will develop cancer in their lifetime. The majority of cancers are epithelial malignancies. Haematological malignancies represent approximately 7% of all malignant disease (Fig. 11.2). There are major geographical variations in occurrence of the diseases; for example, chronic lymphocytic leukaemia (CLL) is the most common leukaemia in the West but rare in the Far East.

The aetiology of haemopoietic malignancy

Exactly how genetic mutations accumulate in haemopoietic malignancies is largely unknown. As in most diseases it is the combination of genetic background and environmental influence that determines the risk of developing a malignancy. For example, single nucleotide polymorphism (SNP) analysis has identified polymorphisms in germline genes, some of which code for proteins involved in B-cell development, that predispose to risk of B-cell acute lymphoblastic leukaemia (B-ALL) (see Chapter 17). However, in the majority of cases neither a genetic susceptibility nor an environmental agent is apparent.

Inherited factors

The incidence of leukaemia is greatly increased in some genetic diseases, particularly Down's syndrome (where acute leukaemia occurs with a 20- to 30-fold increased frequency), Bloom's syndrome, Fanconi's anaemia, ataxia telangiectasia, neurofibromatosis, Klinefelter's syndrome and Wiskott–Aldrich syndrome. There is also a weak familial tendency in diseases such as acute myeloid leukaemia (AML), CLL, Hodgkin lymphoma and non-Hodgkin lymphoma (NHL) although the genes predisposing to this increased risk are largely unknown.

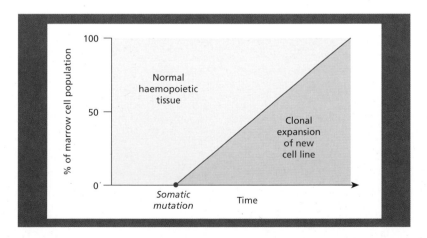

Figure 11.1 Theoretical graph to show the replacement of normal bone marrow cells by a clonal population of malignant cells arising by successive mitotic divisions from a single cell with an acquired genetic alteration.

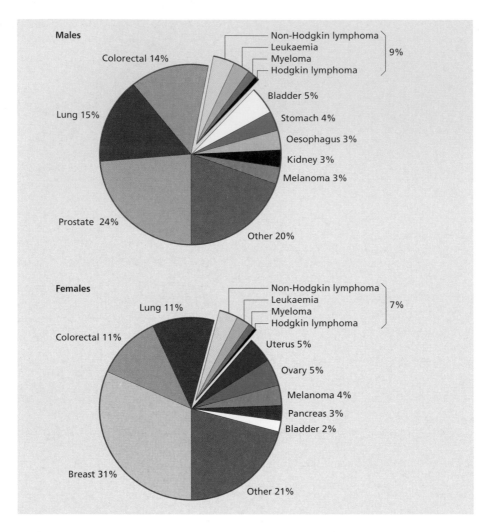

Figure 11.2 The relative frequency of the haematological malignancies as a proportion of malignant disease. (From Smith A. *et al.* (2009) *Br J Haematol* **148**,739–53, with permission.)

Environmental influences

Chemicals

Chronic exposure to benzene is an unusual cause of myelodysplasia or AML. Other industrial solvents and chemicals less commonly cause leukaemia.

Drugs

The alkylating agents (e.g. chlorambucil, melphalan, procarbazine and nitrosoureas – BCNU, CCNU) predispose to AML, especially if combined with radiotherapy. Etoposide is associated with a risk of the development of secondary leukaemias associated with balanced translocations including that of the *MLL* gene at 11q23.

Radiation

Radiation, especially to the marrow, is leukaemogenic. This is illustrated by an increased incidence of all types of leukaemia (except CLL) in survivors of the atom bomb explosions in Japan.

Infection

Children may have a predisposition to acute lymphoblastic leukaemia (ALL) from their germline constitution. A proportion of cases of childhood ALL are then initiated by genetic mutations that occur during development *in utero* (Fig. 11.3). Studies in identical twins have shown that both may be born with the same chromosomal abnormality, e.g. t(12; 21). This has presumably arisen spontaneously in a progenitor cell that has passed from one twin to the other as a result of the shared placental circulation. Environmental exposure during pregnancy may be important for this first event. One twin may develop ALL early (e.g. at age 4) because of a second transforming event affecting the copy numbers of several genes including those in B-cell development and relevant to the leukaemogenesis. The other twin remains well or may develop ALL later. The *TEL-AML1* translocation is present in the blood of approximately 10% of newborn infants but only 1 in 100 of these go on to develop ALL at a later date. The mechanism of the 'second genetic hit' within the tumour cell is unclear but an abnormal response of the immune system to infection is suggested by epidemiological studies. Children with a high level of social activity, notably those attending early nursery daycare, have a reduced incidence of ALL, whereas those living in more isolated communities and who have a reduced exposure to common infections in the first years of life have a higher risk.

Viruses

Viral infection is associated with several types of haemopoietic malignancy, especially different subtypes of lymphoma (see Table 20.2). The retrovirus human T-lymphotropic virus type 1 is the cause of adult T-cell leukaemia/lymphoma (see p. 243) although most people infected with this virus do not develop the tumour. Epstein–Barr virus (EBV) is associated with almost all cases of endemic (African) Burkitt lymphoma, post-transplant lymphoproliferative disease (which develops during

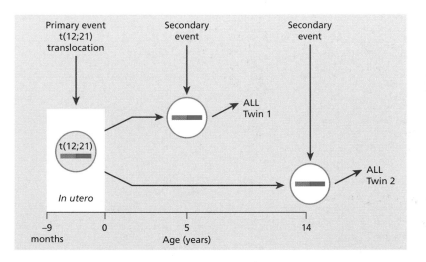

Figure 11.3 Prenatal origin of acute lymphoblastic leukaemia (ALL) in a pair of identical twins. ALL was diagnosed in the first twin at age 5 years and in the second at age 14 years. Both tumours had an identical t(12; 21) translocation indicating probable origin of the leukaemic clone *in utero* and dissemination to both twins via a shared placental blood supply. Because of the prolonged latency of the ALL it is presumed that a secondary event is required to initiate the development of frank leukaemia. At the time of the diagnosis of ALL in twin 1 the t(12; 21) translocation could be detected in the bone marrow of twin 2. It is likely that such a 'fetal origin' of childhood ALL occurs in a significant number of sporadic ALL cases. (After Wiemels J.L. *et al.* (1999) *Blood* **94**,1057–62.)

immunosuppressive therapy after solid organ transplantation (see p. 312)) and a proportion of patients with Hodgkin lymphoma. Human herpes virus 8 (Kaposi's sarcoma-associated virus) is associated with Kaposi's sarcoma and primary effusion lymphoma (see Table 20.2).

HIV infection is associated with an increased incidence of lymphomas at unusual sites such as the central nervous system. The HIV-associated lymphomas are usually of B-cell origin and of high-grade histology.

Bacteria

Helicobacter pylori infection has been implicated in the pathogenesis of gastric mucosa B-cell (MALT) lymphoma (see p. 265).

Protozoa

Endemic Burkitt lymphoma occurs in the tropics, particularly in malarial areas. It is thought that malaria may alter host immunity and predispose to tumour formation as a result of EBV infection.

The genetics of haemopoietic malignancy

Malignant transformation occurs as a result of the accumulation of genetic mutations in cellular genes. The genes that are involved in the development of cancer can be divided broadly into two groups: **oncogenes** and **tumour-suppressor genes**.

Oncogenes

Oncogenes arise because of gain-of-function mutations in normal cellular genes called **proto-oncogenes** (Fig. 11.4). Proto-oncogenes are involved in a variety of important cellular processes, often in the pathway by which external signals are transduced to the cell nucleus to activate genes. Oncogenic versions are generated when the activity of proto-oncogenes is increased or they acquire a novel function. This can occur in a number of ways including translocation, mutation or duplication. One of the striking features of haematological malignancies (in contrast to most solid tumours) is their high frequency of chromosomal translocations. A subset of proto-oncogenes are involved in

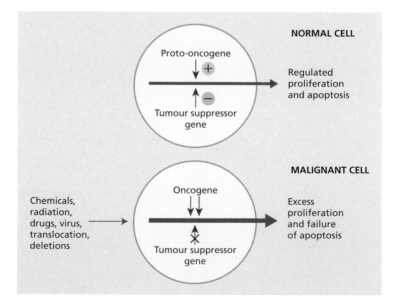

Figure 11.4 Proliferation of normal cells depends on a balance between the action of proto-oncogenes and tumour-suppressor genes. In a malignant cell this balance is disturbed leading to uncontrolled cell division.

control of apoptosis (e.g. *BCL-2* which is overexpressed in follicular lymphoma) (see p. 266).

Tyrosine kinases

These enzymes, which phosphorylate proteins on tyrosine residues, are important as cell receptors and intracellular signalling. Mutations of them underlie a large number of haematological malignancies (see Chapters 13, 14 and 15).

Tumour-suppressor genes

Tumour-suppressor genes may acquire loss-of-function mutations, usually by point mutation or deletion, which lead to malignant transformation (Fig.

11.4). Tumour-suppressor genes commonly act as components of control mechanisms that regulate entry of the cell from the G_1 phase of the cell cycle into the S phase or passage through the S phase to G_2 and mitosis (see Fig. 1.8). Examples of oncogenes and tumour-suppressor genes involved in haemopoietic malignancies are shown in Table 11.1. The most significant tumour-suppressor gene in human cancer is p53 which is mutated or inactivated in over 50% of cases of malignant disease, including many haemopoietic tumours.

Clonal progression

Malignant cells appear to arise as a multistep process with acquisition of mutations in different intracel-

Table 11.1 Some of the more frequent genetic abnormalities within haematological tumours affecting the function of oncogenes.

Disease	Genetic abnormality	Oncogenes involved
AML	t(8; 21)	ETO/AML1 (CBFα)
	t(15; 17)	PML, RARA
	Nucleotide insertion	NPM
	Mutation, ITD	FLT3
	Mutation	TET-2
Secondary AML	11q 23 translocations	MLL
Myelodysplasia	− 5, del (5q)	RPS 14
	− 7, del (7q)	N RAS
CML	t(9; 22)	BCR-ABL1
Myeloproliferative	Point mutation	JAK-2
	Point mutation	TET-2
B-ALL	t(12; 21)	TEL/AML1
	t(9; 22)	BCR-ABL1
	t(4; 11)	AF4/MLL
Follicular lymphoma	t(14; 18)	BCL2
Mantle cell lymphoma	t(11; 14)	Cyclin D1
Burkitt lymphoma	t(8; 14)	MYC
CLL	17p deletion	P53
	11q 22-23 deletion	ATM

AML, acute myeloid leukaemia; B-ALL, B-acute lymphoblastic leukaemia; CLL, chronic lymphocytic leukaemia; CML, chronic myeloid leukaemia; ITD, internal tandem duplication.

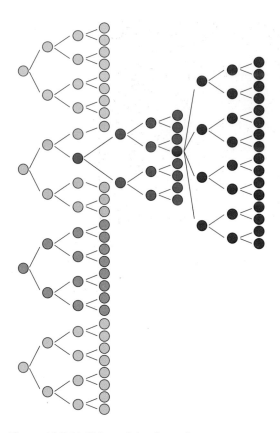

Figure 11.5 Multistep origin of a malignant tumour. Successive mutations lead to a growth advantage of one subclone.

lular pathways (Fig. 11.5). Another feature of malignancy is clonal progression. In many cases the disease develops new characteristics during its clinical course and this may be accompanied by new genetic changes. Selection of subclones may occur during treatment or reflect disease acceleration. Drug resistance can arise through a variety of molecular mechanisms. In one example the cells express a protein that actively pumps a number of different drugs to the outside of the cells (multidrug resistance).

Chromosome nomenclature

The normal somatic cell has 46 chromosomes and is called *diploid*; ova or sperm have 23 chromosomes and are called *haploid*. The chromosomes occur in pairs and are numbered 1–22 in decreasing size order; there are two sex chromosomes, XX in females, XY in males. *Karyotype* is the term used to describe the chromosomes derived from a mitotic cell which have been set out in numerical order (Fig. 11.6). A somatic cell with more or less than 46 chromosomes is termed *aneuploid*; more than 46 is *hyperdiploid*, less than 46 *hypodiploid*; 46 but with chromosome rearrangements, *pseudodiploid*.

Each chromosome has two arms: the shorter called 'p', the longer called 'q'. These meet at the *centromere* and the ends of the chromosomes are called *telomeres*. On staining each arm divides into regions numbered outwards from the centromere and each region divides into bands (Fig. 11.7).

When a whole chromosome is lost or gained, a − or + is put in front of the chromosome number. If part of the chromosome is lost it is prefixed with del (for deletion). If there is extra material replacing part of a chromosome the prefix add (for additional material) is used. Chromosome translocations are denoted by t, the chromosomes involved placed in brackets with the lower numbered chromosome first. The prefix inv describes an inversion where part of the chromosome has been inverted to run in the opposite direction. An *isochromosome*, denoted by i, describes a chromosome with identical chromosome arms at each end; for example, i(17q) would consist of two copies of 17q joined at the centromere.

Telomeres

Telomeres are repetitive sequences at the ends of chromosomes. They decrease by approximately 200 base pairs of DNA with every round of replication. When they decrease to a critical length, the cell exits from cell cycle. Germ cells and stem cells, which need to self-renew and maintain a high proliferative potential, contain the enzyme *telomerase* which can add extensions to the telomeric repeats and compensate for loss at replication and so enable the cells to continue proliferation. Telomerase is also often expressed in malignant cells but this is probably a consequence of the malignant transformation rather than an initiating factor.

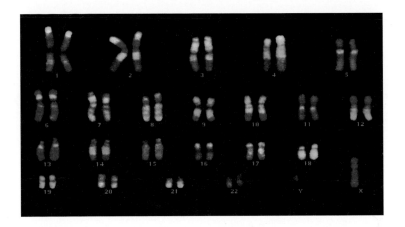

Figure 11.6 A colour-banded karyotype from a normal male. Each chromosome pair shows an individual colour-banding pattern. This involves a cross-species multiple colour chromosome banding technique. Probe sets developed from the chromosomes of gibbons are combinatorially labelled and hybridized to human chromosomes. The success of cross-species colour banding depends on a close homology between host and human conserved DNA, divergence of repetitive DNA and a high degree of chromosomal rearrangement in the host relative to the human karyotype. (Courtesy of Dr C.J. Harrison.)

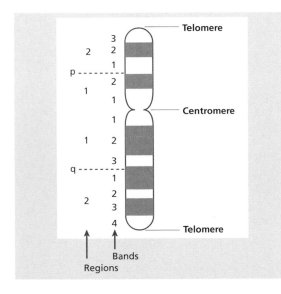

Figure 11.7 A schematic representation of a chromosome. The bands may be divided into subbands according to staining pattern.

Genetic abnormalities associated with haematological malignancies

The genetic abnormalities underlying the different types of leukaemia and lymphoma are described with the diseases which are themselves increasingly classified according to genetic change rather than morphology. The types of gene abnormality include the following (Fig. 11.8).

Point mutation

This is best illustrated by the Val617Phe mutation in the *JAK2* gene which leads to constitutive activation of the JAK2 protein in most cases of myeloproliferative disease (see Chapter 15). Mutations of *TET-2*, a probable tumour-suppressor gene, occur in up to 20% of myeloid neoplasms except chronic myeloid leukaemia (CML) and may be an earlier event than the *JAK2* mutation. Mutations within the *RAS* oncogenes or p53 tumour-suppressor gene are common in many haemopoietic malignancies. The point mutation may involve several base pairs. In 35% of cases of AML the *nucleophosmin* gene shows an insertion of four base pairs resulting in a frameshift change. Internal tandem duplication or point mutations occur in the *FLT-3* gene in 30% of cases of AML.

Translocations

These are a characteristic feature of haematological malignancies and there are two main mechanisms

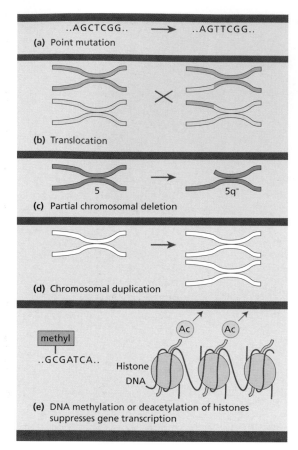

Figure 11.8 Types of genetic abnormality which may lead to haemopoietic malignancy. **(a)** Point mutation; **(b)** chromosomal translocation; **(c)** chromosomal deletion or loss; **(d)** chromosomal duplication; **(e)** DNA methylation or deacetylation of histone tails suppresses gene transcription.

whereby they may contribute to malignant change (Fig. 11.9).

1 Fusion of parts of two genes to generate a chimeric fusion gene that is dysfunctional or encodes a novel '***fusion protein***', e.g. CBF/ETO in the AML t(8;21) (Fig. 11.10), *BCR-ABL1* in t(9; 22) in CML (see Fig. 14.1), *RARα-PML* in t(15; 17) in acute promyelocytic leukaemia (see Fig. 13.7) or *TEL-AML1* in t(12; 21) in B-ALL.

2 Overexpression of a normal cellular gene, e.g. overexpression of *BCL*-2 in the t(14; 18) translocation of follicular lymphoma or of *MYC* in Burkitt lymphoma (Fig. 11.11). Interestingly, this class of translocation nearly always involves a *TCR* or immunoglobulin gene locus, presumably as a result of aberrant activity of the recombinase enzyme which is involved in immunoglobulin or *TCR* gene rearrangement in immature B or T cells.

Deletions

Chromosomal deletions may involve a small part of a chromosome, the short or long arm (e.g. 5q–) or the entire chromosome (e.g. monosomy 7). Losses most commonly affect chromosomes 5, 6, 7, 11, 20 and Y. The critical event is probably loss of a tumour-suppressor gene or of a microRNA as in the 13q14 deletion in CLL (see below). Loss of multiple chromosomes is termed hypodiploidy and is seen frequently in ALL.

Duplication or amplification

In chromosomal duplication (e.g. trisomy 12 in CLL) or gene amplification, gains are common in chromosomes 8, 12, 19, 21 and Y. Gene amplification is not a common feature in haemopoietic malignancy but has been described involving the *MLL* gene.

Epigenetic alterations

Gene expression in cancer may be dysregulated not only by structural changes to the genes themselves but also by alterations in the mechanism by which genes are transcribed. These changes are called ***epigenetic*** and are stably inherited with each cell division so they are passed on as the malignant cell divides. The most important mechanisms are methylation of cytosine residues in DNA and enzymatic alterations, such as acetylation or methylation, of the histone proteins that package DNA within the cell (Fig. 11.8e). Demethylating agents such as aza-cytidine increase gene transcription and are valuable in myelodysplasia (MDS) and AML.

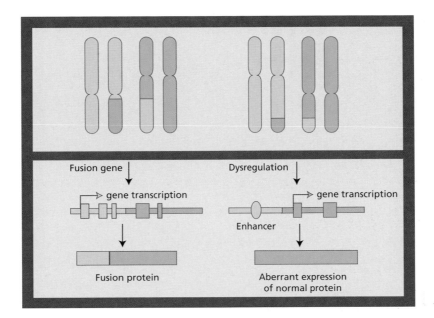

Figure 11.9 The two possible mechanisms by which chromosomal translocations can lead to dysregulated expression of an oncogene.

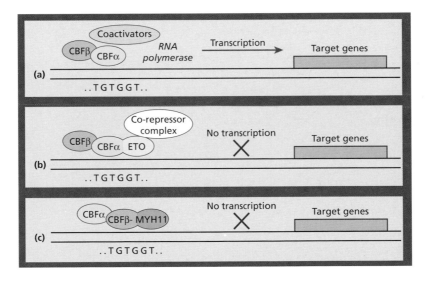

Figure 11.10 Mechanism of action of the core binding factor (CBF) transcription factor and its disruption in two genetic types of acute myeloid leukaemia. CBF consists of two subunits, *CBF*β and *CBF*α (or *AML1*), which together form a heterodimer **(a)**. This complex binds to the DNA sequence TGTGGT in the regulatory region of certain target genes (e.g. IL-3 and GM-CSF). This binding allows recruitment of coactivators which lead to transcription from these genes. **(b)** The t(8; 21) translocation leads to a fusion protein of CBFα with ETO. Although the CBF subunits can still form heterodimers, their binding to DNA leads to recruitment of a co-repressor complex which blocks transcription. **(c)** In the inv(16) mutation, a CBFβ-MYH11 fusion protein is generated, which again can form CBF heterodimers but these do not gain access to DNA. In the t(12;21) translocation associated with B-ALL (not illustrated), the TEL gene is fused to the CBF gene to generate a novel fusion protein. All three translocations involving CBF appear to act as dominant inhibitors of wild type CBF and they are all associated with a relatively good prognosis.

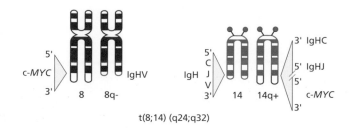

t(8;14) (q24;q32)

Figure 11.11 The genetic events in one of the three translocations found in Burkitt lymphoma and B-cell acute lymphoblastic leukaemia. The oncogene *c-MYC* is normally located on the long arm (q) of chromosome 8. In the (8; 14) translocation, *c-MYC* is translocated into close proximity to the immunoglobulin heavy-chain gene on the long arm of chromosome 14. Part of the heavy-chain gene (the V region) is reciprocally translocated to chromosome 8. C, constant region; IgH, immunoglobulin heavy-chain gene; J, joining region; V, variable region.

MicroRNAs

Chromosomal abnormalities, both deletions and amplifications, can result in loss or gain of short (micro) RNA sequences. These are normally transcribed but not translated. MicroRNAs (miRNAs) control expression of adjacent or distally located genes. Deletion of the miR15a/miR16-1 locus may be relevant to CLL development with the common 13q deletion and deletions of other microRNAs have been described in AML and other haematological malignancies.

Diagnostic methods used to study malignant cells

Karyotype analysis

Karyotype analysis involves direct morphological analysis of chromosomes from tumour cells under the microscope (see Fig. 14.1). This requires tumour cells to be in metaphase and so cells are cultured to encourage cell division prior to chromosomal preparation.

Fluorescence *in situ* hybridization analysis

Fluorescence *in situ* hybridization (FISH) analysis involves the use of fluorescent-labelled genetic probes which hybridize to specific parts of the genome. It is possible to label each chromosome with a different combination of fluorescent labels

(Fig. 11.12). This is a sensitive technique that can detect extra copies of genetic material in both metaphase and interphase (non-dividing) cells (e.g. trisomy 12 in CLL) or, by using two different probes, reveal chromosomal translocations (Fig. 11.12c) or t(9; 22) in CML (see Fig. 14.1e), or reduced chromosome numbers or loss of segments (e.g. monosomy 7 or 5 in myelodysplasia) (Fig. 11.12).

Polymerase chain reaction

Polymerase chain reaction (PCR) (see Fig. 7.23) can be performed on blood or bone marrow for a number of specific translocations such as t(9; 22) and t(15; 17). It can also be used to detect 'clonal' cells of B- or T-cell lineage by immunoglobulin or T-cell receptor (TCR) gene rearrangement analysis. As it is relatively straightforward and extremely sensitive (detecting one abnormal cell in 10^5–10^6 normal cells), it has become of great value in the diagnosis and monitoring of minimal residual disease (see p. 164).

DNA microarray platforms

DNA microarrays allow a rapid and comprehensive analysis of cellular transcription by hybridizing labelled cellular mRNA to DNA probes which are immobilized on a solid support (Fig. 11.13). Oligonucleotides or complementary DNA (cDNA) arrays may be immobilized on the array and RNA from the tissue of interest is used to generate fluo-

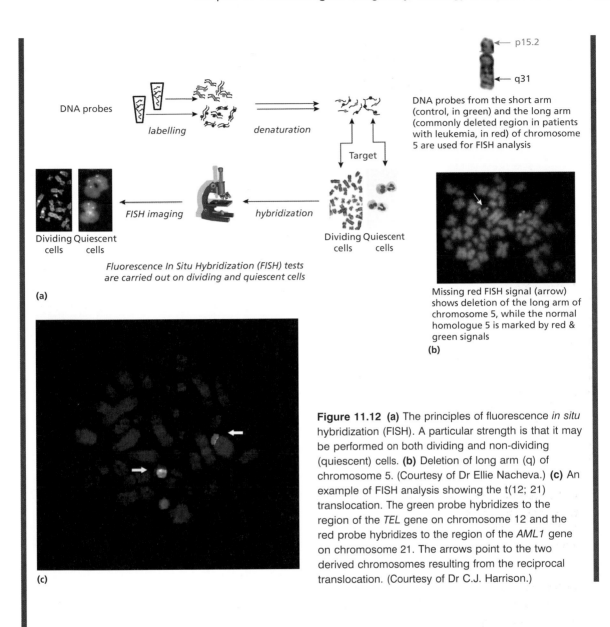

p15.2

q31

DNA probes from the short arm (control, in green) and the long arm (commonly deleted region in patients with leukemia, in red) of chromosome 5 are used for FISH analysis

DNA probes

labelling   *denaturation*

Target

FISH imaging   *hybridization*

Dividing Quiescent   Dividing Quiescent
 cells   cells   cells   cells

Fluorescence In Situ Hybridization (FISH) tests are carried out on dividing and quiescent cells

(a)

Missing red FISH signal (arrow) shows deletion of the long arm of chromosome 5, while the normal homologue 5 is marked by red & green signals

(b)

(c)

Figure 11.12 **(a)** The principles of fluorescence *in situ* hybridization (FISH). A particular strength is that it may be performed on both dividing and non-dividing (quiescent) cells. **(b)** Deletion of long arm (q) of chromosome 5. (Courtesy of Dr Ellie Nacheva.) **(c)** An example of FISH analysis showing the t(12; 21) translocation. The green probe hybridizes to the region of the *TEL* gene on chromosome 12 and the red probe hybridizes to the region of the *AML1* gene on chromosome 21. The arrows point to the two derived chromosomes resulting from the reciprocal translocation. (Courtesy of Dr C.J. Harrison.)

rescent cDNA or RNA which is then annealed to the nucleic acid matrix. This approach can rapidly determine mRNA expression from a large number of genes and may be used to determine the mRNA expression pattern of different leukaemia or lymphoma subtypes (Fig. 11.13b). The technique cannot be used to detect minimal residual disease and is not in routine diagnostic use but it is clear that it can give valuable information, e.g. subclassification of diffuse large B-cell NHL (see Fig. 20.8), or AML without cytogenetic changes.

Flow cytometry

In this technique, antibodies labelled with different fluorochromes recognize the pattern and intensity of expression of different antigens on the surface of normal and leukaemic cells (Fig. 11.14). Normal cells each have a characteristic profile but malignant cells often express an aberrant phenotype that can be useful in allowing their detection (see Figs 13.6 and 17.7). In the case of B-cell malignances (e.g. CLL), expression of only one light chain, κ or λ,

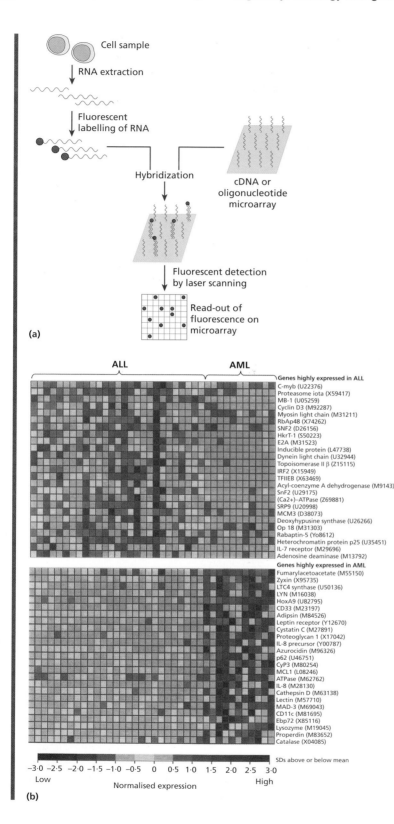

Figure 11.13 **(a)** Principle of transcriptional profiling of RNA expression in leukaemia samples using DNA microarrays. **(b)** Microarray analysis of genes distinguishing acute lymphoblastic leukaemia (ALL) from acute myeloid leukaemia (AML). The 50 genes most highly correlated on gene-expression microarrays with each of these leukaemias are shown. Each row corresponds to a gene; each column corresponds to the expression value in a particular sample. Expression for each gene is normalized across the samples such that the mean is 0 and the SD is 1. Expression greater than the mean is shaded in red, and that below the mean is shaded in blue. Although the genes as a group appear correlated with the type of leukaemia under study, no single gene is uniformly expressed across the class, illustrating the value of a multigene prediction method. (Reproduced courtesy of Golub and colleagues.)

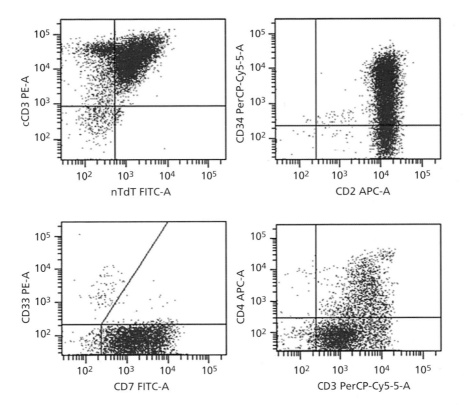

Figure 11.14 FACS analysis of acute lymphoblastic leukaemia, T lineage. The blast cells express cCD3, TdT, CD34, CD7 and CD2. (Courtesy of Immunophenotyping Laboratory, Royal Free Hospital, London.)

by the tumour cells distinguishes them from a normal polyclonal population which express both κ and λ chains, usually in a κ:λ ratio of 2:1 (see Fig. 18.4).

Immunohistology

Antibodies can also be used to stain tissue sections with fluorescent markers and this is known as *immunohistology* or *immunohistochemistry*. The presence and architecture of tumour cells can be identified by visualization of stained tissue sections under the microscope (Fig. 11.15). The clonal nature of B-cell malignancies can be shown in tissue sections by staining for κ or λ chains. A malignant clonal population (e.g. in B-cell NHL) will express one or other light chain but not both (see Fig. 20.5).

Value of genetic markers in management of haematological malignancy

The detection of genetic abnormalities may be important in several aspects of the management of patients with leukaemia or lymphoma.

Initial diagnosis

Many genetic abnormalities are so specific for a particular disease that their presence determines that diagnosis. An example is the t(11; 14) translocation which defines mantle cell lymphoma. Clonal immunoglobulin or TCR gene rearrangements are useful in establishing clonality and determining the lineage of a lymphoid malignancy.

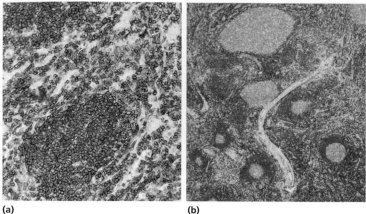

(a)   **(b)**

Figure 11.15 Immunohistologic detection of BCL-2 protein in reactive and neoplastic lymphoid cells. **(a)** A follicular lymphoma is positive, reflecting activation of the BCL-2 gene by the (14;18) translocation. **(b)** In reactive lymphoid tissue unstained germinal centres are surrounded by numerous positive mantle zone B and T cells.

For establishing a treatment protocol

Each major type of haematological malignancy can be further subdivided on the basis of detailed genetic information. For instance, AML is a diverse group of disorders with characteristic genotypes. Individual subtypes respond differently to standard treatment. The t(8; 21) and inv(16) subgroups have a favourable prognosis, whereas monosomy 7 carries a poor prognosis. Treatment strategies are now tailored for the individual and in some instances knowledge of the underlying genetic abnormality can lead to more rational treatment, e.g. the use of all-*trans* retinoic acid in acute promyelocytic leukaemia with t(15; 17) (see p. 186). For BCR–ABL1+ CML and ALL, drugs are now available that target the fusion protein and improve overall survival.

Genetic information is also valuable for giving a prognosis. For instance, hyperdiploidy in ALL is a favourable finding.

Monitoring the response to therapy

The detection of minimal residual disease (disease that cannot be seen by conventional microscopy of the blood or bone marrow) in AML, ALL or CML or other haematological malignancies when the patient is in remission after chemotherapy or stem cell transplantation is possible using the following techniques (in increasing order of sensitivity; Fig. 11.16).

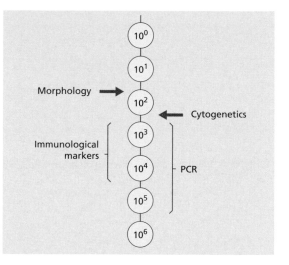

Figure 11.16 Sensitivity of detection of leukaemic cells in bone marrow using four different techniques. 10^1 to 10^6 = 1 cell in 10 to 1 cell in 10^6 detected.

1 Cytogenetic analysis.
2 Fluorescence-activated cell sorting to detect tumour cells using immunological markers that detect 'leukaemia-specific' combinations of antigens (see Fig. 17.7).
3 PCR to amplify tumour-specific translocations or immunoglobulin/TCR sequences specific to the original clone (Fig. 11.17).

These approaches have an important role in determining the treatment of many forms of haemopoietic malignancy.

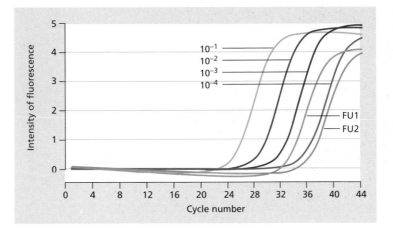

Figure 11.17 Real-time quantitative polymerase chain reaction (PCR) in acute B-lineage lymphoblastic leukaemia for minimal residual disease using the immunoglobulin heavy chain as target. Primers are designed based on DNA from sequence analysis of the presenting leukaemic clone. Bone marrow samples taken in clinical remission are amplified by PCR using these primers and fluorescent labelled using Sybergreen. The intensity of the signal measures the total DNA molecules amplified in successive cycles. In this example, the intensities of amplification of DNA from two follow-up bone marrow samples (FU1 and FU2) are compared with serial deletions of (10^{-1} to 10^{-4}) of the DNA from the presentation bone marrow. FU1 shows a level of residual disease of approximately 1 in 5000 (0.02%) and FU2 of 1 in 12 000 (0.008%). (Courtesy of Dr L. Foroni.)

SUMMARY

■ The haemopoietic malignancies are clonal diseases that derive from a single cell in the marrow or peripheral lymphoid tissue which has undergone genetic alteration.

■ They represent approximately 7% of all malignant disease.

■ Inherited and environmental factors both predispose to tumour development but the relative contribution of these is usually unclear.

■ Infections (viral and bacterial), drugs, radiation and chemicals can all increase the risk of developing a haemopoietic malignancy.

■ Haematological malignances occur because of genetic alterations that lead to increased activation of oncogenes or decreased activity of tumour suppressor genes.

■ These genetic alterations may occur through a variety of mechanisms such as point mutation, chromosomal translocation or gene deletion.

■ Important investigations include study of the chromosomes (karyotype analysis), FISH, PCR, microarray analysis, flow cytometry and immunohistochemistry.

■ These investigations guide the diagnosis, treatment and monitoring for residual disease of individual cases.

Now visit www.wiley.com/go/essentialhaematology
to test yourself on this chapter.

CHAPTER 12
Management of haematological malignancy

Key topics

Essential Haematology, 6th Edition. © A. V. Hoffbrand and P. A. H. Moss. Published 2011 by Blackwell Publishing Ltd.

The treatment of haematological malignancy has improved greatly over the last 40 years. This has resulted from developments in *supportive therapy* and in *specific treatment*. Details of specific treatment are discussed in relation to individual diseases in the appropriate chapter. Support care and general aspects of the agents used in the treatment of haematological malignancy are described here.

General support therapy

Patients with haematological malignancies often present with medical problems related to suppression of normal haemopoiesis and this problem is compounded by the treatments that are given to eradicate the tumour. General supportive therapy for bone marrow failure includes the following.

Insertion of a central venous catheter

A central venous catheter is usually inserted prior to intensive treatment via a skin tunnel from the chest into the superior vena cava (Fig. 12.1). This gives ease of access for administering chemotherapy, blood products, antibiotics and intravenous feeding. In addition, blood may be taken for laboratory tests.

Blood product support (see Chapter 29)

Red cell and platelet transfusions are used to treat anaemia and thrombocytopenia. A number of particular issues apply to the support of patients with haematological malignancy:

1 The threshold haemoglobin for transfusion will depend on clinical factors such as symptoms and speed of onset of anaemia but most units give red cell support for a Hb <8 g/dL, with a higher threshold in older patients. In patients needing both red cells and platelets, platelets are given first to reduce the risk of a further fall in the platelet count.

2 The trigger for platelet transfusion is typically a platelet count $<10 \times 10^9/L$ but this should be doubled in the presence of active bleeding or infection.

3 Fresh frozen plasma (FFP) may be needed to reverse coagulation defects.

4 Cytomegalovirus (CMV) negative blood should be given to all patients until it has been shown that they are either CMV seropositive or that they will never be candidates for stem cell transplantation (SCT). This is to prevent transmission of CMV to uninfected patients as the virus is a

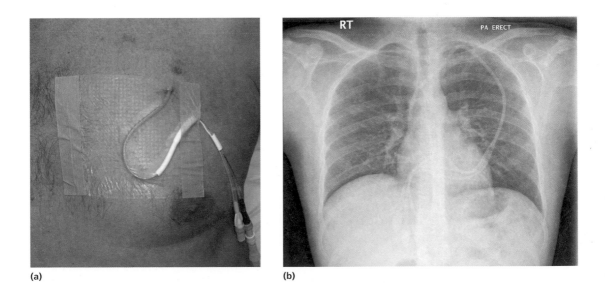

(a)   (b)

Figure 12.1 **(a)** A central venous line in a patient undergoing intensive chemotherapy. **(b)** Chest X-ray showing correct placement of a central venous line, in this case a tunnelled triple lumen left internal jugular line. (Courtesy of Dr P. Wylie.)

significant problem in stem cell transplant recipients (see p. 309).

5 Red cell transfusions should be avoided if at all possible in patients with a very high white cell count ($>100 \times 10^9$/L) because of the hyperviscosity and the risk of precipitating thrombotic episodes as a result of white cell stasis.

6 Large volume transfusions, such as 3 units of blood or more, can precipitate pulmonary oedema in older patients and should be given slowly and with clinical monitoring. Diuretics such as frusemide (furosemide) are often given.

7 Febrile reactions with blood products are not uncommon and should be managed by slowing the infusion and administration of drugs such as antihistamines, pethidine or hydrocortisone. The dosage of steroids should be limited because of concerns with immunosuppression.

8 Blood products given to highly immunosuppressed patients (e.g. from chemotherapy, such as fludarabine, with aplastic anaemia, Hodgkin lymphoma or post-allogeneic SCT) should be irradiated prior to administration to prevent graft-versus-host disease (see p. 306).

9 The use of recombinant erythropoietin to reduce the need for blood transfusion and improve patient well-being (e.g. in myeloma or myelodysplasia) is discussed on p. 18.

Haemostasic support

A coagulation screen should be performed regularly on patients undergoing intensive chemotherapy and support with vitamin K or FFP may be required. Cryoprecipitate may be needed for fibrinogen deficiency (e.g. precipitated by asparaginase in the management of acute lymphoblastic leukaemia; ALL). Antiplatelet drugs such as aspirin or clopidogrel are usually discontinued in patients undergoing intensive chemotherapy and patients on long-term warfarin can be switched to low molecular weight heparin, which can then itself be stopped if the platelet count falls below 50×10^9/L. Progesterones are given to premenopausal women undergoing intensive chemotherapy to prevent menstruation. Tranexamic acid can be given to reduce haemorrhage in patients with chronic low-grade blood loss.

Antiemetic therapy

Nausea and vomiting are common side-effects of chemotherapy. A key objective is to try to prevent nausea occurring early in the treatment as it is more difficult to control once problems have arisen. The 5-HT$_3$ (serotonin) receptor antagonists such as ondansetron or granisetron can control nausea from intensive chemotherapy in over 60% of cases and the addition of dexamethasone can increase this by approximately 20%. Metoclopramide, prochlorperazine or cyclizine, benzodiazepines (e.g. lorazepam), domperidone or cannabinoids (e.g. nabilone) can all have a role.

Tumour lysis syndrome

Chemotherapy may trigger an acute rise in plasma uric acid, potassium and phosphate and cause hypocalcaemia because of rapid lysis of tumour cells. This syndrome is seen most commonly with rapidly dividing tumours such as lymphoblastic lymphoma or acute leukaemia and can cause acute renal failure. Allopurinol, intravenous fluids and electrolyte replacement are the mainstay of prevention and alkalinization of the urine is sometimes used. Rasburicase, an enzyme that oxidises uric acid to allantoin, is highly effective in controlling hyperuricaemia.

Psychological support

Patients with a diagnosis of malignant disease commonly feel concerns about such issues as the discomfort of treatment, finance, sexuality and fear of mortality. Even when patients achieve a clinical remission there is understandable concern about the chance of disease relapse. Psychological support should be an integral part of the relationship between physician and patient, and patients should be allowed to express their fears and concerns at the earliest opportunity. Most patients value the opportunity to read more about their disorder and many excellent booklets or websites are now available. Teamwork is also crucial and the nursing staff and trained counsellors have a vital role in offering support and information during inpatient and outpatient care. Many units have specialist input from clinical psychologists and psychiatric help may occasionally be required. Inadequate communication is perhaps the most common failing of medical teams. The immediate family should be kept informed of the patient's progress whenever possible and appropriate.

Reproductive issues

Men who are to receive cytotoxic drugs should be offered sperm storage, ideally before treatment commences or, if impossible, within a short period of time thereafter. Ethical issues relating to storage or potential usage of tissue in the event of treatment failure will need to be addressed. Permanent infertility in women is less common after chemotherapy although premature menopause may occur. Storage of fertilized ova is usually impractical and storage of unfertilized ova is currently very difficult and, despite some recent progress, is not offered as a routine service.

Nutritional support

Some degree of weight loss is virtually inevitable in patients undergoing inpatient chemotherapy because of the combination of a poor nutritional intake, malabsorption caused by drugs and a catabolic disease state. If a weight loss of >10% occurs, support with total nutrition is often given, either enterally via a nasogastric tube or parenterally through a central venous catheter.

Pain

Pain is rarely a major problem in haematological malignancies except myeloma although bone pain can be a presenting feature. The mucositis that follows intensive chemotherapy can cause severe discomfort and continuous infusions of opiate analgesia are often required. Pain is often a considerable issue in patients with multiple myeloma and can be managed by a combination of analgesia and chemotherapy/radiotherapy. Advice from palliative care teams or specialist pain management practitioners should be sought when required.

Prophylaxis and treatment of infection

Patients with haematological malignancy are at great risk of infection which remains the major cause of morbidity and mortality. Immunosuppression may result from neutropenia, hypogammglobulinaemia and impaired cellular function. These can be secondary to the primary disease or its treatment. Neutropenia is a particular concern and in many patients neutrophils are totally absent from the blood for periods of 2 weeks or more. The use of granulocyte colony-stimulating factor (G-CSF) to reduce periods of neutropenia is discussed on p. 112. One potential protocol for the management of infection in an immunosuppressed patient is illustrated in Fig. 12.2.

Bacterial infection

This is the most common problem and usually arises from the patient's own commensal bacterial flora. Gram-positive skin organisms (e.g. *Staphylococcus* and *Streptococcus*) commonly colonize central venous lines, whereas Gram-negative gut bacteria (e.g. *Pseudomonas aeruginosa*, *Escherichia coli*, *Proteus*, *Klebsiella* and anaerobes) can cause overwhelming septicaemia. Even organisms not normally considered pathogenic, such as *Staphyloccus epidermidis*, may cause life-threatening infection. In the absence of neutrophils, local superficial lesions can rapidly cause severe septicaemia.

Prophylaxis of bacterial infection

Protocols used to limit bacterial infection vary from unit to unit and may include the use of a prophylactic antibiotic such as ciprofloxacin. During periods of neutropenia, topical antiseptics for bathing and chlorhexidine mouthwashes and a 'clean diet' are recommended. The patient is nursed in a reverse-barrier room. The severity and length of mucositis may be reduced by treatment with recombinant human keratinocyte growth factor (palifermin) which reduces the severity of oral mucositis. Oral non-absorbed antimicrobial agents such as neomycin and colistin reduce gut commensal flora but their value is unclear. Regular surveillance cultures are taken to document the patient's bacterial flora and its sensitivity.

Treatment of bacterial infection

Fever is the main indication that infection is present because if neutropenia is present pus will not be

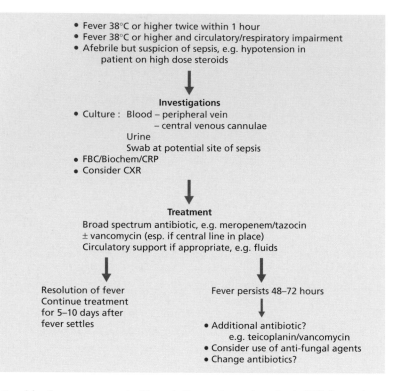

Figure 12.2 A protocol for the management of fever in the neutropenic patient. CRP, C-reactive protein; CXR, chest X-ray; FBC, full blood count.

formed and infections are often not localized. Fever may be caused by blood products or drugs, but infection is the most common cause and fever of over 38°C in neutropenic patients should be investigated and treated within hours. Cultures should be taken from any likely focus of infection including blood from central venous lines and peripheral veins, from urine and mouth swabs. The mouth and throat, intravenous catheter site, and perineal and perianal areas are particularly likely foci. A chest X-ray is indicated as chest infections are frequent.

Antibiotic therapy must be started immediately after blood and other cultures have been taken; in many febrile episodes no organisms are isolated.

There are many different antibiotic regimes in use and a close link with the microbiology team is essential. A typical regimen might be based on a single agent such as a broad-spectrum penicillin (e.g. Tazocin®), meropenem or a broad-spectrum cephalosporin. Teicoplanin, vancomycin or an aminoglycoside such as gentamicin may be indi-

cated. *Staphylococcus epidermidis* is a common source of fever in patients with intravenous lines and an agent such as teicoplanin, vancomycin or linezolid may be needed. If an infective agent and its antibiotic sensitivities become known, appropriate changes in the regimen are made. If no response occurs within 48–72 hours, changing the antibiotics or treating a fungal or viral infection are considered.

Viral infection

Prophylaxis and treatment of viral infection

Herpes viruses, such as herpes simplex, varicella zoster, CMV and Epstein–Barr virus (EBV), undergo latency following primary infection and are never eradicated from the host. Most patients with haematological malignancy have already been infected with these agents and viral reactivation is therefore the most common problem. Aciclovir or valaciclovir is frequently given prophylactically. Herpes simplex is a common cause of oral ulcers but is usually controlled easily by aciclovir. Varicella zoster frequently reactivates in patients with lymphoproliferative diseases to cause shingles which requires treatment with high doses of aciclovir or valaciclovir. Primary infection, usually in children, can be very serious and immunoglobulin can be used to prevent infection following recent exposure. Reactivation of CMV infection is particularly important following SCT (see Chapter 23) but may occur following intensive chemotherapy. Failure of immune control of EBV following allogeneic transplantation can lead to outgrowth of a B-cell tumour known as post-transplant lymphoproliferative disease (see p. 312).

Fungal infection

Prophylaxis and treatment of fungal infection

Because of the intensity of current chemotherapy, fungal infections are a major cause of morbidity and mortality. The two major subtypes are yeasts such as *Candida species* and moulds of which *Aspergillus fumigatus* is the most common.

Invasive aspergillosis is a common cause of infectious death in intensively immunocompromised patients. Infection occurs through inhalation of *Aspergillus* spores (conidia) (Fig. 12.3) and air filtration systems are used in many haematology wards. The major risk factor is neutropenia – nearly 70% of patients become infected if they are neutropenic for over 34 days. Steroid use is also important, as is age, chemotherapy and antimicrobial history.

The diagnosis of invasive aspergillosis can be difficult. Definitive diagnosis requires demonstration of invasive growth on a biopsy specimen but such evidence is rarely available. Polymerase chain reaction for fungal DNA or enzyme-linked immunosorbent assay (ELISA) for *Aspergillus* galactomannan or β1–3 d-glucan are useful. High resolution computed tomography (HRCT) chest scan is valuable and early features are nodular lesions with a 'ground glass' halo appearance. Later on, wedge lesions and the air crescent sign are seen (Fig. 12.4).

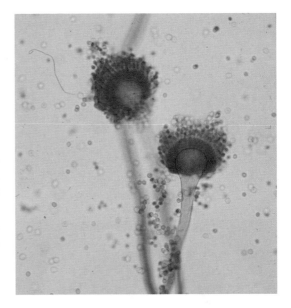

Figure 12.3 Sporing heads of *Aspergillus fumigatus*. (Courtesy of Dr Elizabeth Johnson.)

A high index of suspicion for fungal infection should be maintained and treatment is often started empirically for a fever that has failed to resolve after 3–4 days of antibiotic treatment.

Prophylaxis for patients at risk of *Aspergillus* infection is usually performed with fluconazole, itraconazole, posaconazole or lipid formulation amphotericin.

Treatment of established *Aspergillus* infection is with voriconazole, lipid formulation amphotericin, posaconazole or caspofungin. Surgery to remove lung lesions may be needed.

Candida species are a common hospital pathogen and frequently cause oral infection. *Candida* can be significant when isolated from normally sterile body fluids such as blood or urine. Prophylaxis or treatment is usually with fluconazole, itraconazole or caspofungin. Anidulafungin and micafungin are also licensed. *Pneumocystis jirovecii (carinii)* is an important cause of pneumonitis. Prophylaxis with co-trimoxazole or nebulized pentamidine is highly effective and is given to those who have received intensive (combination) chemotherapy or fludarabine. Treatment is with high dose co-trimoxazole.

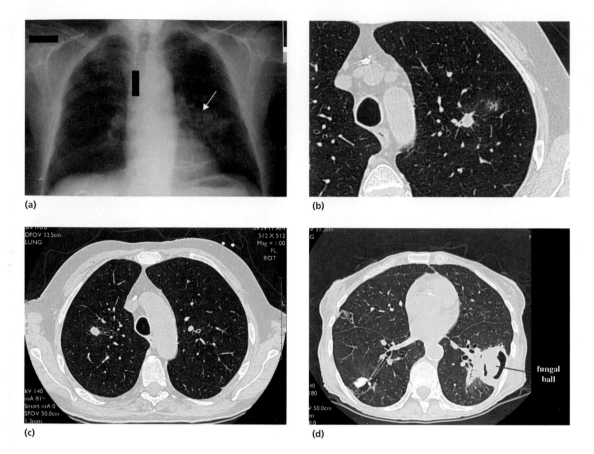

(a)

(b)

(c)

(d)

Figure 12.4 (a) Chest X-ray of patient with pulmonary aspergillosis which shows an area of cavitation containing a central fungal ball (arrow) leading to the typical 'air-crescent' sign. CT scans in *Aspergillus* show hazy ground-glass shadowing with bronchiolar dilatation **(b)** and **(c)**. Nodules are seen in early aspergillosis, whereas a fungal ball with surrounding air is typical of more advanced disease **(d)**.

Specific therapies for haematological malignancy

Specific therapy is aimed at reducing the tumour cell burden by the use of drugs or radiotherapy. The hope in some diseases is to eradicate the tumour completely and cure rates for haematological malignancy are gradually improving. However, cure is often not achievable so palliation can also be an important aim.

A wide variety of drugs are used in the management of haemopoietic malignancies and several drugs acting at different sites (Fig. 12.5) are often combined together in regimens that minimize the potential for resistance to occur against a single agent. Many act specifically on dividing cells and their selectivity is dependent on the high proliferation rate within the tumour. Not all tumour cells will be killed by a single course of treatment and it is usual to give several courses of treatment which gradually eradicate the tumour burden. This 'log kill' hypothesis also gives the residual normal haemopoietic cells the opportunity to recover between treatment courses.

Drugs used in the treatment of haemopoietic malignancies

Cytotoxic drugs (Table 12.1)

Alkylating agents such as chlorambucil, cyclophosphamide and melphalan are activated to expose

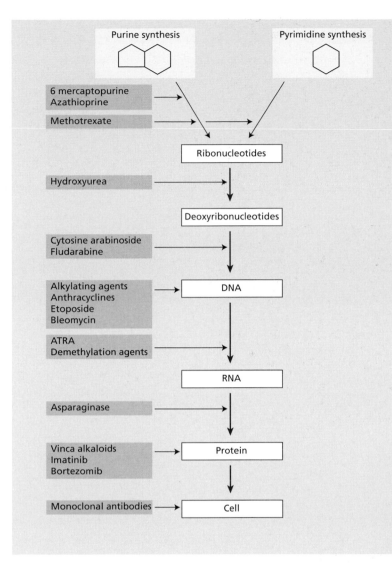

Figure 12.5 The site of action of drugs used in the management of haemopoietic malignancies. ATRA, all-*trans* retinoic acid.

reactive alkyl groups which make covalent bonds to molecules within the cell. These have a particular affinity for purines and are thus able to cross-link DNA strands and impair DNA replication, resulting in a block at G_2 (see Fig. 1.8) and death of the cell by apoptosis (see Fig. 1.11). Bendamustine is a unique drug in this class as it also appears to have activity associated with purine analogue function.

Antimetabolites block metabolic pathways used in DNA synthesis. There are four major groups:

1 Inhibitors of *de novo* DNA synthesis. *Hydroxyurea* (hydroxycarbamide) is used widely in the treatment of myeloproliferative disorders. It inhibits the enzyme ribonucleotide reductase which converts ribonucleotides to deoxyribonucleotides. It is not thought to permanently damage DNA and is used in non-malignant disorders such as sickle cell anaemia (see p. 103).

2 *Folate antagonists*, such as methotrexate (see Fig. 5.5). Methotrexate is widely used alone or in

Table 12.1 Drugs used in the treatment of leukaemia and lymphoma.

	Mechanism of action	Particular side-effects*
Alkylating agents		
Bendamustine	Alylating agent *and* purine analogue	Myelosuppression
Cyclophosphamide	Cross-link DNA, impede RNA formation	Haemorrhagic cystitis, cardiomyopathy, loss of hair
Chlorambucil		Marrow aplasia, hepatic toxicity, dermatitis
Busulfan		Marrow aplasia, pulmonary fibrosis, hyperpigmentation
Melphalan		Marrow aplasia
Nitrosoureas (BCNU, CCNU)		Renal and pulmonary toxicity
Cisplatin	Intrastrand DNA linkage	Renal dysfunction, neurotoxicity, ototoxicity
Antimetabolites		
Hydroxycarbamide (hydroxyurea)	Inhibits ribonucleotide reductase	Pigmentation, nail dystrophy, skin ulceration
Methotrexate	Inhibit pyrimidine or purine synthesis or incorporation into DNA	Mouth ulcers, gut toxicity
Cytosine arabinoside	Inhibits DNA synthesis	CNS especially cerebellar toxicity and conjunctivitis at high doses
6-Mercaptopurine[†], 6-thioguanine[†]	Purine analogue	Jaundice, gut toxicity
Clofarabine	Purine analogue	Myelosuppression
Fludarabine	Inhibit adenosine deaminase or other purine pathways	Immunosuppression (low CD4 counts); renal and neurotoxicity (at high doses)
2-Chlorodeoxyadenosine		
Deoxycoformycin		
Cytotoxic antibiotics		
Anthracyclines (e.g. daunorubicin)	Bind to DNA and interfere with mitosis	Cardiac toxicity, hair loss
Hydroxodaunorubicin (Adriamycin)		
Mitoxantrone		
Idarubicin		
Bleomycin	DNA breaks	Pulmonary fibrosis, skin pigmentation
Plant derivatives		
Vincristine (Oncovin®)	Spindle damage	Neuropathy (peripheral or bladder or gut)
Vinblastine		myelosuppression
Vindesine		
Etoposide	Mitotic inhibitor	Hair loss, oral ulceration

Table 12.1 *Continued*

	Mechanism of action	Particular side-effects*
Demethylating agents		
Azacytidine, decytabine	Inhibit DNA methlytransferase	Myelosuppression
Signal transduction inhibitors		
Imatinib, dasatinib, nilotinib	Inhibit tyrosine kinase	Myelosuppression, fluid retention
Miscellaneous		
Corticosteroids	Lymphoblast lysis	Peptic ulcer, obesity, diabetes, osteoporosis, psychosis, hypertension
Trans-retinoic acid	Induces differentiation	Liver dysfunction, skin hyperkeratosis, leucocytosis and hyperviscosity, pleural or pericardial effusion
Arsenic	Induces differentiation or apoptosis	Hyperleucocytosis, cardiac
α-Interferon	Activation of RNAase and natural killer activity	Flu-like symptoms, thrombocytopenia, leucopenia, weight loss
Bortezomid	Proteasome inhibition	Neuropathy
L-Asparaginase	Deprive cells of asparagine	Hypersensitivity, low albumin and coagulation factors, pancreatitis
Thalidomide Lenalidomide	Immuno-modulation	Neuropathy, constipation, thrombosis
Monoclonal antibodies		
Rituximab (anti-CD20)	Induction of apoptosis	Infusion reactions, immunosuppression
Alemtuzumab (anti-CD52)	Lysis of target cell by complement fixation	Infusion reactions, immunosuppression
Lumiliximab (anti-CD23)	Induction of apoptosis	Infusion reactions, immunosuppression
Ibritumomab (Zevalin®) (anti-CD20^{+90}Y)	Toxicity to bound cell	Myelosuppression, nausea
Mylotarg® (anti-CD33)	Kills myeloid cells	Myelosuppression

*Many of the drugs cause nausea, vomiting, mucositis and bone marrow toxicity, and in large doses infertility. Tissue necrosis is a problem if the drugs are extravasated during infusion.
†Allopurinol potentiates the action and side-effects of 6-mercaptopurine.

combination with cytosine arabinoside as intrathecal prophylaxis of CNS disease in patients with ALL, acute myeloid leukaemia (AML) or high grade non-Hodgkin lymphoma. High systemic doses may also prenetrate the CNS. Folinic acid (formyl THF) is able to overcome the activity of methotrexate and is sometimes administered to 'rescue' normal cells after high-dose methotrexate therapy.

3 *Pyrimidine analogues* include cytosine arabinoside (cytarabine; ara-C) which is an analogue of 2′-deoxycytidine and is incorporated into DNA where it inhibits DNA polymerase and blocks replication.

4 *Purine analogues* include fludarabine (which inhibits DNA synthesis in a manner similar to ara-C), mercaptopurine, azathioprine, bendamustine, clofarabine and pentostatin.

Cytotoxic antibiotic drugs include the anthracyclines such as doxorubicin, hydroxodaunorubicin, epirubicin and mitozantrone. These are able to intercalate into DNA and then bind strongly to topoisomerases which are critical for relieving torsional stress in replicating DNA by nicking and resealing DNA strands. If topoisomerase activity is blocked, DNA replication cannot take place.

Bleomycin is a metal chelating antibiotic that generates superoxide radicals within cells that degrade preformed DNA. It is active on non-cycling cells.

Plant derivatives include the vinca alkaloids such as vincristine which is derived from the periwinkle plant. It binds to tubulin and prevents its polymerization to microtubules. This blocks cell division in metaphase. Etoposide inhibits topisomerase action.

Other agents

Imatinib, dasatinib and nilotinib bind to the BCR-ABL1 fusion protein. They block binding of adenosine triphosphate (ATP) and thus prevent the tyrosine kinase from phosphorylating substrate proteins leading to apoptosis of the cell (see Fig. 14.4).

Corticosteroids have a potent lymphocytotoxic activity and have an important role in many chemotherapeutic regimens used in the treatment of lymphoid malignancy and myeloma.

All-trans retinoic acid (ATRA) is a vitamin A derivative that acts as a differentiation agent in acute promyelocytic leukaemia (APML). Tumour cells in APML are arrested at the promyelocyte stage as a result of transcriptional repression resulting from the PML-RARA fusion protein (see p. 182). ATRA relieves this block and may lead to a brisk neutrophila within a few days of treatment with other side-effects known as the 'ATRA' or 'differentiation' (see p. 183).

Demethylation agents (e.g. azacytidine, decitabine) act to increase transcription by reducing methylation on cytosine resides within DNA.

Interferon-α is an antiviral and antimitotic substance produced in response to viral infection and inflammation. It has proven useful in chronic myeloid leukaemia, myeloma and myeloproliferative diseases.

Monoclonal antibodies are highly effective against B-cell malignancies. Rituximab binds to CD20 on B cells and appears to mediate cell death, primarily through direct induction of apoptosis and opsonization (see p. 265). Alemtuzumab binds to CD52 and is highly efficient at fixing complement which lyzes the target B and T cells. Lumiliximab is an anti-CD23 in trial for treatment of chronic lymphocytic leukaemia. Antibodies may also carry attached toxins (e.g. Mylotarg®), (anti-CD33) or radioactive isotopes (e.g. Zevalin®).

Bortezomid is a proteasome inhibitor widely used in the treatment of myeloma and some lymphomas.

Asparaginase is an enzyme derived from bacteria that breaks down the amino acid asparagine within the circulation. ALL cells lack asparagine synthase and thus need a supply of exogenous asparagine for protein synthesis. Intramuscular asparaginase is an important agent in the treatment of ALL, although hypersensitivity reactions are not uncommon and blood clotting may be disturbed.

Platinum derivatives (e.g. cisplatin) are used in combinations for treating lymphoma.

Arsenic is useful in treatment of acute promyelocytic leukaemia. It induces differentiation and apoptosis.

SUMMARY

- Progress in the treatment of haemopoietic malignancies has been the result of improvements in both supportive therapy and specific tumour treatments.
- Supportive treatments often include:
  insertion of a central venous catheter;
  appropriate use of red cell and platelet transfusions;
  early administration of drugs to treat infection;
  optimization of the blood coagulation system;
  drugs to reduce side effects such as nausea or pain;
  psychological support.
- Gram-positive skin organisms such as *Staphyloccus* are common infections and often colonize central venous catheters.
- Gram-negative bacteria are usually derived from the gut and can cause severe septicaemia.
- The use of air filters, handwashing and antibiotics can reduce infection rates.
- Neutropenic patients who develop a fever should be treated urgently with broad-spectrum antibiotics.
- Herpes viruses are a common cause of infection in patients who are significantly immunosuppressed.
- Fungal infections are a major clinical problem for patients undergoing chemotherapy. Antifungal drugs may be used for either prevention or treatment of disease.
- A wide range of drugs is now available for the treatment of haemopoietic malignancy:
  alkylating agents;
  antimetabolites;
  anthracyclines;
  folate antagonists;
  signal transduction inhibitors;
  steroids;
  monoclonal antibodies;
  immune modulators;
  proteasome inhibitors; and
  inhibitors of mitosis.

Now visit www.wiley.com/go/essentialhaematology to test yourself on this chapter.

Acute myeloid leukaemia

Essential Haematology, 6th Edition. © A. V. Hoffbrand and P. A. H. Moss. Published 2011 by Blackwell Publishing Ltd.

The leukaemias are a group of disorders characterized by the accumulation of malignant white cells in the bone marrow and blood. These abnormal cells cause symptoms because of: (i) bone marrow failure (e.g. anaemia, neutropenia, thrombocytopenia); and (ii) infiltration of organs (e.g. liver, spleen, lymph nodes, meninges, brain, skin or testes).

Classification of leukaemia

The main classification is into four types: acute and chronic leukaemias, which are further subdivid[ed] into lymphoid or myeloid.

Acute leukaemias are usually aggressive disea[se] in which malignant transformation occurs in [a] haemopoietic stem cell or early progenitors. Gen[etic] damage is believed to involve several key biochemical steps resulting in (i) an increased rate of proliferation, (ii) reduced apoptosis and (iii) a block in cellular differentiation. Together these events cause accumulation in the bone marrow of early haemopoietic cells known as **blast cells**. The dominant clinical feature of acute leukaemia is usually bone marrow failure caused by accumulation of blast cells although organ infiltration also occurs. If untreated, acute leukaemias are usually rapidly fatal but, paradoxically, they may be easier to cure than chronic leukaemias.

Diagnosis of acute leukaemia

Acute leukaemia is normally defined as the presence of over 20% of blast cells in the blood or bone marrow at clinical presentation. However, it can be diagnosed with less than 20% blasts if specific leukaemia-associated cytogenetic or molecular genetic abnormalities are present (Table 13.1).

The lineage of the blast cells is defined by microscopic examination (morphology), immunophenotypic (flow cytometry), cytogenetic and molecular analysis. This will define whether the blasts are of myeloid or lymphoid lineage and also localize the stage of cellular differentiation (Table 13.2). The typical 'myeloid immunophenotype' is CD13$^+$, CD33$^+$, CD117$^+$ and TdT$^-$ (Table 13.2; Fig. 13.1) and special antibodies are helpful in the diagnosis of the rare undifferentiated, erythroid or megakaryoblastic subtypes (Table 13.2).

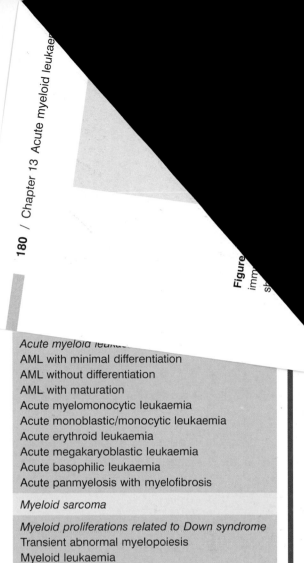

Acute myeloid leuka[emia]
AML with minimal differentiation
AML without differentiation
AML with maturation
Acute myelomonocytic leukaemia
Acute monoblastic/monocytic leukaemia
Acute erythroid leukaemia
Acute megakaryoblastic leukaemia
Acute basophilic leukaemia
Acute panmyelosis with myelofibrosis

Myeloid sarcoma

Myeloid proliferations related to Down syndrome
Transient abnormal myelopoiesis
Myeloid leukaemia

Cytogenetic and **molecular** analysis is essential and is usually performed on marrow cells although blood may be used if the blast cell count is particularly high. Cytochemistry can be useful in determining the blast cell lineage but is no longer performed in centres where the newer and more definitive tests are available.

Acute myeloid leukaemia

Incidence

Acute myeloid leukaemia (AML) is the most common form of acute leukaemia in adults and

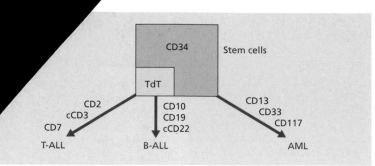

13.1 Development of three cell lineages from pluripotential stem cells giving rise to the three main
unological subclasses of acute leukaemia. The immunological characterization using pairs of markers is
own, as well as the three markers characterizing the early 'stem' cells. AML, acute myeloid leukaemia; B-ALL,
B-cell acute lymphoblastic leukaemia; c, cytoplasmic; HLA, human leucocyte antigen; T-ALL, T-cell acute
lymphoblastic leukaemia; TdT, terminal deoxynucleotidyl transferase.

Table 13.2 Specialized tests for acute myeloid leukaemia.

Cytochemistry

Myeloperoxidase	+ (including Auer rods)
Sudan black	+ (including Auer rods)
Non-specific esterase	+ in M_4, M_5

Immunological markers (flow cytometry)

CD13, CD33, CD117	+
Glycophorin	+ (erythroid)
Platelet antigens (e.g. CD41)	+ (megakaryoblastic)
Myeloperoxidase	+ (undifferentiated)

Chromosome and genetic analysis (Tables 13.1 & 13.3)

becomes increasingly common with age with a median onset of 65 years. It forms only a minor fraction (10–15%) of the leukaemias in childhood. Cytogenetic abnormalities and response to initial treatment have a major influence on prognosis (Table 13.3).

Classification

AML is classified according to the World Health Organization (2008) scheme. There is an increasing focus on the genetic abnormalities within the malignant cells and it is likely that ultimately almost all AML cases will be classified by specific genetic subtype. Currently this is not possible but many genetic subtypes have been determined. Approximately 60% of cases exhibit karyotypic abnormalities on cytogenetic analysis and many cases with a normal karyotype carry mutations in genes such as nucleophosmin (*NPM*), *FLT3* and *CEBPA* detected only by molecular methods.

Six main groups of AML are recognized (Table 13.1) and these are discussed below.

1 **AML with recurrent genetic abnormalities** encompasses subtypes with specific chromosomal translocations or gene mutations. The detection of these abnormalities defines the tumour as AML and so the diagnostic criteria for this subgroup are relaxed in that the bone marrow blast cell count does not need to exceed 20% in order to make a diagnosis. In general these disorders have a good prognosis.

2 **AML with myelodysplasia-related changes.** In this group the AML is associated with microscopic features of dysplasia in at least 50% of cells in at least two lineages. The clinical outcome of these patients is impaired in relation to the first subgroup.

3 **Therapy-related myeloid neoplasms (t-AML)** arise in patients who have been previously treated with drugs such as etoposide or alkylating agents. They commonly exhibit mutations in the *MLL* gene and the clinical response is usually poor.

Table 13.3 Prognostic factors in acute myeloid leukaemia (AML).

	Favourable	Intermediate	Unfavourable

Cytogenetics	t(15; 17)
	t(8; 21)
	inv(16)
	NPM mutation
	CEBPA mutation
		Normal
		Other non-complex
		  changes
			Deletions of chromosome 5
			  or 7
			Abnormal (3q)
			t(6; 11)
			t(10; 11)
			t(9; 22)
			Complex rearrangements (>3
			  unrelated abnormalities)
			FLT3 internal tandem repeat

Bone marrow response to remission induction	<5% blasts after first course		>20% blasts after first course
Age			>60 years

4 **AML, not otherwise specified.** This group is defined by the absence of cytogenetic abnormalities and comprises around 30% of all cases. Mutations in the *NPM* and *FLT3* genes are seen in approximately 50% and 30% of AML cases, respectively, and are more frequent in those with normal cytogenetics.

5 **Myeloid sarcoma** is rare but refers to a disease that resembles a solid tumour but is composed of myeloid blast cells.

6 **Myeloid proliferations related to Down's syndrome.** Children with Down's syndrome have a greatly increased risk of acute leukaemia. Two myeloid variants are recognized: (i) transient abnormal myelopoiesis in which there is a self-limiting leucocytosis; and (ii) AML.

Clinical features

The clinical features of AML are dominated by the pattern of bone marrow failure caused by the accumulation of malignant cells within marrow (Fig. 13.2). Infections are frequent and anaemia and thrombocytopenia are often profound. A bleeding tendency caused by thrombocytopenia and disseminated intravascular coagulation (DIC) is characteristic of the promyelocytic variant of AML. Tumour cells can infiltrate a variety of

tissues. Gum hypertrophy and infiltration (Fig. 13.3), skin involvement and CNS disease are characteristic of the myelomonocytic and monocytic subtypes.

Investigations

Haematological investigations reveal a normochromic normocytic anaemia with thrombocytopenia in most cases. The total white cell count is usually increased and blood film examination typically shows a variable numbers of blast cells. The bone marrow is hypercellular and typically contains many leukaemic blasts (Fig. 13.4). Blast cells are characterized by morphology, cytochemistry (Fig. 13.5), immunological (flow cytometric) (Fig. 13.6) and cytogenetic analysis. As discussed above, cytogenetic and molecular analysis is critical for determining the prognosis and developing a treatment plan (Table 13.3).

Tests for DIC are often positive in patients with the promyelocytic variant of AML (see below). Biochemical tests are performed as a baseline before treatment begins and may reveal raised uric acid or lactate dehydrogenase.

The differential diagnosis includes acute lymphoid leukaemia (ALL) or marrow infiltration by other malignancies (e.g. carcinoma).

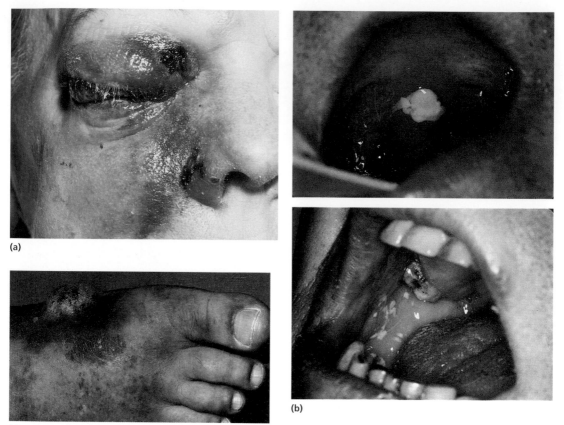

(a)

(b)

(c)

Figure 13.2 (a) An orbital infection in a female patient (aged 68 years) with acute myeloid leukaemia and severe neutropenia (haemoglobin 8.3 g/dL, white cells 15.3 × 10⁹/L, blasts 96%, neutrophils 1%, platelets 30 × 10⁹/L). **(b)** Acute myeloid leukaemia: top: plaque *Candida albicans* on soft palate; lower: plaque *Candida albicans* in the mouth, with lesion of herpes simplex on the upper lip. **(c)** Skin infection (*Pseudomonas aeruginosa*) in a female patient (aged 33 years) with acute lymphoblastic leukaemia receiving chemotherapy and with severe neutropenia (haemoglobin 10.1 g/dL, white cells 0.7 × 10⁹/L, neutrophils <0.1 × 10⁹/L, lymphocytes 0.6 × 10⁹/L, platelets 20 × 10⁹/L).

Cytogenetics and molecular genetics

Cytogenetic abnormalities are used to classify the majority of cases of AML (Table 13.1). Two of the most common affect the core binding factor genes *CBFα* or *CBFβ* (see Fig. 11.10). CBF is a heterodimeric transcription factor important in regulating genes such as interleukin 3 (IL-3) and granulocyte–macrophage colony-stimulating factor (GM-CSF). They are t(8; 21) in which the *CBFα* gene (also known as *AML1*) is translocated to the

ETO gene on chromosome 8 and inv(16) in which the *CBFβ* gene is fused to the *SMMHC* (*MYH11*) gene. Both are associated with a relatively good prognosis.

Acute promyelocytic leukaemia is a variant of AML that contains the t(15; 17) translocation in which the promyelocytic leukaemia gene *PML* on chromosome 15 is fused to the retinoic acid receptor α gene, *RARα*, on chromosome 17 (Fig. 13.7). The resultant PML-RARα fusion protein functions as a transcriptional repressor whereas normal (wild-

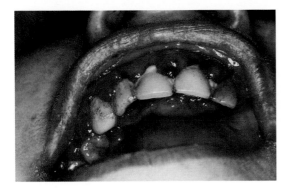

Figure 13.3 Monocytic acute myeloid leukaemia: the gums are swollen and haemorrhagic because of infiltration by leukaemic cells.

type) *RARα* is an activator. Normally, the PML protein forms homodimers with itself whereas the RARα protein forms heterodimers with the retinoid X receptor protein, RXR. The PML-RARα fusion protein binds to PML and RXR, preventing them from linking with their natural partners. This results in the cellular phenotype of arrested differentiation.

Point mutations affecting the genes *NPM, FLT-3, CEBPA, TET2, WT1, IDH1, IDH2* and others are frequent in AML, especially in those cases without a cytogenetic abnormality. They may be used to subclassify the disease (Table 13.1) and have prognostic significance.

Treatment

Management is both supportive and specific.

1 **General supportive therapy** for bone marrow failure is described in Chapter 12 and includes the insertion of a central venous cannula, blood product support and prevention of tumour lysis syndrome. The platelet count is generally maintained above 10×10^9/L and the haemoglobin above 8 g/dL. Any episode of fever must be treated promptly. Acute promyelocytic leukaemia needs special support as described below.

2 **The aim of treatment** in acute leukaemia is to induce complete remission (<5% blasts in the bone marrow, normal blood counts and clinical status) and then to consolidate this with intensive therapy, hopefully eliminating the disease (Fig.

13.8). Allogeneic stem cell transplantation is considered in poor prognosis cases or patients who have relapsed.

3 **Specific therapy of AML** is determined by the age and performance status of the patient as well as the genetic lesions within the tumour. In younger patients treatment is primarily with the use of intensive chemotherapy. This is usually given in four blocks each of approximately 1 week and the most commonly used drugs are cytosine arabinoside and daunorubicin (both in conventional or high doses). Idarubicin, mitoxantrone and etoposide are also used in various regimens (Figs 13.8 and 13.9).

A typical good response in AML is shown in Figure 13.10. The drugs are myelotoxic with limited selectivity between leukaemic and normal marrow cells and so marrow failure resulting from the chemotherapy is severe, and prolonged and intensive supportive care is required. Maintenance therapy is of no value except in promyelocytic AML and CNS prophylaxis is not usually given. New drugs such as FLT3 inhibitors are now being introduced for tumours with *FLT3* mutations. Monoclonal immunoconjugates targeted against CD33 (e.g. Mylotarg®) or CD45 provide an additional therapeutic option for initial or consolidation AML therapy.

Problems unique to AML include the haemorrhagic syndrome associated with promyelocytic variant. The disease may present with catastrophic haemorrhage or this may develop in the first few days of treatment. It is treated as for DIC with multiple platelet transfusions and replacement of clotting factors with fresh frozen plasma (see p. 358). In addition, all-*trans* retinoic acid (ATRA) therapy is given in conjunction with chemotherapy for this disease subtype. The ***differentiation syndrome*** (also known as ATRA syndrome) is a specific complication that may arise after ATRA treatment. Clinical problems, which are thought to result from the neutrophilia that follows differentiation of promyelocytes from the bone marrow, include fever, hypoxia with pulmonary infiltrates and fluid overload. Treatment is with 10 mg dexamethasone intravenously twice daily. ATRA is only discontinued in very severe cases.

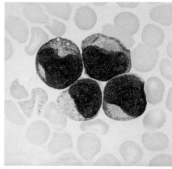

(a)

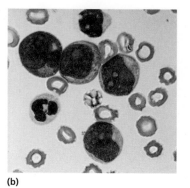

(b)

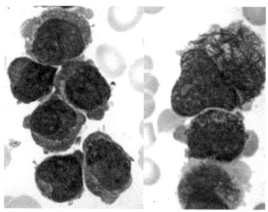

(c)

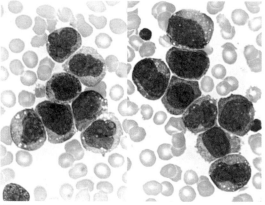

(d)

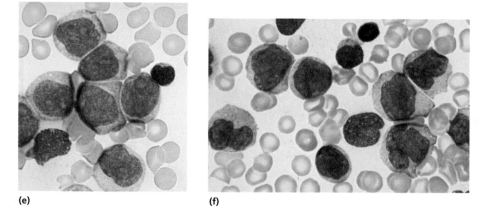

(e)

(f)

Figure 13.4 Morphological examples of acute myeloid leukaemia. **(a)** Blast cells without differentiation show few granules but may show Auer rods, as in this case; **(b)** cells in differentiation show multiple cytoplasmic granules or **(c)** M$_3$ blast cells contain prominent granules or multiple Auer rods; **(d)** myelomonocytic blasts have some monocytoid differentiation; **(e)** monoblastic leukaemia in which >80% of blasts are monoblasts; **(f)** monocytic with <80% of blasts monoblasts.

(*Continued*)

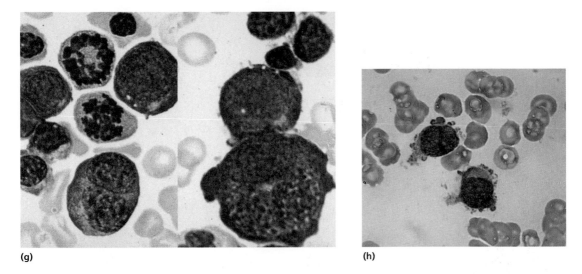

(g) (h)

Figure 13.4 *Continued* **(g)** Erythroid showing preponderance of erythroblasts; **(h)** megakaryoblastic showing cytoplasmic blebs on blasts.

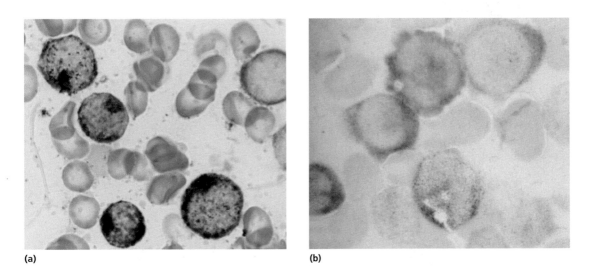

(a) (b)

Figure 13.5 Cytochemical staining in acute myeloid leukaemia. **(a)** Sudan black B shows black staining in the cytoplasm. **(b)** Myelomonocytic: non-specific esterase/chloracetate staining shows orange-staining monoblast cytoplasm and blue-staining (myeloblast) cytoplasm.

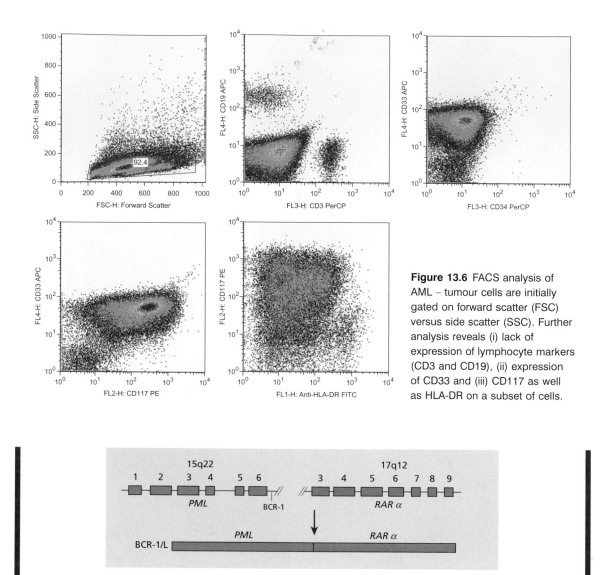

Figure 13.6 FACS analysis of AML – tumour cells are initially gated on forward scatter (FSC) versus side scatter (SSC). Further analysis reveals (i) lack of expression of lymphocyte markers (CD3 and CD19), (ii) expression of CD33 and (iii) CD117 as well as HLA-DR on a subset of cells.

Figure 13.7 Generation of the t(15; 17) translocation. The *PML* gene at 15q22 may break at one of three different breakpoint cluster regions (BCR-1, -2 and -3) and joins with exons 3–9 of the *RARα* gene at 17q12. Three different fusion mRNAs are generated (termed long (L), variable (V) or short (S)) and these give rise to fusion proteins of different size. In this diagram only the long version resulting from a break at BCR-1 is shown.

Promyelocytic leukaemia with the t(15; 17) translocation responds to treatment with high doses of ATRA which causes differentiation of the abnormal promyelocytes and results in improved prognosis. Interestingly, in rare variants of *RARα* is fused to other genes and in these cases ATRA treatment is not successful.

Prognosis and treatment stratification

The outcome for an individual patient with AML will depend on a number of factors including age and white cell count at presentation. However, the genetic abnormalities in the tumour are the most important determinant.

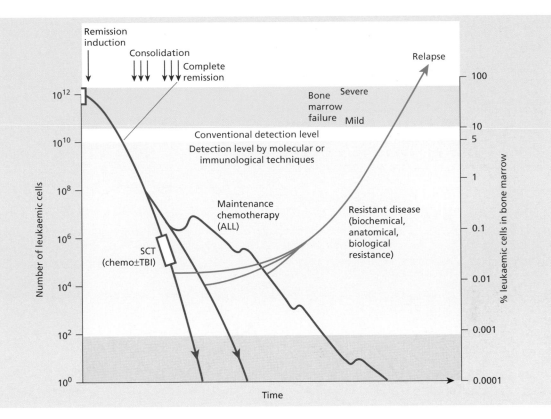

Figure 13.8 Acute leukaemia: principles of therapy. ALL, acute lymphoblastic leukaemia; SCT, stem cell transplantation; TBI, total body irradiation.

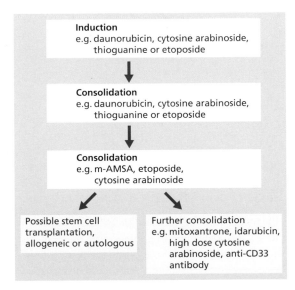

Figure 13.9 Acute myeloid leukaemia: flow chart illustrating typical treatment regimen.

An important concept developing in AML therapy is that of basing the treatment schedule of individual patients on their risk group. Favourable cytogenetics and remission after one course of chemotherapy both predict for a better prognosis. In contrast, monosomy 5 or 7 abnormalities, blast cells with the *FLT3* internal tandem duplication mutation or poorly responsive disease places patients into poor risk groups which need more intensive treatments (Table 13.3).

Monitoring of **minimal residual disease** during and after chemotherapy is being investigated as a means to guide appropriate treatment. It may be performed by polymerase chain reaction (PCR) or flow cytometric analysis of the abnormal 'leukaemia-associated immunophenotype' that is seen in over 90% of cases.

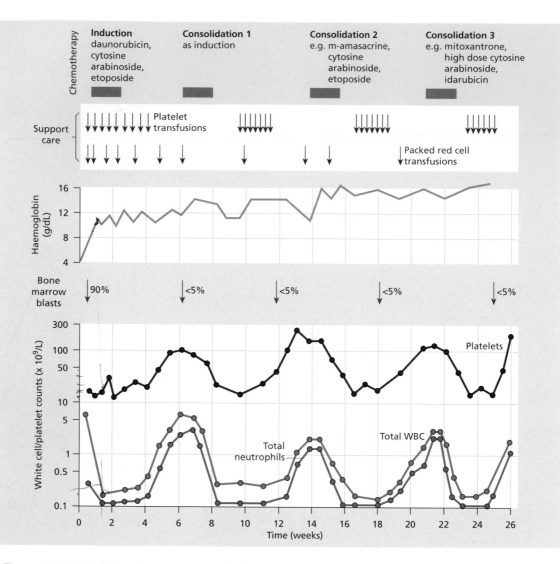

Figure 13.10 Typical flow chart for the management with chemotherapy of acute myeloid leukaemia. WBC, white blood cells.

Stem cell transplantation

Allogeneic stem cell transplantation (SCT) reduces the rate of AML relapse but carries risk of morbidity and mortality. It is therefore not used for patients in the favourable risk group unless they have disease relapse. SCT is used for some patients with standard or poor risk AML in first remission. Clinical trials are continuing to establish firm indications.

Patients over 70 years of age

The median age for presentation of AML is approximately 65 years and treatment outcomes in the elderly are poor because of primary disease resistance and poor tolerability of intensive treatment protocols. Death from haemorrhage, infection or failure of the heart, kidneys or other organs is more frequent than in younger patients. In elderly patients

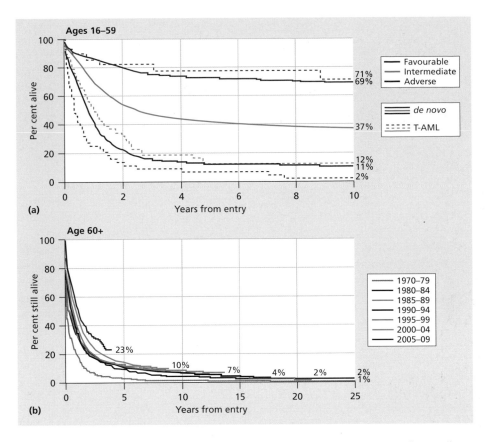

Figure 13.11 Overall survival for adult patients: **(a)** aged 16–59 years and grouped according to disease karyotype and whether de novo or therapy-related (T-AML); and **(b)** over 60 years with AML treated in UK trials. (Courtesy of Professor A.K. Burnett.)

with serious disease of other organs, the decision may be made to use supportive care with or without gentle single-drug chemotherapy. However, in those otherwise well, combination chemotherapy similar to that used in younger patients may produce long-term remissions and reduced-intensity SCT may be considered.

Treatment of relapse

Most patients suffer relapse and the outlook will then depend on age, the duration of the first remission and the cytogenetic risk group. In addition to further chemotherapy, allogeneic SCT with either standard or reduced-intensity conditioning is usually performed in those patients who can tolerate the procedure and who have a suitable human leucocyte antigen (HLA) matching related or unre-

lated donor. Arsenic trioxide is useful in management of relapse in the promyelocytic variant.

Outcome

The prognosis for patients with AML has been improving steadily, particularly for those under 60 years of age, and approximately one-third of this group can expect to achieve long-term cure (Fig. 13.11a). Cytogenetic abnormalities and initial response to treatment are major predictors of favourable, intermediate or adverse prognosis. Tracking of minimal residual disease using molecular cytogenetic markers or aberrant phenotypes may be helpful in predicting long-term remission or relapse. For the elderly the situation is poor and less than 10% of those over 70 years of age can expect long-term remission (Fig. 13.11b).

SUMMARY

- The leukaemias are a group of disorders characterized by the accumulation of malignant white cells in the bone marrow and blood. They can be classified into four subtypes on the basis of being either *acute* or *chronic*, and *myeloid* or *lymphoid*.
- Acute leukaemias are aggressive diseases in which transformation of a haemopoietic stem cell leads to accumulation of >20% blast cells in the bone marrow.
- The clinical features of acute leukaemia result from bone marrow failure and include anaemia, infection and bleeding. Tissue infiltration can also occur.
- AML is rare in childhood but becomes increasingly common with age with a median onset of 65 years.
- The diagnosis is made by analysis of blood and bone marrow using microscopic examination (morphology) as well as immunophenotypic, cytogenetic and molecular studies.
- Cytogenetic and molecular abnormalities are used to classify and indicate prognosis in the majority of cases of AML.

- In younger patients treatment is primarily with the use of intensive chemotherapy. This is usually given in four blocks each of approximately 1 week using drugs such as cytosine arabinoside and daunorubicin.
- Acute promyelocytic leukaemia is a variant of AML that carries a t(15; 17) chromosomal translocation. It commonly presents with bleeding and is treated with retinoic acid and chemotherapy.
- The prognosis for patients with AML has been improving steadily, particularly for those under 60 years of age, and approximately one-third of this group can expect to achieve long-term cure. The outcome for elderly people remains disappointing.
- Allogeneic stem cell transplantation is useful in treating some subsets of patients and may also be curative for patients with relapsed disease.

Now visit www.wiley.com/go/essentialhaematology to test yourself on this chapter.

CHAPTER 14
Chronic myeloid leukaemia

Key topics

Essential Haematology, 6th Edition. © A. V. Hoffbrand and P. A. H. Moss. Published 2011 by Blackwell Publishing Ltd.

The chronic leukaemias are distinguished from acute leukaemias by their slower progression. Chronic leukaemias can be broadly subdivided into myeloid (Table 14.1) and lymphoid groups (see Chapter 18).

Chronic myeloid (myelogenous) leukaemia BCR-ABL1 positive

Chronic myeloid leukaemia BCR-ABL1+ (CML) is a clonal disorder of a pluripotent stem cell. The disease accounts for around 15% of leukaemias and

Table 14.1 Chronic myeloid leukaemia (CML) and myelodysplastic myeloproliferative neoplasms (see Chapter 16).

Type	Molecular genetics
BCR-ABL-1 rearrangement positive CML	>95% BCR-ABL-1 p210 <5% p190 or p230
BCR-ABL-1 rearrangement negative CML	Various cytogenetic abnormalities
Chronic neutrophilic leukaemia	Deletions of chromosome 20q and trisomy 21 or 9 in some
Chronic eosinophilic leukaemia	FIPILI–PDGFR-α (in those who respond to imatinib) generated by interstitial deletion on chromosome 4q12
Chronic monocytic leukaemia	Very rare
Chronic myelomonocytic leukaemia	PDGFR-β rearrangement in a minority who respond to imatinib
Juvenile myelomonocytic leukaemia	30% PTPN11 (encodes SHP-2) mutations 20% K-RAS or N-RAS mutations 10% NF1 mutation
Refractory anaemia with ringed sideroblasts and thrombocytosis	Somatic mutations of JAK2 and MPL

may occur at any age. The diagnosis of CML is rarely difficult and is assisted by the characteristic presence of the Philadelphia (Ph) chromosome. This results from the t(9; 22) (q34; q11) transloca-tion between chromosomes 9 and 22 as a result of which part of the oncogene ABL1 is moved to the BCR gene on chromosome 22 (Fig. 14.1a) and part of chromosome 22 moves to chromosome 9. The abnormal chromosome 22 is the Ph chromosome. In the Ph translocation 5′ exons of BCR are fused to the 3′ exons of ABL1 (Fig. 14.1b,c). The resulting chimeric BCR-ABL1 gene codes for a fusion protein of size 210 kDa (p210). This has tyrosine kinase activity in excess of the normal 145-kDa ABL1 product. The Ph translocation is also seen in a minority of cases of acute lymphoblastic leukaemia (ALL) and in some of these the breakpoint in BCR occurs in the same region as in CML. However, in other cases the breakpoint in BCR is further upstream, in the intron between the first and second exons, leaving only the first BCR exon intact. This chimeric BCR-ABL1 gene is expressed as a p190 protein which, like p210, has enhanced tyrosine kinase activity.

In most patients the Ph chromosome is seen by karyotypic examination of tumour cells (Fig. 14.1d) but in a few the Ph abnormality cannot be seen under the microscope but the same molecular rear-rangement is detectable by more sensitive tech-niques: fluorescence *in situ* hybridization (FISH) (Fig. 14.1e) or polymerase chain reaction (PCR). Ph-negative BCR-ABL1 positive CML behaves clin-ically like Ph-positive CML. As the Ph chromosome is an acquired abnormality of haemopoietic stem cells it is found in cells of both the myeloid (granulocytic, erythroid and megakaryocytic) and lymphoid (B and T cell) lineages. Ph–, BCR-ABL1– chronic myeloid leukaemia is classified with the myelodysplastic/myeloproliferative syndromes (see Chapter 16).

Clinical features

This disease occurs in either sex (male : female ratio of 1.4 : 1), most frequently between the ages of 40 and 60 years. However, it may occur in children and neonates, and in the very old. In most cases there are no predisposing factors but the incidence was

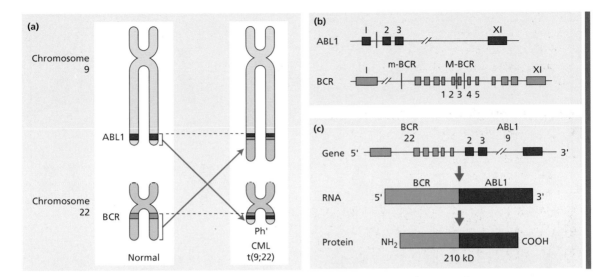

Figure 14.1 The Philadelphia chromosome. **(a)** There is translocation of part of the long arm of chromosome 22 to the long arm of chromosome 9 and reciprocal translocation of part of the long arm of chromosome 9 to chromosome 22 (the Philadelphia chromosome). This reciprocal translocation brings most of the *ABL* gene into the *BCR* region on chromosome 22 (and part of the *BCR* gene into juxtaposition with the remaining portion of *ABL* on chromosome 9). **(b)** The breakpoint in *ABL* is between exons 1 and 2. The breakpoint in *BCR* is at one of the two points in the major breakpoint cluster region (M-BCR) in chronic myeloid leukaemia (CML) or in some cases of Ph+ acute lymphoblastic leukaemia (ALL). **(c)** This results in a 210-kDa fusion protein product derived from the *BCR-ABL* fusion gene. In other cases of Ph+ ALL, the breakpoint in *BCR* is at a minor breakpoint cluster region (m-BCR) resulting in a smaller *BCR-ABL* fusion gene and a 190-kDa protein. (*Continued*)

increased in survivors of the atom bomb exposures in Japan. Its clinical features include the following:

1 Symptoms related to hypermetabolism (e.g. weight loss, lassitude, anorexia or night sweats).
2 Splenomegaly is nearly always present and is frequently massive. In some patients splenic enlargement is associated with considerable discomfort, pain or indigestion.
3 Features of anaemia may include pallor, dyspnoea and tachycardia.
4 Bruising, epistaxis, menorrhagia or haemorrhage from other sites because of abnormal platelet function.
5 Gout or renal impairment caused by hyperuricaemia from excessive purine breakdown may be a problem.

6 Rare symptoms include visual disturbances and priapism.
7 In up to 50% of cases the diagnosis is made incidentally from a routine blood count.

Laboratory findings

1 Leucocytosis is usually $>50 \times 10^9/L$ and sometimes $>500 \times 10^9/L$ (Fig. 14.2). A complete spectrum of myeloid cells is seen in the peripheral blood. The levels of neutrophils and myelocytes exceed those of blast cells and promyelocytes (Fig. 14.3).
2 Increased circulating basophils.
3 Normochromic normocytic anaemia is usual.
4 Platelet count may be increased (most frequently), normal or decreased.

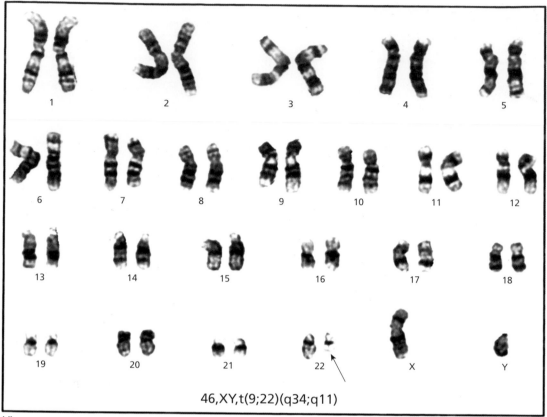

46,XY,t(9;22)(q34;q11)

(d)

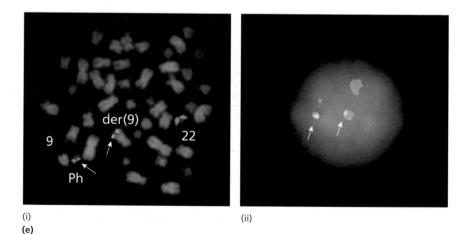

(i)

(ii)

(e)

Figure 14.1 (*Continued*) **(d)** Karyotype showing the t(9; 22) (q34; q11) translocation. The Ph chromosome is arrowed. **(e)** Visualization of the Philadelphia chromosome on: (i) dividing (metaphase); and (ii) quiescent (interphase) cells by fluorescence *in situ* hybridization (FISH) analysis (ABL probe in red and BCR probe in green) with fusion signals (red/green) on the Ph and der(9) chromosomes. (Courtesy of Dr Ellie Nacheva)

5 Bone marrow is hypercellular with granulopoietic predominance.
6 Presence of the *BCR-ABL1* gene fusion by PCR analysis and in 98% of cases Ph chromosome on cytogenetic analysis (Fig. 14.1d).
7 Serum uric acid is usually raised.

Treatment

Treatment of chronic phase

Tyrosine kinase inhibitors

Imatinib (Glivec®) was designed as a specific inhibitor of the BCR-ABL1 fusion protein and blocks tyrosine kinase activity by competing with adenosine triphosphate (ATP) binding (Fig. 14.4). It is the first-line drug in the management of chronic phase disease. At 400 mg/day it can produce a complete haematological response in virtually all patients (Fig. 14.5). Side-effects include skin rash, fluid retention, muscle cramps and nausea. Neutropenia and thrombocytopenia may occur and in some cases, dose reduction or cessation may be required.

Monitoring of response to imatinib

Imatinib is highly effective at reducing the number of tumour cells in the bone marrow and should be monitored by karyotypic analysis of the bone marrow together with PCR analysis for *BCR-ABL1* transcripts in marrow or blood. Assessment of response starts with regular (3–6 monthly) bone

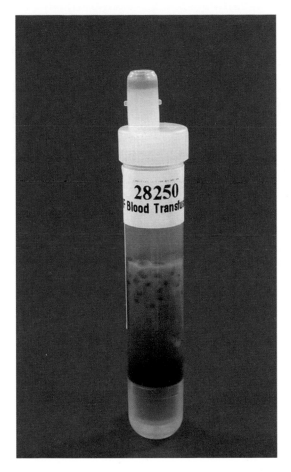

Figure 14.2 Chronic myeloid leukaemia: peripheral blood film showing a vast increase in buffy coat. The white cell count was 532 × 10⁹/L.

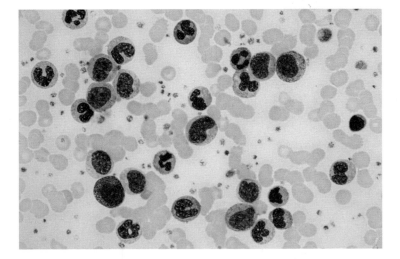

Figure 14.3 Chronic myeloid leukaemia: peripheral blood film showing various stages of granulopoiesis including promyelocytes, myelocytes, metamyelocytes and band and segmented neutrophils.

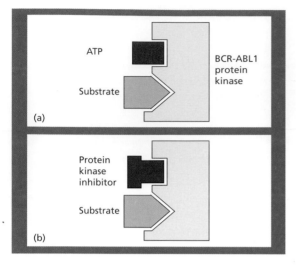

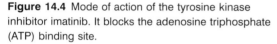

Figure 14.4 Mode of action of the tyrosine kinase inhibitor imatinib. It blocks the adenosine triphosphate (ATP) binding site.

marrow analysis to assess marrow metaphase cytogenetics. A *complete cytogenetic response (CCyR)* is defined as the absence of Ph-positive metaphases within bone marrow and once CCyR is achieved monitoring continues with PCR quantification of *BCR-ABL1* transcripts within blood at regular intervals.

The response of CML to imatinib can be defined as *optimal*, *suboptimal* or treatment *failure*.

An *optimal response* to is defined by:

- Complete haematological response (normal blood count) and at least minimal cytogenetic response (CyR) (Ph+ <95%) at 3 months;
- At least partial CyR (Ph+ <35%) at 6 months;
- Complete CyR at 12 months; and
- Major molecular response with at least a 3-log reduction in *BCR-ABL1* transcripts at 18 months (i.e. to 0.1% or less of pre-treatment level).

Failure of response is defined by:

- Incomplete haematological response at 3 months;
- No CyR (Ph+ >95%) at 6 months;
- Less than partial CyR (Ph+ >35%) at 12 months;
- Less than complete CyR at 18 months; and
- Loss of a previous complete haematological or cytogenetic response.

In any other situation, the response is defined as *suboptimal*.

Patients with optimal responses continue imatinib whereas those with treatment failure are treated with second generation tyrosine kinase inhibitor (TKI) therapy or stem cell transplantation (SCT). Patients with suboptimal responses can be treated with an increase in the dose of imatinib to 600 or 800 mg/day, change in TKI therapy or early allogeneic SCT.

BCR-ABL1 mutation screening

One mechanism of disease resistance to imatinib treatment is the development of mutations within the *BCR-ABL1* fusion gene. These mutations may be detected by sequencing the *BCR-ABL1* gene and this is performed in many centres for patients who fail to respond adequately to imatinib treatment. The pattern of mutation can be useful for determining which treatment to choose as second-line therapy.

Second generation tyrokinase kinase inhibitors

Dasatinib is a broad multikinase inhibitor that is effective in many cases in which *BCR-ABL1* has acquired mutations that render it resistant to imatinib. It is widely used in this setting although fluid retention can be a troublesome side effect.

Nilotinib has a mechanism of action similar to imatinib but has a higher affinity for the BCR-ABL1 kinase and can be effective in cases with imatinib-resistant mutations. Both nilotinib and dasatinib are currently being assessed in comparison with imatinib for first-line treatment of CML and early results suggest they may be superior.

Overall response to imatinib therapy

The IRIS study recruited 553 patients to study efficacy of imatinib therapy in chronic phase CML and reported 7-year clinical follow-up in 2008. This showed that 60% of patients remained on treatment with imatinib whereas 40% has discontinued treatment because of disease progression or intolerance of therapy. Overall survival was excellent with 84% of patients still alive at 7 years (Fig. 14.6).

If patients become negative for *BCR-ABL1* transcripts and imatinib is discontinued, some patients remain negative. For those who become positive again, imatinib will usually produce a further

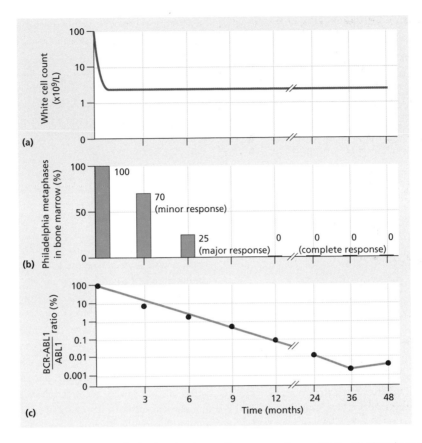

Figure 14.5 Example of the haematological and cytogenetic response in a patient with chronic myeloid leukaemia who achieves complete remission with imatinib therapy. **(a)** The white cell count returns to normal within days. **(b)** Karyotypic examination of the bone marrow reveals a gradual reduction in the number of Philadelphia chromosomes over the first year. **(c)** Polymerase chain reaction (PCR) analysis of the bone marrow or blood shows a reduction in the number of BCR-ABL1 transcripts in comparision with the normal ABL1 transcript. BCR-ABL1 transcripts continue to be detected at a very low level but can become negative in some patients. In this case analysis was performed on bone marrow for the first 12 months and on peripheral blood thereafter.

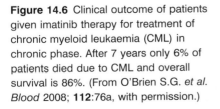

Figure 14.6 Clinical outcome of patients given imatinib therapy for treatment of chronic myeloid leukaemia (CML) in chronic phase. After 7 years only 6% of patients died due to CML and overall survival is 86%. (From O'Brien S.G. *et al.* *Blood* 2008; **112**:76a, with permission.)

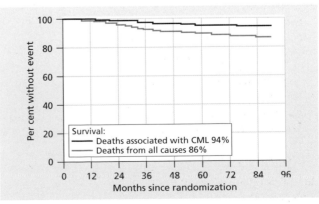

negative remission. It is possible that imatinib, and similar drugs in development, may cure some patients with CML but this will need much longer clinical follow-up than is available at the present time.

Chemotherapy

Hydroxyurea treatment can control and maintain the white cell count in the chronic phase but does not reduce the percentage of *BCR-ABL1* positive cells. A typical regimen is to start with 1.0–2.0 g/day and then to reduce this in weekly increments to a maintenance dosage of 0.5–1.5 g/day. The alkylating agent busulfan is also effective in controlling the disease but has considerable long-term side-effects and is now rarely used. Imatinib has now largely replaced both drugs.

α-Interferon

This was often used after the white cell count had been controlled by hydroxyurea but has now been superceded by imatinib. A typical regimen would be 3–9 megaunits between three to seven times each week given as a subcutaneous injection. The aim is to keep the white cell count low (around 4×10^9/L). Almost all patients have symptoms of a 'flu-like' illness in the first few days of treatment which responds to paracetamol and gradually wears off. More serious complications include anorexia, depression and cytopenias (see Table 12.1). A minority (approximately 15%) of patients may achieve long-term remission with loss of the Ph chromosome on cytogenetic analysis although the *BCR-ABL1* fusion gene can usually still be detected by PCR. Interferon produces an overall prolongation of the chronic phase with increased life expectancy.

Stem cell transplantation

Allogeneic SCT is a proven curative treatment for CML but, because of the risk, is usually reserved for imatinib failures. The results are better when it is performed in chronic rather than acute or accelerated phases. The 5-year survival is approximately 50–70% although this is reduced by approximately 10% if transplantation is delayed for more than 1 year following diagnosis. Although international bone marrow donor panels are playing an increas-

ingly important part in providing human leucocyte antigen (HLA) matching unrelated donors, allogeneic SCT can only be offered to a minority of patients. Relapse of CML after the transplant is a significant problem but donor leucocyte infusions are highly effective in CML (see p. 311), particularly if relapse is diagnosed early by molecular detection of the *BCR-ABL1* transcript.

Accelerated phase disease and blastic transformation

Acute transformation (20% or more blasts in the marrow) may occur rapidly over days or weeks (Fig. 14.7). More commonly, the patient has an *accelerated phase* with anaemia, thrombocytopenia and an increase in basophils, eosinophils or blast cells in the blood and marrow. The spleen may be enlarged despite control of the blood count and the marrow may become fibrotic. The patient may be in this phase for several months during which the disease is less easy to control than in the chronic phase. In both the accelerated and acute phases, new chromosome abnormalities are often present. In approximately one-fifth of cases, acute transformation is lymphoblastic and patients may be treated in a similar way to ALL with a number of patients returning to the chronic phase for months or even

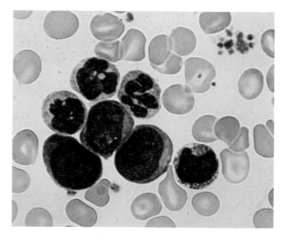

Figure 14.7 Chronic myeloid leukaemia: acute myeloblastic transformation. Peripheral blood film showing frequent myeloblasts.

a year or two. In the majority, transformation is into acute myeloid leukaemia (AML) or mixed types. These are more difficult to treat and survival is rare beyond a few months. Imatinib is valuable in the management of blastic transformation but resistance to treatment usually occurs within a few weeks. New tyrosine kinase inhibitors aimed at overcoming resistance to imatinib include dasatinib and nilotinib (see p. 196). Allogeneic SCT may be tried in younger subjects with an HLA-matching donor.

Chronic neutrophilic leukaemia

These patients have no inflammatory or other causes of neutrophilia and no evidence for any other myeloproliferative disease. They may have mild splenomegaly. Cytogenetics are usually normal; the prognosis is variable.

Chronic eosinophilic leukaemia

Chronic eosinophilic leukaemia is a clonal persistent eosinophilia ($>1.5 \times 10^9$/L). There may be an interstitial lesion in chromosome 4 resulting in *FIP1L1-PDGFRA* fusion gene (in which case there is a response to imatinib) or other less frequent cytogenetic or molecular defects. There may be >5% but <20% blasts in the marrow. The cells may infiltrate various organs causing damage (e.g. endomyocardial fibrosis, lung, CNS, skin and gastrointestinal tract). If clonality cannot be shown and blasts are <5%, the condition is diagnosed as hypereosinophilic syndrome (see p. 121).

SUMMARY

- Chronic myeloid leukaemia is a clonal disorder of a pluripotent stem cell. The disease accounts for around 15% of leukaemias and may occur at any age.
- All cases of CML have a translocation between chromosomes 9 and 22. This leads to the oncogene *ABL1* being moved to the *BCR* gene on chromosome 22 and generates the Philadelphia chromosome.
- The resulting chimeric *BCR-ABL1* gene codes for a fusion protein with tyrosine kinase activity.
- In most patients the Philadelphia chromosome is seen by karyotypic examination of tumour cells but the molecular rearrangement may sometimes only be detected by FISH or PCR.
- The disease can occur at any age but is most common between the ages of 40 and 60 years.
- The clinical features include anaemia, bleeding and splenomegaly. There is usually a marked neutrophilia with myelocytes and basophils seen in the blood film.
- Transformation to an accelerated phase or acute leukaemia may occur.
- Treatment is with tyrosine kinase inhibitors such as imatinib, dasatinib or nilotinib. Tumour cells can acquire resistance to treatment and drug therapy is tailored in response to this.
- Stem cell transplantation can be curative and may also be useful for advanced disease.
- The clinical outlook is now very good and patients can expect long-term control of disease.
- Chronic eosinophilic and neutrophil leukaemias are much rarer.

Now visit www.wiley.com/go/essentialhaematology to test yourself on this chapter.

CHAPTER 15
The non-leukaemic myeloproliferative neoplasms

Key topics

Essential Haematology, 6th Edition. © A. V. Hoffbrand and P. A. H. Moss. Published 2011 by Blackwell Publishing Ltd.

The term myeloproliferative neoplasms (MPN) describes a group of conditions arising from marrow stem cells and characterized by clonal proliferation of one or more haemopoietic components in the bone marrow and, in many cases, the liver and spleen. The three major non-leukaemic disorders included in this classification are:

1 Polycythaemia vera (PV);
2 Essential thrombocythaemia (ET); and
3 Primary myelofibrosis.

Mastocytosis is also discussed in this chapter; BCR-ABL1 positive chronic myeloid leukaemia in Chapter 14 and the myelodysplastic syndromes and mixed myelodysplastic/myeloproliferative diseases in Chapter 16.

The non-leukaemic myeloproliferative disorders are closely related to each other and transitional forms can occur with evolution from one entity into another during the course of the disease (Fig. 15.1). These diseases are associated with clonal abnormalities involving genes that encode cytoplasmic or receptor tyrosine kinase (Table 15.1). A single acquired mutation of the cytoplasmic tyrosine kinase Janus-associated kinase 2 (JAK2) (Val617Phe)

occurs (heterozygous or homozogous) in the marrow and blood of almost all patients with PV and in approximately 50% of those with ET and primary myelofibrosis, showing the common aetiology of these three diseases (Fig. 15.2). The mutation occurs

Table 15.1 Myeloproliferative diseases and other myeloid neoplasms associated with point mutation or rearrangement of tyrosine kinase genes.	
Disease	**Tyrosine kinase gene mutated**
Chronic myeloid leukaemia	*ABL1*
Polycythaemia vera	*JAK2 V617F; JAK2 exon12*
Primary myelofibrosis	*JAK2 V617F; MPL W151L/K*
Essential thrombocythaemia	*JAK2 V617F; MPL W151L/K*
Mastocytosis	*KIT D816V*
Myeloid neoplasm with eosinophilia	*PDGFRA, PDGFRB, FGFR1*

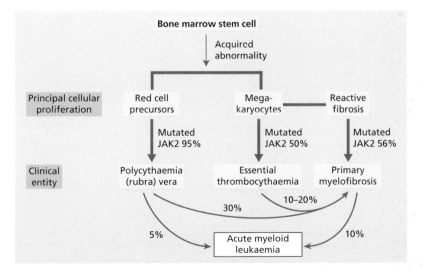

Figure 15.1 Relationship between the three myeloproliferative diseases. They may all arise by somatic mutation in the pluripotential stem and progenitor cells. Many transitional cases occur showing features of two conditions and, in other cases, the disease transforms during its course from one of these diseases to another or to acute myeloid leukaemia. The three diseases, polycythaemia rubra vera, essential thrombocythaemia and primary myelofibrosis, are characterized by *JAK2* mutation in a varying proportion of cases (see text).

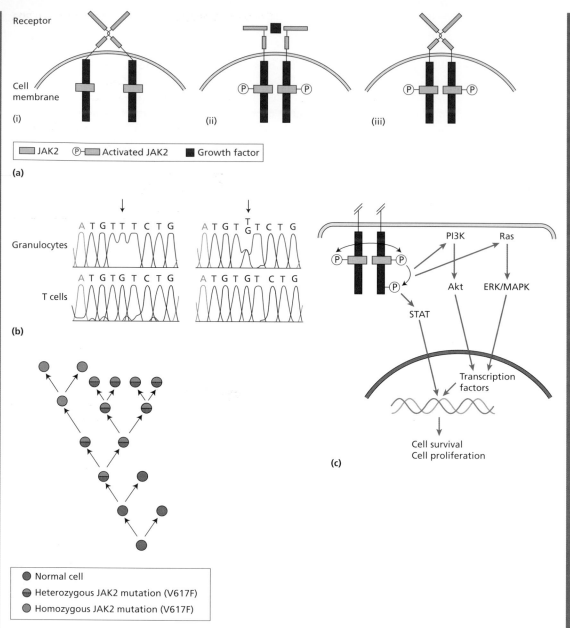

Figure 15.2 The role of *JAK2* mutation in the generation of myeloproliferative diseases. **(a)** (i) Most haemopoietic growth factor receptors do not have intrinsic kinase activity but associate with a protein kinase such as JAK2 in the cytoplasm. (ii) When the receptor binds a growth factor the cytoplasmic domains move closer together and the JAK2 molecules can activate each other by phosphorylation. (iii) The V617F *JAK2* mutation allows the JAK protein to become activated even when no growth factor is bound. **(b)** DNA sequencing shows homozygous G → T mutation in *JAK2* in granulocytes but not in T lymphocytes (left-hand panel) and heterozygous mutation in right-hand panel. (After Kralovic R. *et al*. *N Engl J Med* 2005, **352**, 1779–90.) **(c)** JAK2 activation leads to cell survival and proliferation through activation of three major pathways; the STAT transcription factors, the PI3K pathway acting through Akt and Ras activation which subsequently activate ERK and MAPK. The net result is production of a diverse range of proteins that promote cell survival and proliferation. **(d)** A model for the development of myeloproliferative disease following *JAK2* mutation. The primary event appears to predispose to an acquired heterozygous mutation of *JAK2* (V617F). This leads to a survival advantage. In some patients, a mitotic recombination event leads to a homozygous *JAK2* mutation state.

in a highly conserved region of the pseudokinase domain, which is believed to negatively regulate JAK2 signalling. JAK2 has a major role in normal myeloid development by transducing signals from diverse cytokines and growth factors including interleukin-3 (IL-3), erythropoietin, granulocyte–macrophage colony-stimulating factor (GM-CSF), granulocyte colony-stimulating factor (G-CSF) and thrombopoietin (see Fig. 1.8). Why the same mutation is associated with different myeloproliferative diseases is unclear. The exact cell in which the mutation arises, the number of stem cells involved, the genetic background of individual subjects including polymorphism of the *JAK2* gene, and other factors may be relevant.

Polycythaemia

Polycythaemia is defined as an increase in the haemoglobin concentration above the upper limit of normal for the patient's age and sex.

Classification of polycythaemia

Polycythaemia is classified according to its pathophysiology but the major subdivision is into **absolute polycythaemia** or erythrocytosis, in which the red cell mass (volume) is raised to greater than 125% of that expected for body mass and gender, and **relative** or **pseudopolycythaemia** in which the red cell volume is normal but the plasma volume is reduced. If the haematocrit is >0.60 then there will always be a raised red cell mass. Hb >18.5 g/dL or haematocrit >0.52 in men, and Hb >16.5 g/dL or haematocrit >0.48 in women, indicate that erythrocytosis is likely but isotope studies may be required (Table 15.2).

Once established, absolute polycythaemia can then be subdivided into **primary polycythaemia** (in which the erythroid progenitor cell shows an enhanced response to cytokines) or **secondary polycythaemia** (driven by factors outside the erythroid compartment) (Table 15.3).

Primary polycythaemia (erythrocytosis)

Congenital

(See below.)

Acquired

This is caused by the acquisition of mutations in the *JAK2* gene leading to PV.

Polycythaemia vera

In PV, the increase in red cell volume is caused by a clonal malignancy of a marrow stem cell. The disease results from somatic mutation of a single haemopoietic stem cell which gives its progeny a proliferative advantage. The Val617Phe *JAK2* mutation is present in haemopoietic cells in over 95% of patients and a mutation in exon 12 is seen in some of the remainder. Although the increase in red cells is the diagnostic finding, in many patients there is also an overproduction of granulocytes and platelets. Some families have an inherited predisposition to myeloproliferative disease and, interestingly, although affected individuals acquire *JAK2* mutations in the marrow, these are not present in the germline.

Table 15.2 Radiodilution methods for measuring red cell and plasma volume.

	Normal	Primary or secondary polycythaemia	Relative polycythaemia
Total red cell volume (^{51}Cr)	Men 25–35 mL/kg Women 22–32 mL/kg	Increased	Normal
Total plasma volume (^{125}I-albumin)	40–50 mL/kg	Normal	Decreased

Table 15.3 Causes of polycythaemia (erythrocytosis).

Primary erythrocytosis
Congenital
Erythropoietin receptor mutations

Acquired
Polycythaemia vera

Secondary erythrocytosis
Congenital
Defects of the oxygen-sensing pathway
  VHL gene mutation (Chuvash erythrocytosis)
  PHD2 mutations
  HIF-2α mutations
Other congenital defects
  High oxygen-affinity haemoglobin

Acquired
Erythropoietin-mediated
  Central hypoxia
  Chronic lung disease
  Right to left cardiopulmonary vascular shunts
  Carbon monoxide poisoning
  Smoking
  Obstructive sleep apnoea
  High altitude
Local hypoxia
  Renal artery stenosis
  End-stage renal disease
  Hydronephrosis
  Renal cysts (polycystic kidney disease)
  Post-renal transplant erythrocytosis
Pathologic erythropoietin production
  Tumours – cerebellar haemangioblastoma,
    meningioma, parathyroid tumours,
    hepatocellular carcinoma, renal cell cancer,
    phaeochromocytoma, uterine leiomyoma
Drug-associated
  Erythropoietin administration
  Androgen administration

Table 15.4 Criteria for diagnosis of polycythaemia vera. (From McMullin M.F. et al., (2007) *B J Haem* **138**: 821.)

JAK2-positive polycythaemia vera

A1	High haematocrit (>0.52 in men, >0.48 in women) *or* raised red cell mass (>25% above predicted)*
A2	Mutation in *JAK2*

Diagnosis requires both criteria to be present

JAK2-negative polycythaemia vera

A1	Raised red cell mass (>25% above predicted) *or* haematocrit >0.60 in men, >0.56 in women.
A2	Absence of mutation in *JAK2*
A3	No cause of secondary erythrocytosis
A4	Palpable splenomegaly
A5	Presence of an acquired genetic abnormality (excluding *BCR-ABL*) in the haematopoietic cells
B1	Thrombocytosis (platelet count >450 × 10^9/L)
B2	Neutrophil leucocytosis (neutrophil count >10 × 10^9/L in non-smokers; >12.5 × 10^9/L in smokers)
B3	Radiological evidence of splenomegaly
B4	Endogenous erythroid colonies or low serum erythropoietin

Diagnosis requires A1 + A2 + A3 + either another A or two B criteria

*WHO (2008) uses haemoglobin >18.5 g/dL in men and 16.5 g/dL in women as a major criterion, in JAK2+ cases and hypercellular marrow as a minor criterion as well as criteria A2 and B4 above.

Diagnosis

Making the diagnosis of PV in a patient who presents with polycythaemia can be difficult and two subsets are recognized based on the presence of the *JAK2* mutation (Table 15.4).

Clinical features

This is a disease of older subjects with an equal sex incidence. Clinical features are the result of hyper-viscosity, hypervolaemia or hypermetabolism.

1 Headaches, dyspnoea, blurred vision and night sweats. Pruritus, characteristically after a hot bath, can be a severe problem.
2 Plethoric appearance: ruddy cyanosis (Fig. 15.3), conjunctival suffusion and retinal venous engorgement.

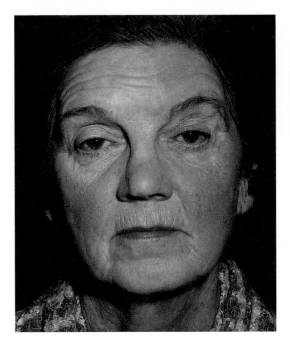

Figure 15.3 Polycythaemia vera: facial plethora and conjunctival suffusion in a 63-year-old woman. Haemoglobin 18 g/dL; total red cell volume 45 mL/kg.

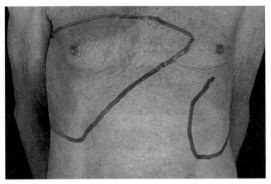

(a)

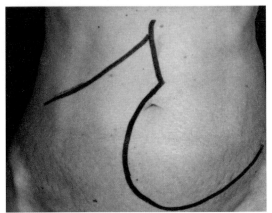

(b)

Figure 15.4 Splenomegaly: enlarged spleens in male patients with **(a)** polycythaemia vera and **(b)** myelofibrosis.

3 Splenomegaly in 75% of patients (Fig. 15.4).

4 Haemorrhage (e.g. gastrointestinal, uterine, cerebral) or thrombosis either arterial (e.g. cardiac, cerebral, peripheral) or venous (e.g. deep or superficial leg veins, cerebral, portal or hepatic veins) are frequent.

5 Hypertension in one-third of patients.

6 Gout (as a result of raised uric acid production; Fig. 15.5a).

Laboratory findings

1 The haemoglobin, haematocrit and red cell count are increased. The total red cell volume (Table 15.1) is increased.

2 A neutrophil leucocytosis is seen in over half of patients, and some have increased circulating basophils.

3 A raised platelet count is present in about half of patients.

4 The *JAK2* mutation is present in the bone marrow and peripheral blood granulocytes in over 95% of patients.

5 The bone marrow is hypercellular with trilineage growth (panmyelosis), best assessed by a trephine biopsy (Fig. 15.6a).

6 Serum erythropoietin is low.

7 Plasma urate is often increased; the serum lactate dehydrogenase (LDH) is normal.

8 Circulating erythroid progenitors (erythroid colony-forming unit, CFU_E, and erythroid burst-forming unit, BFU_E; see p. 16) are increased compared to normal and grow *in vitro* independently of added erythropoietin (endogenous erythroid colonies).

9 Chromosome abnormalities (e.g. deletions of 9p or 20q) are found in a minority of subjects and mutations in *TET-2* occur in 10–20%.

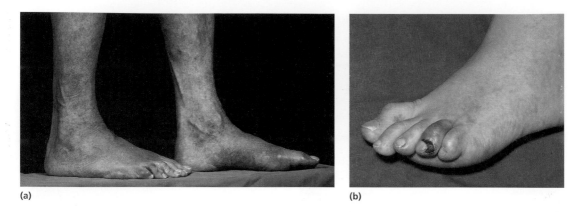

(a)   (b)

Figure 15.5 (a) The feet of a 72-year-old man with polycythaemia rubra vera. There is inflammation of the right metatarsophalangeal and other joints caused by uric acid deposits. **(b)** Gangrene of the left fourth toe in essential thrombocythaemia.

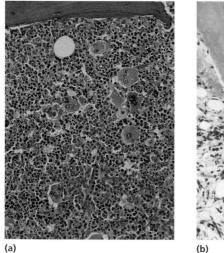
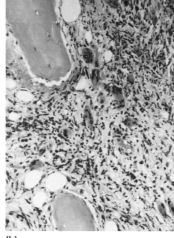

(a)   (b)

Figure 15.6 Iliac crest trephine biopsies. **(a)** Polycythaemia vera: fat spaces are almost completely replaced by hyperplastic haemopoietic tissue. All haemopoietic cell lines are increased with megakaryocytes particularly prominent. **(b)** Primary myelofibrosis: normal marrow architecture is lost and haemopoietic cells are surrounded by increased fibrous tissue and intercellular substance.

Treatment

Treatment is aimed at maintaining a normal blood count. The haematocrit should be maintained at about 0.45 and the platelet count below 400×10^9/L.

Venesection

Venesection to reduce the haematocrit to less than 0.45 is particularly useful when a rapid reduction of red cell volume is required (e.g. at the start of therapy). It is especially indicated in younger patients and those with mild disease. The resulting iron deficiency may limit erythropoiesis. Unfortunately, venesection does not control the platelet count.

Cytotoxic myelosuppression

This is considered if there is poor tolerance of venesection, symptomatic or progressive splenomegaly, or night sweats. Daily ... ...rea) is valuable in con... ...d may need to be continued ... ... (Fig. 15.7). Side-effects of hydroxyurea in...de myelosuppression, nausea and skin toxicity. Busulfan, which can be used intermittently, is sometimes used in older patients. Pipobroman is similar to alkylating agents and is used in Europe but not in the UK. The concern with cytotoxic drugs, especially busulfan, is that they may be associated with an increased rate of progression to leukaemia. This risk is low and there is probably no increased risk with hydroxyurea.

Phosphorus-32 therapy

This is only used for older patients with severe disease. ^{32}P is a β-emitter, with a half-life of 14.3 days. It is concentrated in bone and is a most effective myelosuppressive agent. The usual remission time after a single dose is 2 years. Concern about late development of leukaemia limits its use.

Interferon

α-Interferon suppresses excess proliferation in the marrow and has produced good haematological responses. It is less convenient than the oral agents and side-effects are frequent. It may be particularly valuable in controlling itching and is often used for patients less than 40 years old to avoid early exposure to chemotherapy drugs.

Aspirin

Low-dose aspirin reduces thrombotic complications without an increased risk of major haemorrhage.

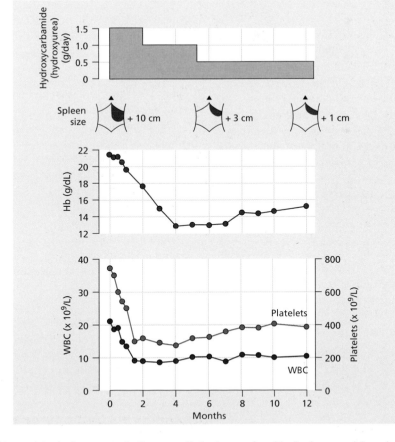

Figure 15.7 Haematological response to therapy with hydroxycarbamide (hydroxyurea) in polycythaemia vera. Hb, haemoglobin; WBC, white blood cells.

JAK2 inhibitors

Drugs which inhibit JAK2 activity are in clinical trials and are showing great promise, in both JAK2 wild type and mutated cases. It is anticipated that they may become first-line agents.

Course and prognosis

Typically, the prognosis is good with a median survival of 10–16 years. Thrombosis and haemorrhage are the major clinical problems. Increased viscosity, vascular stasis and high platelet levels may all contribute to thrombosis, whereas defective platelet function may promote haemorrhage.

Transition from PV to myelofibrosis occurs in approximately 30% of patients and approximately 5% of patients progress to acute leukaemia. ^{32}P and busulfan are generally avoided, particularly in younger subjects as they may increase this risk.

Congenital causes

Congenital causes are relatively rare and include cases caused by mutations in the genes that regulate oxygen sensing (*VHL*, *PHD2* or *HIF2A*) (see Chapter 2) as well as mutation of the erythropoietin receptor and haemoglobin mutations that lead to high oxygen affinity variants with subsequent tissue hypoxia. These patients often have a family history of polycythaemia and present at a young age.

Secondary polycythaemia

The causes of secondary polycythaemia are listed in Table 15.3.

Acquired causes are due to an increase in the erythropoietin level. Hypoxia caused by chronic obstructive airways disease is one of the most frequent, and measurement of arterial oxygen saturation is a valuable test. Renal and tumour causes of inappropriate erythropoietin secretion are rare.

There is very little evidence on which to guide a treatment plan. Some would advise venesection if the haematocrit is above 0.54 with the aim of reducing to a target around 0.5. A lower target for venesection may be used if there is hypertension, diabetes, dyspnoea, angina or a previous thrombotic episode. Low dose aspirin may be of benefit for many patients.

Apparent polycythaemia

Apparent polycythaemia, also known as pseudopolycythaemia, is the result of plasma volume contraction. By definition, the red cell mass is normal. The cause is uncertain but it is far more common than PV. It occurs particularly in young or middle-aged men and may be associated with cardiovascular problems, e.g. hypertension (Gaisböck's syndrome), myocardial ischaemia or cerebral transient ischaemic attacks. Diuretic therapy, heavy smoking, obesity and alcohol consumption are frequent associations. Venesection to maintain a haematocrit around 0.45–0.47 is recommended in those with a recent history of thrombosis, or with additional risk factors for this.

Differential diagnosis of polycythaemia

The identification of the *JAK2* mutation has rationalized the approach to diagnosis of polycythaemia. A three-stage approach to diagnosis has been suggested:

1 **Stage 1** History and examination
   Full blood count/film
   JAK2 mutation
   Serum ferritin
   Renal and liver function tests
   If JAK2 is negative and there is no clear secondary cause, proceed to stage 2.
2 **Stage 2** Red cell mass
   Arterial oxygen saturation
   Abdominal ultrasound
   Serum erythropoietin level
   Bone marrow aspirate and trephine
   Cytogenetic analysis
   BFU_E culture
   Specialized tests may then be required.
3 **Stage 3** Arterial oxygen dissociation
   Sleep study
   Lung function studies
   Gene mutations *EPOR, VHL, PHD2*

Essential thrombocythaemia

In this condition there is a sustained increase in platelet count, because of megakaryocyte proliferation and overproduction of platelets. The haematocrit is normal and the Philadelphia chromosome or *BCR-ABL1* rearrangement are absent. The bone marrow shows no collagen fibrosis. A persisting platelet count of $>450 \times 10^9$/L is the central diagnostic feature but other causes of a raised platelet count (particularly iron deficiency, inflammatory or malignant disorder and myelodysplasia) need to be fully excluded before the diagnosis can be made.

Half of patients show the *JAK2* (Val617Phe) mutation and these cases tend to resemble more closely PV with higher haemoglobin and white cell counts than *JAK2* negative cases. Mutations within the *MPL* gene are seen in 4% of cases. Rare primary familial cases in children have been associated with mutations in the genes for thrombopoietin or its receptor MPL.

Diagnosis

This used to be based on the exclusion of other causes of chronic thrombocytosis but now that specific genetic lesions have been identified a positive diagnosis can be made in approximately 50% of cases.

Suggested diagnostic criteria for essential thrombocythaemia

(From Beer P.A. and Green A.R. (2009) *Hematology Am Soc Hematol Educ Program*, 621–8.)

Diagnosis requires A1–A3 or A1 + A3–A5:

A1 Sustained platelet count $>450 \times 10^9$/L.

A2 Presence of an acquired pathogenetic mutation (e.g. in *JAK2* or *MPL*).

A3 No other myeloid malignancy, PV, primary myelofibrosis, chronic myeloid leukaemia (CML) or myelodysplastic syndrome.

A4 No reactive cause for thrombocytosis and normal iron stores.

A5 Bone marrow trephine histology showing increased megakaryocytes with prominent large hyperlobulated forms; reticulin is generally not increased.

Clinical and laboratory findings

The dominant clinical features are thrombosis and haemorrhage. Most cases are symptomless and diagnosed on routine blood counts. Thrombosis may occur in the venous or arterial systems (Fig. 15.5b) whereas haemorrhage, as a result of abnormal platelet function, may cause either chronic or acute bleeding. Some patients (JAK2+) present with Budd–Chiari syndrome when the platelet count may be normal because of the splenomegaly. A characteristic symptom is erythromelalgia, a burning sensation felt in the hands or feet and promptly relieved by aspirin. Up to 40% of patients will have palpable splenomegaly whereas in others there may be splenic atrophy because of infarction.

Abnormal large platelets and megakaryocyte fragments may be seen on the blood film (Fig. 15.8). The bone marrow is similar to that in PV but an excess of abnormal megakaryocytes is typical. Cytogenetics and molecular analysis are analysed to exclude BCR-ABL1+ CML. The condition must be distinguished from other causes of a raised platelet count (Table 15.5). Platelet function tests (see p. 328) are consistently abnormal, failure of aggregation with adrenaline being particularly characteristic.

Prognosis and treatment

The principle is to reduce the risk of thrombosis or haemorrhage which are the major clinical problems.

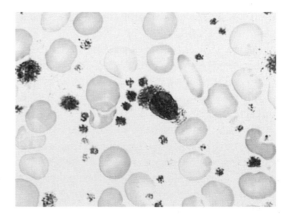

Figure 15.8 Peripheral blood film in essential thrombocythaemia showing increased numbers of platelets and a nucleated megakaryocytic fragment.

Table 15.5 Causes of a raised platelet count.

Reactive
Haemorrhage, trauma, postoperative
Chronic iron deficiency
Malignancy
Chronic infections
Connective tissue diseases (e.g. rheumatoid
  arthritis)
Post-splenectomy

Endogenous
Essential thrombocythaemia (*JAK2* mutation +
  or −)
Some cases of polycythaemia vera, primary
  myelofibrosis, BCR-ABL1+ chronic myeloid
  leukaemia, myelodysplasia (5q- or refractory
  anaemia with ring sideroblasts)

The patients most at risk of thrombosis are those over 60 years old or with previous thrombotic episodes. Additional risk factors include presence of *JAK2* mutation, smoking history and hypertension; the importance of the absolute platelet count is uncertain.

Standard cardiovascular risk factors such as cholesterol, smoking, diabetes, obesity and hypertension should be identified and treated. Low dose aspirin at 75 mg/day is generally recommended in all cases.

Patients at **high risk** include those over 60 years of age, with previous thrombosis or with platelet count over 1500×10^9/L and this group should be treated with drugs to reduce the platelet count. **Low risk** patients are those aged <40 years and here aspirin alone is sufficient. Optimum control of the **medium risk** group (age 40–60 years) is uncertain.

Hydroxyurea is the most widely used treatment and is well tolerated although some patients develop skin ulceration or pigmentation. Anagrelide is a good second-line treatment but has more side-effects, particularly on the cardiovascular system, and a possible increased risk of myelofibrosis is also of concern. These two drugs can be combined at low doses to reduce side-effects. α-Interferon is also effective and is often used in younger patients or

during pregnancy. A long-acting Pegylated preparation is preferred. JAK2 inhibitors are now being introduced into clinical trials.

Course

Often the disease is stationary for 10–20 years or more. The disease may transform after a number of years to myelofibrosis but the risk of transformation to acute leukaemia is relatively low (<5%).

Primary myelofibrosis

The predominant feature of primary myelofibrosis is a progressive generalized reactive fibrosis of the bone marrow in association with the development of haemopoiesis in the spleen and liver (known as myeloid metaplasia). Clinically this leads to anaemia and massive splenomegaly. In some patients there is osteosclerosis. Myelofibrosis is a clonal stem cell disease. The fibrosis of the bone marrow is secondary to hyperplasia of abnormal megakaryocytes. It is thought that fibroblasts are stimulated by platelet-derived growth factor and other cytokines secreted by megakaryocytes and platelets.

The *JAK2* mutation occurs in approximately 50% of patients, whereas around 15% have a mutation of *TET-2* and some patients carry mutations in the *MPL* gene (the receptor for thrombopoietin). Non-specific cytogenetic abnormalities may be found in approximately half of patients. One-third of patients with similar features have a previous history of PV or ET and some patients present with clinical and laboratory features of both disorders.

Clinical features

1 An insidious onset in older people is usual with symptoms of anaemia.
2 Symptoms resulting from massive splenomegaly (e.g. abdominal discomfort, pain or indigestion) are frequent; splenomegaly is the main physical finding (Fig. 15.4b).
3 Hypermetabolic symptoms such as loss of weight, anorexia, fever and night sweats are common.
4 Bleeding problems, bone pain or gout occur in a minority of patients.

Primary myelofibrosis and CML are responsible for most cases of massive (>20 cm) splenic enlargement in the UK and North America (see Table 10.1).

Laboratory findings

1 Anaemia is usual but a normal or increased haemoglobin level may be found in some patients.
2 The white cell and platelet counts are frequently high at the time of presentation. Later in the disease leucopenia and thrombocytopenia are common.
3 A leucoerythroblastic blood film is found. The red cells show characteristic 'tear-drop' poikilocytes (Fig. 15.9).
4 Bone marrow is usually unobtainable by aspiration. Trephine biopsy (Fig. 15.6b) shows a fibrotic hypercellular marrow. Increased megakaryocytes are frequently seen. In 10% of cases there is increased bone formation with increased bone density on X-ray.
5 *JAK2* kinase is mutated in approximately 50% of cases.
6 High serum urate and LDH levels reflect the increased but largely ineffective turnover of haemopoietic cells.
7 Transformation to acute myeloid leukaemia occurs in 10–20% of patients.

Treatment

This is usually palliative and aimed at reducing the effects of anaemia and splenomegaly. Blood transfusions and regular folic acid therapy are used in severely anaemic patients. Hydroxyurea may help to reduce splenomegaly and hypermetabolic symptoms. Trials of thalidomide, lenalidomide, azacytidine and histone deacetylase inhibitors are in progress. JAK2 inhibitors (in clinical trials) reduce spleen size, and can be effective in both *JAK2* mutated and wild-type cases. Danazol, an androgen derivative, may improve anaemia in approximately 30% of patients. Erythropoietin can also be tried but may cause splenic enlargement.

Splenectomy is considered for patients with severe symptomatic splenomegaly – mechanical discomfort, thrombocytopenia, portal hypertension, excessive transfusion requirements or hypermetabolic symptoms. Splenic irradiation is an alternative but usually provides relief only for 3–6 months. Allopurinol is indicated in virtually all patients to prevent gout and urate nephropathy from hyperuricaemia. Allogeneic stem cell transplantation may be curative for young patients.

The median survival is less than 5 years and causes of death include heart failure, infection and leukaemic transformation. A haemoglobin level of <10 g/dL, a white cell count of less than 4 or greater than 30×10^9/L and the presence of abnormal chromosomes are associated with a worse prognosis.

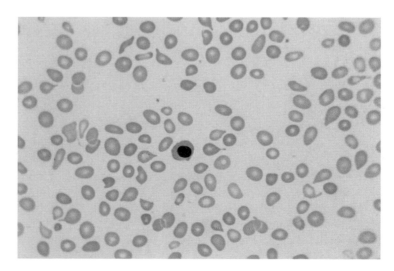

Figure 15.9 Peripheral blood film in primary myelofibrosis. Leucoerythroblastic change with 'tear-drop' cells and an erythroblast.

Mastocytosis

Mastocytosis is a clonal neoplastic proliferation of mast cells that accumulate in one or more organ systems. Mast cells (tissue basophils) are derived from haemopoietic stem cells. Mature cells survive for months or years in vascular tissues and most organs. Systemic mastocytosis is a clonal myeloproliferative disorder involving usually the bone marrow, heart, spleen, lymph nodes and skin.

The somatic *KIT* mutation Asp816Val is detected in the majority of patients and may be partly responsible for autonomous growth and enhanced survival of the neoplastic mast cells. In many patients this mutation is also detected in other haemopoietic cells.

Symptoms are related to histamine and prostaglandin release and include flushing, pruritus, abdominal pain and bronchospasm. H_1 and H_2 antihistamine blocking drugs are valuable. The skin usually shows urticaria pigmentosa (Fig. 15.10). Serum tryptase is increased and can be used to monitor treatment. Interferon, chlorodeoxyadenosine and tyrosine kinase inhibitors can be helpful. In many patients the disease runs a chronic indolent course. In others an aggressive course may be associated with acute myeloid leukaemia, mast cell leukaemia or other haemopoietic proliferative or dysplastic conditions (see Appendix 2).

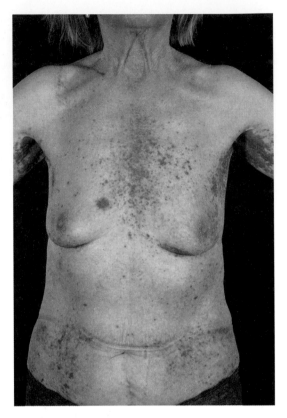

Figure 15.10 Systemic mastocytosis: female 72 years; widespread erythematous, confluent plaques of urticaria pigmentosa over chest, abdomen and upper arms. (Courtesy of Dr M. Rustin.)

SUMMARY

- Myeloproliferative neoplasms are a group of conditions arising from marrow stem cells and characterized by clonal proliferation of one or more haemopoietic components in the bone marrow. The three major subtypes are: polycythaemia vera (PV); essential thrombocythaemia (ET); and primary myelofibrosis.
- These subtypes are closely related to each other and mutation of the *JAK2* gene is detected in almost all patients with PV and in approximately 50% of those with ET and primary myelofibrosis.

- Polycythaemia is defined as an increase in the haemoglobin concentration and the major subdivision is into *absolute polycythaemia,* in which the red cell mass is raised, and *relative polycythaemia* in which the red cell volume is normal but the plasma volume is reduced.
- Absolute polycythaemia is divided into primary polycythaemia, known as polycythaemia vera (PV), or secondary polycythaemia.
- The diagnosis of PV is made by finding polycythaemia together with a *JAK2* mutation. It occurs in older patients and

the increase in blood viscosity leads to headaches, plethoric appearance and splenomegaly.

■ Treatment aims to maintain the haematocrit around 0.45. Useful approaches include venesection or hydroxyurea and aspirin is also given. *JAK2* inhibitors are being assessed in clinical trials. Survival is usually over 10 years but there may be progression to leukaemia or myelofibrosis.

■ Secondary polycythaemia can arise from rare congenital causes or acquired disorders such as lung disease or tumours that secrete erythropoietin. Venesection may be needed.

■ Essential thrombocythaemia is diagnosed by persistent raised platelet count in the absence of other causes. *JAK2* is mutated in approximately 50% of cases.

■ The predominant feature of primary myelofibrosis is a progressive generalized reactive fibrosis of the bone marrow in association with the development of haemopoiesis in the spleen and liver. Symptoms usually result from anaemia and a grossly enlarged spleen.

■ Diagnosis is made on blood film, which shows a leucoerythroblastic appearance, together with bone marrow biopsy and *JAK2* mutation screen. Treatment is with red cell transfusion. Splenectomy is sometimes used and *JAK2* inhibitors appear encouraging.

■ Systemic mastocytosis is a clonal proliferation of mast cells with involvement of bone marrow, skin (as uticaria pigmentosa) and other organs.

Now visit www.wiley.com/go/essentialhaematology to test yourself on this chapter.

CHAPTER 16
Myelodysplasia

Key topics

Essential Haematology, 6th Edition. © A. V. Hoffbrand and P. A. H. Moss. Published 2011 by Blackwell Publishing Ltd.

Myelodysplasia (myelodysplastic syndromes)

This is a group of clonal disorders of haemopoietic stem cells characterized by increasing bone marrow failure in association with quantitative and qualitative abnormalities of cells in peripheral blood (Table 16.1). A hallmark of the disease is simultaneous proliferation and apoptosis of haemopoietic cells (*ineffective haemopoiesis*) leading to the paradox of a hypercellular bone marrow but pancytopenia in peripheral blood. There is a tendency to progress to acute myeloid leukaemia (AML), although death often occurs before this develops.

Table 16.1 The World Health Organization (2008) classification of myelodysplasia.

Subtype	Peripheral blood	Bone marrow	Relative proportion (%)
Refractory cytopenia with unilineage dysplasia (RCUD)			
Refractory anaemia (RA)	Anaemia, <1% blasts	Unilineage erythroid dysplasia (in >10% cells), <5% blasts	10–20
Refractory neutropenia (RN)	Neutropenia, <1% blasts	Unilineage granulocytic dysplasia, <5% blasts	<1
Refractory thrombocytopenia (RT)	Thrombocytopenia, <1% blasts	Unilineage megakaryocytic dysplasia, <5% blasts	<1
Refractory anaemia with ring sideroblasts (RARS)	Anaemia, no blasts	Unilineage erythroid dysplasia, >15% erythroid precursors are ring sideroblasts, <5% blasts	3–10%
Refractory cytopenia with multilineage dysplasia (RCMD)	Cytopenia(s), <1% blasts. No Auer rods	Multilineage dysplasia +/– ring sideroblasts, <5% blasts. No Auer rods	30
Refractory anaemia with excess blasts type 1 (RAEB-1)	Cytopenia(s), 2–9% blasts. No Auer rods	Unilineage or multilineage dysplasia, 5–9% blasts. No Auer rods	40
Refractory anaemia with excess blasts type 2 (RAEB-2)	Cytopenia(s), 5–19% blasts +/– Auer rods	Unilineage or multilineage dysplasia, 10–19% blasts. +/– Auer rods	
Myelodysplastic syndrome associated with isolated del(5q)	Anaemia Normal or high platelet count, <1% blasts	5q31 deletion Anaemia, hypolobulated megakaryocytes, <5% blasts	<5%
Myelodysplastic syndrome, unclassifiable (MDS-U)	Cytopenia(s), <1% blasts	Does not fit in other groups	Rare
Childhood myelodysplastic syndrome	Pancytopenia	<5% blasts	<1%

In most cases, the disease is *primary* but in a significant proportion of patients it is *secondary* to chemotherapy and/or radiotherapy that has been given for treatment of another malignancy. This latter type is termed **therapy-related MDS (t-MDS)** and is now classified with therapy-related AML.

The **pathogenesis** of myelodysplastic syndromes (MDS) is unclear but is presumed to start following genetic damage to a multipotent haemopoietic progenitor cell. The immune system may have a minor role in suppressing bone marrow function and immunosuppression is sometimes used in treatment (see below).

Classification

The myelodysplastic syndromes are classified on the basis of the blood count, their morphological appearance, the number of blast cells in blood or bone marrow and cytogenetics (Table 16.1). Although the classification appears complex, the principles are as follow:

- Dysplasia may be present solely in a single lineage – red cells (*refractory anaemia*), neutrophils or platelets – or present in two or more myeloid lineages (*refractory cytopenia with multilineage dysplasia*; RCMD).
- Erythroid dysplasia can also be associated with **ring sideroblasts** to define a unique subtype. The definition of a pathological ring sideroblast is an erythroid precursor with five or more iron granules encircling at least one-third of the nucleus. A rare condition, refractory anaemia with ring sideroblasts and thrombocytosis (platelets $> 450 \times 10^9$/L) in which the *JAKV617F* mutation is often present, is classified with the myelodysplastic–myeloproliferative diseases (Table 16.4).
- If the blast cell count is increased in blood or bone marrow, the diagnosis is made of *refractory anaemia with excess blasts* and these subtypes have a poor prognosis.
- *5q-Syndrome* receives its own classification. The gene that is deleted is *RPS14*, encoding a ribosomal protein (see Fig. 22.3). It is more common in women and typically there is anaemia with

Table 16.2 Cytogenetic abnormalities in myelodysplastic syndromes.

1 Chromosome deletion or loss (e.g. del 5q, monosomy 5, del 7q. monosomy 7, del 11q)

2 Chromosome gain (e.g. trisomy 8, trisomy 11)

3 Chromosome rearrangement (e.g. t3q26, t(1; 7), t11q23)

4 Complex karyotypes: three or more abnormalities

Table 16.3 Classification of risk group in myelodysplastic syndromes (MDS).

Lower risk MDS	Higher risk MDS
Survival of 3–10 years	Survival <1.5 years
Low rate of transformation to AML	High rate of AML transformation
RA, RARS	RAEB
RCUD, RCMD	
MDS-U, MDS del(5q)	
IPSS low	IPSS high

AML, acute myeloid leukaemia; IPSS, International Prognostic Scoring System; RA, refractory anaemia; RAEB, refractory anaemia with excess blasts; RARS, refractory anaemia with ring sideroblasts; RCUD, refractory cytopenia with unilineage dysplasia; RCMD, refractory cytopenia with multilineage dysplasia; MDS, myelodysplastic syndrome; MDS-U, myelodysplastic syndrome, unclassifiable.

thrombocytosis in 50% of cases. It has a particularly good prognosis (Table 16.3).

Clinical features

The disease has an incidence of 4 in 100 000 and a slight male predominance. Over half of patients are over 70 years and fewer than 25% are less than 50 years old. The evolution is often slow and the disease may be found by chance when a patient has a blood count for some unrelated reason. The symptoms, if present, are those of anaemia, infections or of easy bruising or bleeding (Fig. 16.1). In some patients transfusion-dependent anaemia dominates the course, while in others recurring infections or spontaneous bruising and bleeding are the major clinical

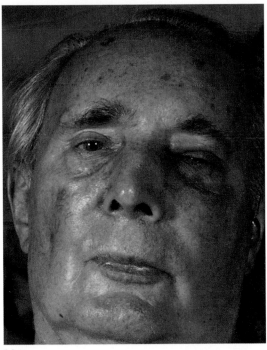

(a)

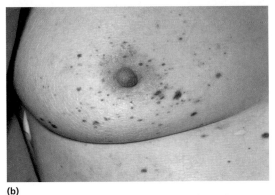

(b)

Figure 16.1 Myelodysplasia. **(a)** A 78-year-old male patient with refractory anaemia had recurring infections of the face and maxillary sinuses associated with neutropenia (haemoglobin 9.8 g/dL; white cells 1.3 × 10⁹/L; neutrophils 0.3 × 10⁹/L; platelets 38 × 10⁹/L). **(b)** Purpura in a 58-year-old female with refractory anaemia (haemoglobin 10.5 g/dL; white cells 2.3 × 10⁹/L; platelets 8 × 10⁹/L).

problems. The function of the neutrophils, monocytes and platelets is often impaired so that infections and bleeding may occur out of proportion to the severity of the cytopenia. The spleen is not usually enlarged.

It is important to remember that dysplastic features in bone marrow may be seen in a wide range of conditions such as excess alcohol intake, megaloblastic anaemia, parvovirus, recovery from cytotoxic chemotherapy and granulocyte colony-stimulating factor (G-CSF) therapy. These must be ruled out before making a diagnosis of MDS and diagnostic tests may need to be repeated over time in some patients.

Laboratory findings

Peripheral blood

Pancytopenia is a frequent finding. The red cells are usually macrocytic or dimorphic but occasionally hypochromic; normoblasts may be present. The reticulocyte count is low. Granulocytes are often reduced in number and frequently show lack of granulation (Fig. 16.2). Their chemotactic, phagocytic and adhesive functions are impaired. The Pelger abnormality (single or bilobed nucleus) is often present. The platelets may be unduly large or small and are usually decreased in number but in 10% of cases are elevated. In poor prognosis cases variable numbers of myeloblasts are present in the blood.

Bone marrow

The cellularity is usually increased. Multinucleate normoblasts and other dyserythropoietic features (e.g. internuclear bridges, nuclear budding) are seen (Fig. 16.2). The appearance of ring sideroblasts is caused by iron deposition in the mitochondria of erythroblasts. The granulocyte precursors often show defective granulation and may be difficult to distinguish from monocytes. Megakaryocytes are abnormal with micronuclear, small binuclear or polynuclear forms (Fig. 16.2). A small number of dysplastic cells may be seen in marrow from healthy elderly individuals so at least 10% of the cells in a lineage should be dysplastic in order to consider the

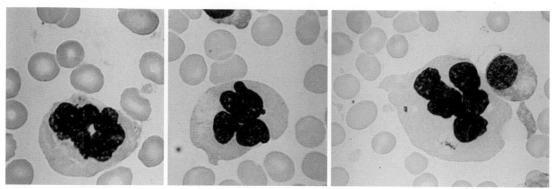

(a)

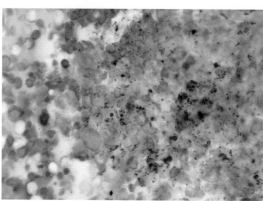

(b)

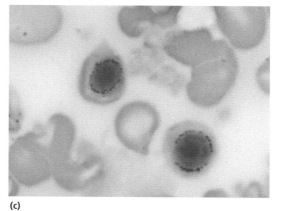

(c)

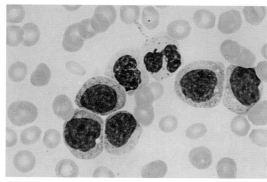

(d)

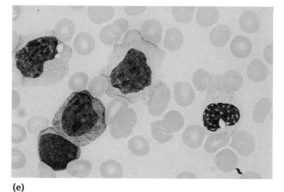

(e)

Figure 16.2 Myelodysplasia: appearances of the peripheral blood and bone marrow. **(a)** Multinucleate polychromatic erythroblasts. **(b)** Perls' stain showing iron overload in macrophages of a bone marrow fragment. **(c)** Ring sideroblasts. **(d)** White cells showing pseudo-Pelger cells, agranular myelocytes and neutrophils. **(e)** Monocytoid cells and an agranular neutrophil. **(f)** Mononuclear megakaryocyte.

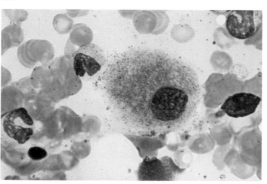

(f)

diagnosis of MDS. In a minority of cases (about 20%) the marrow is hypocellular and may resemble aplastic anaemia; in others there is fibrosis.

Cytogenetic abnormalities

Cytogenetic abnormalities are more frequent in secondary than primary MDS and most commonly constitute partial or total loss of chromosomes 5 or 7 or trisomy 8 (Table 16.2). Several cytogenetic abnormalities are considered so diagnostic of MDS that they allow diagnosis of MDS even in the absence of morphological abnormalities within cells. Mutations may also be found with molecular testing (e.g. of *TET-2* or *N-RAS*).

The classification of MDS can be confusing and flow charts are helpful in the approach to diagnosis (Fig. 16.3).

Treatment

Treatment for MDS has improved significantly in recent years. A key subdivision is into patients with low risk or high risk disease. An International Prognostic Scoring System (IPSS) classifies the patients according to percentage of marrow blasts, type of karyotype abnormality, and number and severity of cytopenias (Table 16.3).

Low-risk myelodysplastic syndromes

Patients with less than 5% of blasts in the marrow and only one cytopenia and favourable cytogenetics are defined as having low-grade MDS. Intensive chemotherapy is rarely used for these patients. Instead they are not treated or, if necessary, attempts may be made to improve marrow function with haemopoietic growth factors, either singly or in combination. Erythropoietin may improve anaemia although the haemoglobin should not be raised above 12 g/dL. G-CSF shows synergy with erythropoietin and may increase the response rate. Ciclosporin or antilymphocyte globulin occasionally help, particularly for those with a hypocellular bone marrow.

Tranfusion support with red cells and platelets as well as appropriate use of antibiotics is often required. In the long term, iron overload may be a problem after multiple transfusions; iron chelation therapy should be started after 30–50 units have been transfused if the anaemia and the need for transfusion continues to be the dominant problem. Lenalidomide is particularly effective in MDS associated with del(5q) where it can often reduce the size of the del(5q) clone and reduce transfusion requirements. Myelosuppression is a common side-effect.

In selected patients standard or low-intensity allogeneic stem cell transplantation (SCT) offers a permanent cure.

High-risk myelodysplastic syndromes

In these patients a variety of treatments have been attempted to improve the overall prognosis, with varying degrees of success.

Single-agent chemotherapy
Hydroxyurea, clofarabine, mercaptopurine, etoposide or low-dose cytosine arabinoside may be given with some benefit to patients with refractory anaemia with excess blasts (RAEB).

DNA methyl-transferase inhibitors
5-Azacytidine (azacitidine) and 5-aza-2'-deoxycitidine (decitabine) improve blood counts in a minority of high risk MDS patients. Azacitidine is given for 7 days every month and improves survival by approximately 9 months.

Intensive chemotherapy
Chemotherapy as given in AML (see p. 183) may be tried in high-risk patients. Although the majority of patients may obtain a remission, relapse is almost inevitable and frequently occurs within a few months. The risks of intensive chemotherapy are great because prolonged pancytopenia may occur in some cases without normal haemopoietic regeneration, presumably because normal stem cells are not present.

Stem cell transplantation
SCT offers the prospect of complete cure for MDS and the advent of non-myeloablative conditioning is increasing the age range of patients that may be treated. SCT is usually carried out in MDS without

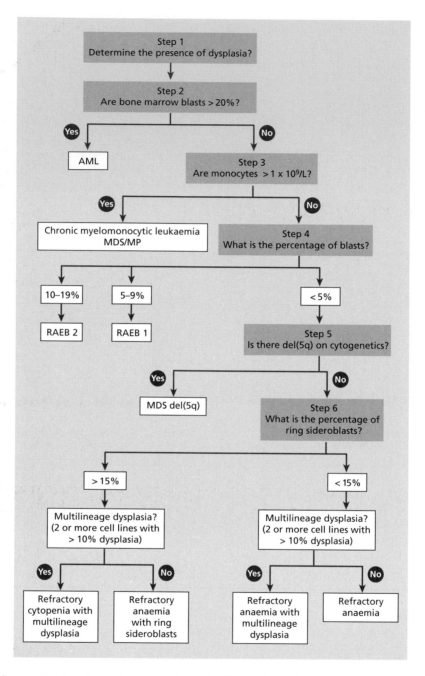

Figure 16.3 Approach to the diagnosis of myelodysplasia. MP, myeloproliferative. (Based on Bennett J.M. and Komrokji R.S. (2006) *Hematology* **10**, Suppl 1:258–69.)

a complete remission being first obtained with chemotherapy, although in high-risk cases initial chemotherapy may be tried to reduce the blast proportion and the risk of recurrence of the MDS.

General support care only

This is most suitable in elderly patients with other major medical problems. Transfusions of red cells and platelets, and therapy with antibiotics and antifungals, are given as needed.

Myelodysplastic/myeloproliferative neoplasms

A group of disorders are classified between myelodysplasia and myeloproliferative disorders as they show the presence of dysplastic features but also increased number of circulating cells in one or more lineage (Table 16.4). There are some common clinical and genetic features between these disorders. Mutations of the *TET2* tumour suppressor gene on chromosome 4 are found in about 20% of cases, and of *JAK2* in a smaller proportion.

Chronic myelomonocytic leukaemia

This is defined by a persistent monocytosis of $>1.0 \times 10^9$/L with blasts <20% in the marrow, dys-

plasia in other lineages and negative for the BCR-ABL1 translocation. The total white cell count is usually raised and may exceed 100×10^9/L. Patients may develop skin rashes and around half have splenomegaly. Bruising is frequent and gum hypertrophy and lymphadenopathy may also be present. *TET-2* mutations are frequent. Treatment is difficult although oral hydroxyurea or etoposide may be useful. SCT may be tried in younger patients. Median survival is approximately 2 years, with increased marrow blasts a predictor of poor outcome.

Atypical chronic myeloid leukaemia

These patients have an increased white cell count with mainly granulocytes and granulocyte precursors in the blood and hypercellular bone marrow but the Philadelphia chromosome and *BCR-ABL1* fusion gene are not present. There are usually some morphological features in the blood or bone marrow of myelodysplasia. Treatment is difficult and the outlook is poor.

Juvenile myelomonocytic leukaemia

This presents in the first 4 years of life and has features of both myelodysplasia and a myeloproliferative disease. There is often an eczematous, skin

Table 16.4 Classification of myelodysplastic/myeloproliferative neoplasms.

	Diagnostic features
Chronic myelomonocytic leukaemia	Monocytosis $>1 \times 10^9$/L
Atypical chronic myeloid leukaemia *BCR-ABL1* negative	WBC $>13 \times 10^9$/L *BCR-ABL1* absent
Juvenile myelomonocytic leukaemia	
Myelodysplastic/ myeloproliferative neoplasm, unclassifiable	
Refractory anaemia with ring sideroblasts associated with marked thrombocytosis	Platelet count $>450 \times 10^9$/L Large atypical megakaryocytes

rash, hepatosplenomegaly and lymphadenopathy. There is a monocytosis to >1.0 × 10⁹/L and clonal cytogenetic change. The only curative treatment is allogeneic SCT. If untreated, death usually occurs within 4 years, often from acute transformation with leukaemic infiltration (e.g. of the lungs). Children with two genetic disorders, Noonan's syndrome and neurofibromatosis, are at increased risk of juvenile myelomonocytic leukaemia (JMML) and mutations in the marrow of the genes *PTPN11* and *NF1*, which in the germline underlie these genetic disorders, are frequent in the bone marrow in cases of JMML not associated with Noonan's syndrome or neurofibromatosis.

SUMMARY

- Myelodysplasia includes a group of clonal disorders of haemopoietic stem cells that lead to bone marrow failure and low blood cell counts. A hallmark of the disease is simultaneous proliferation and apoptosis of haemopoietic cells leading to the paradox of a hypercellular bone marrow but pancytopenia in peripheral blood. There is a tendency to progress to acute myeloid leukaemia.

- In most cases, the disease is *primary* but it may be *secondary* to chemotherapy given for treatment of another malignancy.

- The main clinical features of anaemia, infection and bleeding, are caused by reduction in the blood count. Most patients are over 70 years of age.

- Diagnosis is made by examination of the blood and bone marrow together with genetic studies of the tumour cells.

- They are classified into eight major subtypes.

- Scoring systems can divide patients in those with low-grade or high-grade disease.

- Low-grade disease may not need treatment. Haemopoietic growth factors, lenalidomide or blood product support may be useful when required.

- High-grade myelodysplasia may be treated by intensive chemotherapy, demethylating drugs or stem cell transplantation. Allogeneic transplantation is the only curative procedure.

- Myelodysplastic/myeloproliferative neoplasms are a group of disorders classified between myelodysplasia and myeloproliferative disorders and show the presence of dysplastic features but also increased number of circulating cells.

Now visit www.wiley.com/go/essentialhaematology to test yourself on this chapter.

CHAPTER 17
Acute lymphoblastic leukaemia

Key topics

Acute lymphoblastic leukaemia (ALL) is caused by an accumulation of lymphoblasts in the bone marrow and is the most common malignancy of childhood.

Incidence and pathogenesis

The incidence of ALL is highest at 3–7 years with 75% of cases occurring before the age of 6. There is a secondary rise after the age of 40 years. Eighty-five per cent of cases are of B-cell lineage and have an equal sex incidence; there is a male predominance for the 15% of T-cell ALL (T-ALL).

The pathogenesis is varied. Certain germline polymorphism in a group of genes mainly involved in B-cell development (e.g. IKZF1) are more frequent in patients with B-cell ALL (B-ALL) than controls. Interestingly, IKZF1 is also deleted in the leukaemic cells in 30% of high risk B-ALL and 95% of ALL BCR-ABL1 positive cases. In a proportion of cases the first event occurs in the fetus *in utero*, with a secondary event possibly precipitated by infection in childhood (see Fig. 11.3). The first event is a translocation (e.g. t(12; 21)) or point mutation. The second event involves genome-wide copy number alterations, some of which encode for functions relevant to leukaemogenesis. This is discussed further in Chapter 11. In other cases, the disease seems to arise as a postnatal mutation in an early lymphoid progenitor cell.

Classification

Acute lymphoblastic leukaemia, B cell or T cell, is subclassified by WHO (2008) according to the underlying genetic defect (Table 17.1). Within B-ALL there are several specific genetic subtypes such as those with the t(9; 22) or t(12; 21) translocations, rearrangements of the *MLL* gene or alteration in chromosome number (diploidy) (Table 17.1). The subtype is an important guide to the optimal treatment protocol and to prognosis. In T-ALL an abnormal karyotype is found in 50–70% of cases and the NOTCH sig-

Table 17.1 Classification of acute lymphoblastic leukaemia (ALL) according to the World Health Organization (WHO) classification (modified).

Precursor lymphoid neoplasms
B lymphoblastic leukaemia/lymphoma
B lymphoblastic leukaemia/lymphoma, NOS
B lymphoblastic leukaemia/lymphoma with recurrent genetic abnormalities
B lymphoblastic leukaemia/lymphoma with t(9; 22)(q34; q11.2); *BCR-ABL1*
B lymphoblastic leukaemia/lymphoma with t(v; 11q23); *MLL* rearranged
B lymphoblastic leukaemia/lymphoma with t(12; 21)(p13; q22); *TEL-AML1* (*ETV6-RUNX1*)
B lymphoblastic leukaemia/lymphoma with hyperdiploidy
B lymphoblastic leukaemia/lymphoma with hypodiploidy (hypodiploid ALL)

T lymphoblastic leukaemia/lymphoma

NOS, not otherwise specified.

nalling pathway is activated in most cases (see below).

Clinical features

Clinical features are a result of the following.

Bone marrow failure

- Anaemia (pallor, lethargy and dyspnoea);
- Neutropenia (fever, malaise, features of mouth, throat, skin, respiratory, perianal or other infections);
- Thrombocytopenia (spontaneous bruises, purpura, bleeding gums and menorrhagia).

Organ infiltration

Tender bones, lymphadenopathy (Fig. 17.1a), moderate splenomegaly, hepatomegaly and meningeal

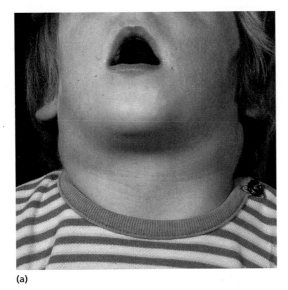
(a)

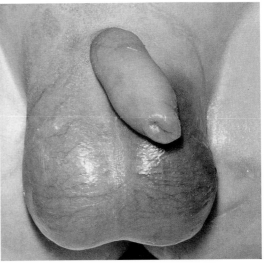
(b)

Figure 17.1 Acute lymphoblastic leukaemia. **(a)** Marked cervical lymphadenopathy in a boy. **(b)** Testicular swelling and erythema on the left-hand side of the scrotum caused by testicular infiltration. (Courtesy of Professor J.M. Chessels.)

syndrome (headache, nausea and vomiting, blurring of vision and diplopia). Fundal examination may reveal papilloedema and sometimes haemorrhage. Many patients have a fever which usually resolves after starting chemotherapy. Less common manifestations include testicular swelling (Fig. 17.1b) or signs of mediastinal compression in T-ALL (Fig. 17.2).

If lymph node or solid extranodal masses predominate with <20% blasts in the marrow the disease is called lymphoblastic lymphoma but is treated as ALL.

Investigations

Haematological investigations reveal a normochromic normocytic anaemia with thrombocytopenia in most cases. The total white cell count may be decreased, normal or increased to 200×10^9/L or more. The blood film typically shows a variable numbers of blast cells. The bone marrow is hypercellular with >20% leukaemic blasts. The blast cells are characterized by morphology (Fig. 17.3), cytochemisty (Table 17.2), immunological tests (Table 17.3) and cytogenetic analysis (Table 17.1).

Table 17.2 Specialized tests for acute lymphoblastic leukaemia (ALL).

Cytochemistry	
Myeloperoxidase	–
Sudan black	–
Non-specific esterase	–
Periodic acid–Schiff	+ (coarse block positivity in ALL)
Acid phosphatase	+ in T-ALL (Golgi staining)
Immunoglobulin and TCR genes	B-ALL: clonal rearrangement of immunoglobulin genes T-ALL: clonal rearrangement of TCR genes
Chromosomes and genetic analysis	(Table 17.1)
Immunological markers (flow cytometry)	(Table 17.3)

B-ALL, B-cell acute lymphoblastic leukaemia; T-ALL, T-cell acute lymphoblastic leukaemia; TCR, T-cell receptor.

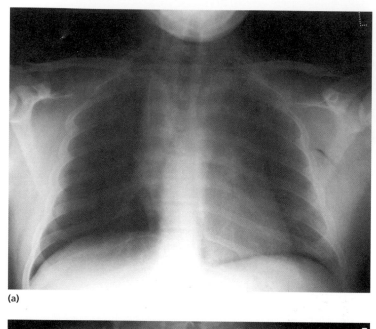

(a)

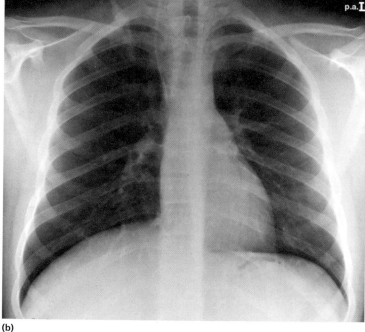

(b)

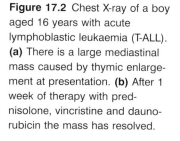

Figure 17.2 Chest X-ray of a boy aged 16 years with acute lymphoblastic leukaemia (T-ALL). **(a)** There is a large mediastinal mass caused by thymic enlargement at presentation. **(b)** After 1 week of therapy with prednisolone, vincristine and daunorubicin the mass has resolved.

Identification of the immunoglobulin or T-cell receptor (TCR) gene rearrangement, (aberrant) immunophenotype and molecular genetics of the tumour cells is important to determine treatment and to detect minimal residual disease (MRD) during follow-up.

Lumbar puncture for cerebrospinal fluid (CSF) examination is not generally performed as it may promote the spread of tumour cells to the CNS. Biochemical tests may reveal a raised serum uric acid, serum lactate dehydrogenase or, less commonly, hypercalcaemia. Liver and renal function

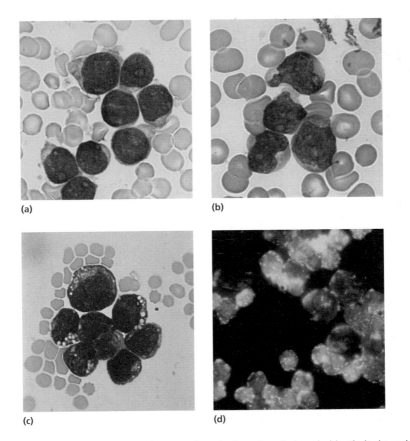

(a)

(b)

(c)

(d)

Figure 17.3 Morphology, cytochemistry and immunophenotyping of acute lymphoblastic leukaemia (ALL).
(a) Lymphoblasts show scanty cytoplasm without granules. **(b)** Lymphoblasts are large and heterogeneous with abundant cytoplasm. **(c)** Lymphoblasts are deeply basophilic with cytoplasmic vacuolation. **(d)** Indirect immunofluorescence reveals nuclear terminal deoxynucleotidyl transferase (TdT) (green) and membrane CD10 (orange). (Courtesy of Professor G. Janossy.)

tests are performed as a baseline before treatment begins. Radiography may reveal lytic bone lesions and a mediastinal mass caused by enlargement of the thymus and/or mediastinal lymph nodes characteristic of T-ALL (Fig. 17.2).

The differential diagnosis includes acute myeloid leukaemia (AML), aplastic anaemia (with which ALL sometimes presents), marrow infiltration by other malignancies (e.g. rhabdomyosarcoma, neuroblastoma and Ewing's sarcoma), infections such as infectious mononucleosis and pertussis, juvenile rheumatoid arthritis and immune thrombocytopenic purpura.

Cytogenetics and molecular genetics

Cytogenetic analysis shows differing frequencies of abnormalities in infants, children and adults which partly explains the different prognoses of these groups (Fig. 17.4). Cases are stratified according to the number of chromosomes in the tumour cell (*ploidy*) or by specific molecular abnormalities.

Hyperdiploid cells have >50 chromosomes and generally have a good prognosis whereas *hypodiploid* cases (<44 chromosomes) carry a poor prognosis. The most common specific abnormality in childhood B-ALL is the t(12; 21)(p13; q22) *TEL-*

AML1 translocation. The AML1 protein plays an important part in transcriptional control of haemopoiesis and is repressed by the TEL-AML1 fusion protein.

The frequency of the Philadelphia translocation t(9; 22) increases with age and carries a poor prognosis. Translocations of chromosome 11q23 involve the *MLL* gene and are seen particularly in cases of infant leukaemia. Using more sensitive molecular genetic tests, as well as fluorescence *in situ* hybridization (FISH) analysis, some cases normal by conventional cytogenetic testing are found to have fusion genes, e.g BCR-ABL1 or other genetic abnormalities. These molecular genetic changes carry prognostic significance whether or not a corresponding chromosomal change is present.

T-ALL accounts for 15% of childhood and 25% of adult ALL and the clinical picture is often dominated by a very high white cell count, mediastinal mass or pleural effusion. TCR (and in 20% the *IGH* gene) show clonal rearrangement. Cytogenetic changes often involve the TCR loci with different partner genes. The majority of cases have acquired genetic abnormalities that lead to constitutive activation of the *NOTCH* signalling pathway and drugs that target these abnormalities are being developed (Fig. 17.5).

Treatment

This may be conveniently divided into *supportive* and *specific* treatment.

General supportive therapy

General supportive therapy for bone marrow failure is described in Chapter 12 and includes the insertion of a central venous cannula, blood product

Table 17.3 Immunological markers for classification of acute lymphoblastic (ALL) leukaemia.

	ALL	
Marker	B	T
B lineage		
CD19	+	–
cCD22	+	–
cCD79a	+	–
CD10	+ or –	–
clg	+ (pre-B)	–
slg	–	–
TdT	+	+
T lineage		
CD7	–	+
cCD3	–	+
CD2	–	+
TdT	+	+

c, Cytoplasmic; S, surface.
*B-ALL resembles precursor B-ALL immunologically but has surface immunoglobulin (Ig) and is terminal deoxynucleotidyl transferase negative (TdT⁻).

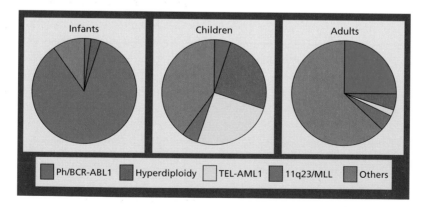

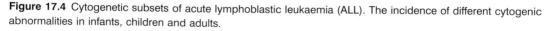

Figure 17.4 Cytogenetic subsets of acute lymphoblastic leukaemia (ALL). The incidence of different cytogenic abnormalities in infants, children and adults.

Figure 17.5 The molecular basis of activation of NOTCH signalling in T-ALL. **(a)** The molecular basis of NOTCH signalling. NOTCH is expressed at the cell membrane and after binding to a ligand (Delta-like or Jagged) on a neighbouring cell, the protein is cleaved in two places – first by extracellular ADAM 10 and then by an intracellular γ-secretase complex. The portion of intracellular NOTCH that is released is then translocated to the nucleus where it leads to activation of NOTCH1 target genes. **(b)** Several types of genetic abnormalities are seen in the NOTCH signalling pathway in patients with T-ALL. These include (1) mutations in the extracellular cleavage site, (2) insertion of an internal tandem duplications in the juxtamembrane region or (3) deletion of the intracellular PEST domain. The net result of all these mutations is to increase the rate of cleavage and nuclear translocation of the NOTCH domain.

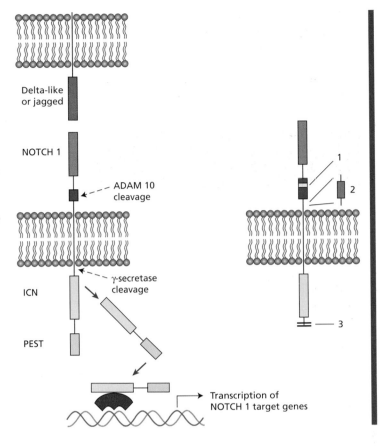

support and prevention of tumour lysis syndrome. Any episode of fever must be treated promptly.

Specific therapy of ALL in children

Specific therapy of ALL is with chemotherapy and sometimes radiotherapy (Fig. 17.6), and treatment protocols are extremely complex. There are several phases in a treatment course which usually has four components (Fig. 17.6). The protocols are *risk adjusted* to reduce the treatment given to patients with good prognosis. The factors that guide treatment include age, gender and white cell count at presentation. The initial response to therapy is also important as slow clearance of blood or marrow blasts after a week or two of induction therapy or persistence of MRD (see below) is associated with a relatively high risk of relapse. ALL in infants (<1 year) has a worse clinical outcome with cure rates of only 20–50%. The disease is associated with

chromosomal translocation involving the *MLL* gene in 80% of cases and is treated by unique protocols.

Minimal residual disease

Even when the blood and bone marrow appear to be clear of leukaemia, small numbers of tumour cells may sometimes be detected by fluorescence activated cell sorter (FACS) analysis or molecular methods (see page 164, Fig. 17.7). A positive result indicates *minimal residual disease* (MRD) and the analysis of children for the presence of MRD at day 29 or adults at 3 months of treatment has prognostic significance and is being used in planning therapy (see below) (Fig. 17.8).

Remission induction
At presentation, the patient with acute leukaemia has a very high tumour burden and is at great risk

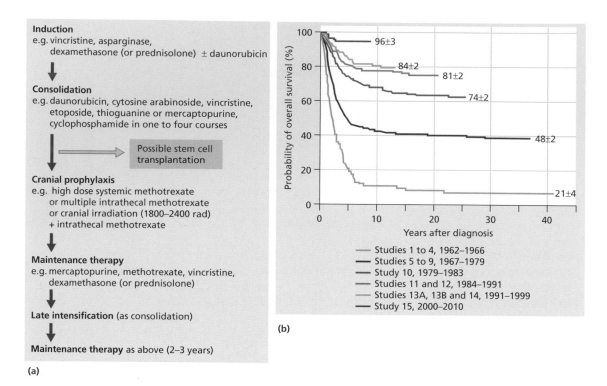

Induction
e.g. vincristine, asparginase,
  dexamethasone (or prednisolone) ± daunorubicin

Consolidation
e.g. daunorubicin, cytosine arabinoside, vincristine,
  etoposide, thioguanine or mercaptopurine,
  cyclophosphamide in one to four courses

  Possible stem cell transplantation

Cranial prophylaxis
e.g. high dose systemic methotrexate
  or multiple intrathecal methotrexate
  or cranial irradiation (1800–2400 rad)
  + intrathecal methotrexate

Maintenance therapy
e.g. mercaptopurine, methotrexate, vincristine,
  dexamethasone (or prednisolone)

Late intensification (as consolidation)

Maintenance therapy as above (2–3 years)

(a)

(b)

Studies 1 to 4, 1962–1966
Studies 5 to 9, 1967–1979
Study 10, 1979–1983
Studies 11 and 12, 1984–1991
Studies 13A, 13B and 14, 1991–1999
Study 15, 2000–2010

Figure 17.6 Acute lymphoblastic leukaemia (ALL). **(a)** Flow chart illustrating typical treatment regimen. **(b)** Kaplan–Meier analyses of overall survival in 2628 children with newly diagnosed ALL. (Updated from Pui C.H. and Evans W.E. (2006) *N Engl J Med* **354**, 169.)

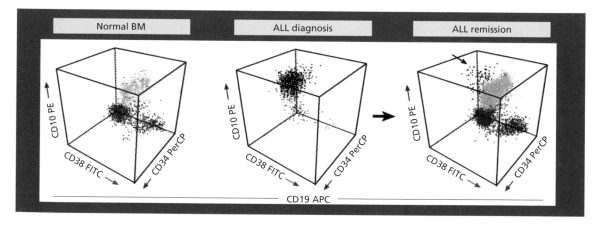

Figure 17.7 Detection of minimal residual disease (MRD) by four-colour flow cytometry in: normal bone marrow mononuclear cells (BM), BM from a patient with B lineage ALL at diagnosis and in remission 6 weeks after diagnosis. The cells were detected with four different antibodies (anti-CD10, anti-CD19, anti-CD34, anti-CD38) attached to fluorescent labels abbreviated as PE, APC, PerCP and FITC, respectively. The tridimensional plot shows the immunophenotype of CD19+ lymphoid cells in the three samples. MRD of 0.03% of cells expressing the leukaemia-associated phenotype (CD10+, CD34+, CD38−) were detected at 6 weeks, confirmed by polymerase chain reaction (PCR) analysis. (From Campana D. and Coustan-Smith E. (1999) *Commun Clin Cytometry* **38**, 139–52, with permission.)

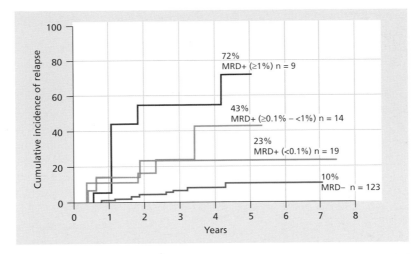

Figure 17.8 Cumulative incidence of relapse according to minimal residual disease (MRD) levels at the end of remission induction in children with acute lymphoblastic leukaemia (ALL) treated at St Jude Children's Research Hospital. (Courtesy of Dr D. Campana.)

from the complications of bone marrow failure and leukaemic infiltration (Fig. 17.1). The aim of **remission induction** is to rapidly kill most of the tumour cells and get the patient into remission. This is defined as less than 5% blasts in the bone marrow, normal peripheral blood count and no other symptoms or signs of the disease. Dexamethasone, vincristine and asparaginase are the drugs usually used and they are very effective – achieving remission in over 90% of children and in 80–90% of adults (in whom daunorubicin is also usually added). However, it should be remembered that remission is not the same as cure. In remission a patient may still be harbouring large numbers of tumour cells and without further chemotherapy virtually all patients will relapse (see Fig. 13.8). Nevertheless, achievement of remission is a valuable first step in the treatment course. Patients who fail to achieve remission need to change to a more intensive protocol.

Intensification (consolidation)

These courses use high doses of multidrug chemotherapy in order to eliminate the disease or reduce the tumour burden to very low levels. The doses of chemotherapy are near the limit of patient tolerability and during intensification blocks patients may need a great deal of support. Typical protocols involve the use of vincristine, cyclophosphamide, cytosine arabinoside, daunorubicin, etoposide or mercaptopurine given as blocks in different combinations. Three blocks of intensification are generally given for children, with more sometimes used in adults.

Central nervous system directed therapy

Few of the drugs given systemically are able to reach the CSF and specific treatment is required to prevent or treat central nervous system (CNS) disease. Options are high-dose methotrexate given intravenously, intrathecal methotrexate or cytosine arabinoside, or cranial irradiation. Cranial irradiation is now avoided as far as possible in children because of substantial side-effects. CNS relapses still occur and present with headache, vomiting, papilloedema and blast cells in the CSF. Treatment is with intrathecal methotrexate, cytosine arabinoside and hydrocortisone, with or without cranial irradiation and systemic reinduction because bone marrow disease is usually also present.

Maintenance

This is given for 2 years in girls and adults and for 3 years in boys, with daily oral mercaptopurine and once-weekly oral methotrexate. Intravenous vincristine with a short course (5 days) of oral dexamethasone is added at monthly or 3-monthly (in adults) intervals. The value of tests for MRD at the end of induction or during consolidation is being explored in trials in which the intensity of consolidation or maintenance therapy is reduced in those who rapidly become MRD negative, whereas more intensified therapy, or even stem cell transplantation (SCT), is given to those with persistent MRD. There is a high risk of varicella or measles during maintenance therapy in children who lack immunity to these viruses. If exposure to these infections occurs, prophylactic immunoglobulin should be given. In addition, oral co-trimoxazole is given to reduce the risk of *Pneumocystis carinii*.

Treatment of relapse

If relapse occurs during or soon after maintenance chemotherapy the outlook is poor. Reinduction with combination chemotherapy including novel drugs such as clofarabine may help. Chemotherapy is usually followed, where possible, by allogeneic SCT. If relapse occurs after years off all therapy the outlook is better and reinduction, consolidation and maintenance therapy are given. Allogeneic SCT may also be indicated.

Specific therapy of ALL in adults

Treatment for ALL in adults has proven challenging compared to the great successes that have been observed in childhood therapy. The initial control of the leukaemia (remission induction) is comparable in both groups but the rate of disease relapse is much higher in adults. Although cure rates in children now approach 90%, no more than 40% of adult patients remain free of leukaemia after 5 years and this rate is much lower in older patients. A significant factor is that the genetic subtypes of the ALL differ according to age. Hyperdiploidy and t(12; 21), which carry a good prognosis and together make up 50% of childhood cases, are both rare in adult patients. In contrast, the presence of the Philadelphia chromosome (Ph+ ALL) becomes more common with age (Fig. 17.4).

An additional factor that has contributed to the relatively poor outcome for ALL in adults is the lower doses of chemotherapy that have traditionally been used in adult patients. This is now being addressed in younger adult patients where high intensity chemotherapy regimens are being introduced. The presence of MRD after 3 months or more of therapy is an unfavourable prognostic sign.

Table 17.4 Prognosis in acute lymphoblastic leukaemia (ALL).

	Good	Poor
WBC	Low	High (e.g. >50 × 10^9/L)
Sex	Girls	Boys
Immunophenotype	B-ALL	T-ALL (in children)
Age	Child	Adult (or infant <1 year)
Cytogenetics	Normal or hyperdiploidy; TEL rearrangement	Ph+, 11q23 rearrangements MLL gene rearrangement Hypodiploidy (<44 chromosomes)
Time to clear blasts from blood	<1 week	>1 week
Time to remission	<4 weeks	>4 weeks
CNS disease at presentation	Absent	Present
Minimal residual disease	Negative at 1 month (children) or 3 months (adults)	Still positive at 3–6 months

CNS, central nervous system; Ph+, Philadelphia chromosome positive; WBC, white blood cell count.

Allogeneic SCT is playing an increasingly important role for ALL in adults and many patients are treated with this if a suitable sibling or matched unrelated donor is available.

Treatment of BCR-ABL1 positive ALL

The introduction of imatinib and other tyrosine kinase inhibitors (TKIs) has transformed the management of patients with BCR-ABL1+ (Ph+) ALL. Imatinib may be used alone or in combination with chemotherapy and is able to obtain remission of the disease in most patients. However, relapse is very common because of the appearance of resistant subclones containing mutations in the *BCR-ABL1* gene. As such, allogeneic SCT is recommended wherever possible once remission has been obtained. Second generation TKIs are now in use but their long-term value is uncertain at present.

Prognosis

There is a great variation in the chance of individual patients achieving a long-term cure based on a number of biological variables (Table 17.4). Approximately 25% of children relapse after first-line therapy and need further treatment but overall 85% of children can expect to be cured. The cure rate in adults drops significantly to less than 5% over the age of 70 years.

SUMMARY

- Acute lymphoblastic leukaemia (ALL) is caused by an accumulation of lymphoblasts in the bone marrow. It is the most common malignant disease of childhood – 75% of cases occur before the age of 6 years. Eighty-five per cent of cases are of B-cell lineage with the rest being of T-cell lineage.
- The first genetic mutation occurs in many cases *in utero*, with a secondary genetic event occurring later in childhood, possibly as a reaction to an infection.
- The clinical presentation is with the features of bone marrow failure (anaemia, infection and bleeding) together with symptoms of tissue infiltration by tumour cells, leading to bone pain or swollen lymph nodes.
- Diagnosis is by examination of blood and bone marrow. Important tests include microscopic examination of the tumour cells, immunophenotyping and genetic analysis.
- ALL is subclassified according to the underlying genetic defect and a wide variety of genetic lesions are seen. The number of chromosomes in the tumour cell has prognostic importance: *Hyperdiploid* cells have >50 chromosomes and generally have a good prognosis whereas *hypodiploid* cases (<44 chromosomes) carry a poor prognosis.
- Treatment protocols for ALL are extremely complex and usually have four components – remission induction, intensification, CNS-directed therapy and maintenance.
- Treatment is *risk adjusted* to reduce the treatment given to patients with good prognosis. This is based on age, gender, white cell count and cytogenetics at presentation.
- Small numbers of tumour cells may sometimes be detected by FACS or molecular analysis even when the blood and bone marrow appear to be clear of leukaemia. This *minimal residual disease* has prognostic significance and is used in planning therapy.
- If relapse occurs during chemotherapy the outlook is poor but if it happens after years off all treatment the outlook is better. Further chemotherapy and allogeneic SCT should be considered.
- Overall, 85% of children can now expect to be cured. The cure rate in adults drops significantly to less than 5% over the age of 70 years.

 Now visit www.wiley.com/go/essentialhaematology to test yourself on this chapter.

CHAPTER 18
The chronic lymphoid leukaemias

Key topics

Essential Haematology, 6th Edition. © A. V. Hoffbrand and P. A. H. Moss. Published 2011 by Blackwell Publishing Ltd.

Table 18.1 Classification of the chronic lymphoid leukaemias.

B-cell	T-cell
Chronic lymphocytic leukaemia (CLL)	Large granular lymphocytic leukaemia
Prolymphocytic leukaemia (PLL)	T-cell prolymphocytic leukaemia (T-PLL)
Hairy cell leukaemia (HCL)	Adult T-cell leukaemia/lymphoma
Plasma cell leukaemia	
	Sézary syndrome (see Chapter 20)

Source: WHO (2008) classification (see p. 426).

Several disorders are included in this group characterized by accumulation in the blood of mature lymphocytes of either B- or T-cell type (Table 18.1). There is some overlap with the non-Hodgkin lymphomas. In many cases of non-Hodgkin lymphoma, lymphoma cells are found in the blood and the distinction between chronic leukaemia and lymphoma is arbitrary, depending on the relative proportion of the disease in soft tissue masses compared to blood and bone marrow. In general, the diseases are incurable but tend to run a chronic and fluctuating course.

Diagnosis

This group is characterized by a chronic persistent lymphocytosis. Subtypes are distinguished by morphology, immunophenotype and cytogenetics. DNA analysis may be useful in showing a monoclonal rearrangement of either immunoglobulin or T-cell receptor genes.

B-CELL DISEASES

Chronic lymphocytic leukaemia

Chronic lymphocytic leukaemia (CLL) is the most common of the chronic lymphoid leukaemias and has a peak incidence between 60 and 80 years of age. The aetiology is unknown but there are geographical variations in incidence. It is the most common of the leukaemias in the Western world but rare in the Far East. In contrast to other forms of leukaemia there is no higher incidence after previous chemotherapy or radiotherapy. There is a sevenfold increased risk of CLL in the close relatives of patients which indicates a genetic predisposition.

The tumour cell appears to be a relatively mature B cell with weak surface expression of immunoglobulin (IgM or IgD). The cells accumulate in the blood, bone marrow, liver, spleen and lymph nodes as a result of increased production and prolonged lifespan with impaired apoptosis. Small lymphocytic lymphoma (SLL) (see Chapter 20) is the tissue equivalent of CLL. The lymphoma cells have the same immunophenotype and cytogenetics but in SLL there is solid tissue disease and fewer than 5×10^9/L circulating monoclonal B cells.

Monoclonal B-cell lymphocytosis Clonal B cells with the same phenotype as CLL are found at low levels in the blood of many older patients. Indeed, this monoclonal B-cell lymphocytosis (MBL) has been demonstrated in 3% of patients over the age of 50 years and it is believed that all cases of clinical CLL progress from this state. Similar genetic changes to these found in CLL may be present. If CLL is to be diagnosed there must be a monoclonal B-cell count of $>5 \times 10^9$/L or tissue involvement outside the bone marrow.

Clinical features

1 The disease occurs in older subjects with only 15% of cases before 50 years of age. The male : female ratio is 2 : 1.
2 Most cases are diagnosed when a routine blood test is performed. With increasing routine medical check-ups, this proportion is rising to >80%.
3 Symmetrical enlargement of cervical, axillary or inguinal lymph nodes is the most frequent clinical sign (Fig. 18.1). The nodes are usually discrete and non-tender. Tonsillar enlargement may be a feature.

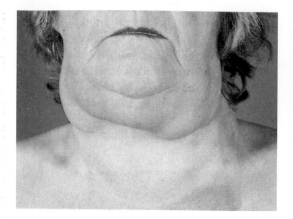

Figure 18.1 Chronic lymphocytic leukaemia: bilateral cervical lymphadenopathy in a 67-year-old woman. Haemoglobin 12.5 g/dL; white blood count 150×10^9/L (lymphocytes 146×10^9/L); platelets 120×10^9/L.

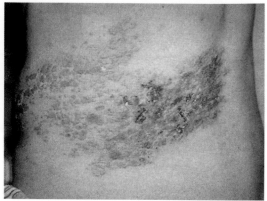

Figure 18.2 Chronic lymphocytic leukaemia: herpes zoster infection in a 68-year-old female.

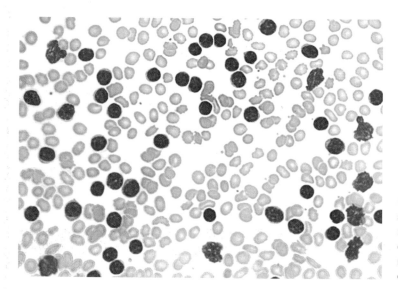

Figure 18.3 Chronic lymphocytic leukaemia: peripheral blood film showing lymphocytes with thin rims of cytoplasm, coarse condensed nuclear chromatin and rare nucleoli. Typical smudge cells are present.

4 Features of anaemia may be present. Patients with thrombocytopenia may show bruising or purpura.

5 Splenomegaly and, less commonly, hepatomegaly are common in later stages.

6 Immunosuppression may be a significant problem resulting from hypogammaglobulinaemia and cellular immune dysfunction. Early in the disease course bacterial infections predominate but with advanced disease viral and fungal infections such as herpes zoster are also seen (Fig. 18.2).

Laboratory findings

1 Lymphocytosis. The absolute clonal B cell lymphocyte count is $>5 \times 10^9$/L and may be up to 300×10^9/L or more. Between 70 and 99% of white cells in the blood film appear as small lymphocytes. Smudge or smear cells are also present (Fig. 18.3).

2 Immunophenotyping of the lymphocytes shows them to be B cells (surface CD19$^+$), weakly expressing surface immunoglobulin (IgM or

IgD). This is shown to be monoclonal because of expression of only one form of light chain (κ or λ; Table 18.2). Characteristically, the cells are also surface CD5$^+$ and CD23$^+$ but are CD79b$^-$ and FMC7$^-$ (Fig. 18.4).

3 Normochromic normocytic anaemia is present in later stages as a result of marrow infiltration or hypersplenism. Autoimmune haemolysis may also occur (see below). Thrombocytopenia occurs in many patients.

4 Bone marrow aspiration shows lymphocytic replacement of normal marrow elements. Lymphocytes comprise 25–95% of all the cells. Trephine biopsy reveals nodular, diffuse or interstitial involvement by lymphocytes (Fig. 18.5).

5 Reduced concentrations of serum immunoglobulins are found and this becomes more marked with advanced disease. Rarely, a paraprotein is present.

6 Autoimmunity directed against cells of the haemopoietic system is common. Autoimmune haemolytic anaemia is most frequent but immune thrombocytopenia (see p. 334), neutropenia and red cell aplasia are also seen.

Prognostic markers

Cytogenetics

The most common chromosome abnormalities are deletion of 13q14, trisomy 12, deletions at 11q23 (affecting the *ATM* gene), structural abnormalities of 17p involving the p53 gene and 6q21 deletion. These abnormalities carry prognostic significance (Table 18.3). The 13q14 deletion leads to loss of microRNAs which normally control expression of proteins that regulate B-cell survival (see p. 160).

Somatic hypermutation of the immunoglobulin genes

When B cells recognize antigen in the germinal centre of secondary lymphoid tissues they undergo a process called *somatic hypermutation* in which random mutations occur in the immunoglobulin heavy-chain gene. In CLL, the *IGVH* gene shows evidence of this hypermutation in approximately 50% of cases whereas in the other cases the *VH* genes are unmutated. CLL with unmutated immunoglobulin genes has an unfavourable prognosis (Table 18.3).

Tumour cell phenotype

ZAP-70 is a protein tyrosine kinase that is involved in cell signalling following recognition of antigen by antigen receptors on lymphocytes. Its expression is normally restricted to T cells but it is also aberrantly expressed in cases of CLL where it is associated with an unfavourable clinical outcome. Strong expression of CD38 also is an unfavourable prognostic feature.

Table 18.2 Immunophenotype of the chronic B-cell leukaemias/lymphomas (all cases CD19$^+$).

	CLL	PLL	HCL	FL	MCL
SIg	Weak	++	++	++	+
CD5	+	–	–	–	+
CD22/FMC7	–	+	+	+	++
CD23	+	–	–	–	–
CD79b	–	++	–/+	++	++
CD103*	–/+	–	+	–	–

CLL, chronic lymphocytic leukaemia; FL, follicular lymphoma; HCL, hairy cell leukaemia; MCL, mantle cell lymphoma; PLL, prolymphocytic leukaemia.
*CD103 is positive only in HCL.

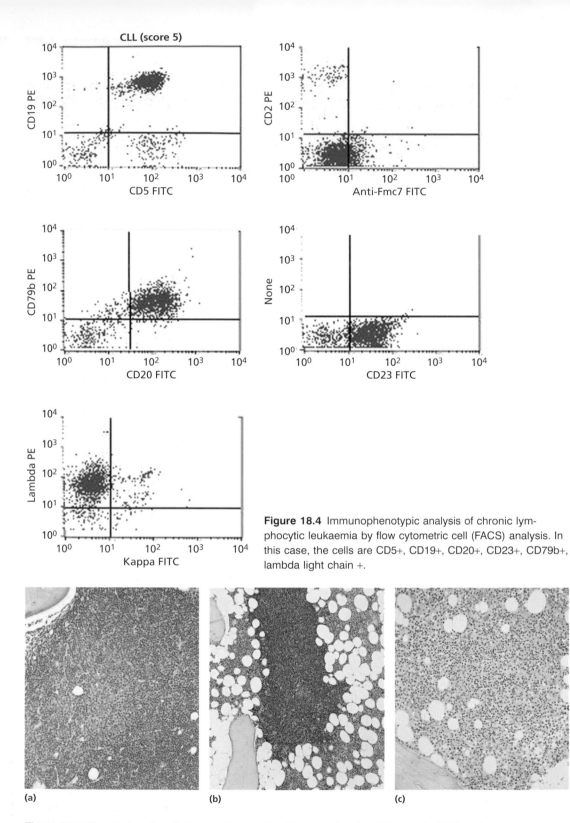

Figure 18.4 Immunophenotypic analysis of chronic lymphocytic leukaemia by flow cytometric cell (FACS) analysis. In this case, the cells are CD5+, CD19+, CD20+, CD23+, CD79b+, lambda light chain +.

Figure 18.5 Chronic lymphocytic leukaemia: trephine biopsies showing: **(a)** a marked diffuse increase in marrow lymphocytes (closely packed cells with small dense nuclei); **(b)** a nodular pattern of lymphocyte accumulation (in a different patient); and **(c)** interstitial infiltration.

Table 18.3 Prognostic factors in chronic lymphocytic leukaemia.

	Good	Bad
Stage	Binet A (Rai 0–I)	Binet B, C (Rai II–IV)
Sex	Female	Male
Lymphocyte doubling time	Slow	Rapid
Bone marrow biopsy appearance	Nodular	Diffuse
Chromosomes	Deletion 13q14	Deletion 17p
VH immunoglobulin genes	Hypermutated	Unmutated Use of VH3.21
ZAP expression	Low	High
CD38 expression	Negative	Positive
LDH	Normal	Raised

LDH, lactate dehydrogenase.

Staging

It is useful to stage patients at presentation both for prognosis and for deciding on therapy. The Rai and Binet staging systems are shown in Table 18.4. Typical survival ranged from 12 years for Rai stage 0 to less than 4 years for stage IV but there is considerable variation between patients, and with current therapies survival rates are improving. Most patients in Stage O have a normal life expectancy.

Treatment

Cures are rare in CLL and so the approach to therapy is conservative, aiming for symptom control rather than a normal blood count. Indeed, chemotherapy given too early in the disease can shorten rather than prolong life expectancy. Many patients never need treatment. Treatment is given for troublesome organomegaly, haemolytic episodes and bone marrow suppression. The lymphocyte count alone is not a good guide to treatment. Usually, patients in Binet stage C will need treatment as will some in stage B.

Chemotherapy

The optimal treatment for patients with CLL is a combination therapy known as R-FC which com-

bines the antibody rituximab (anti-CD20; see p. 265) with fludarabine and cyclophosphamide. These agents are given together every 4 weeks and are able to control the white cell count, and reduce organ swelling, in most cases. Four to six courses are usually given and treatment can be stopped after a satisfactory response has been achieved. It is usually needed again when the disease progresses. The average 'time to disease progression' after treatment with R-FC is approximately 36 months.

This regimen has a number of potential side effects including myelosuppression and immunosuppression. Purine analogues such as fludarabine lead to a prolonged reduction of CD4 (helper) T lymphocytes and co-trimoxazole is typically given during, and for 6 months after treatment as prophylaxis against *Pneumocystis carinii* infection. Aciclovir is also given for prophylaxis against herpes infections.

Chlorambucil

This oral alkylating agent is often used for elderly patients and can be used as a daily treatment (e.g. 4–6 mg/day) or in a monthly cycle (e.g. 10 mg/m^2/day for 7 days). Typically the drug will need to be given for several months after which a remission of variable duration will be obtained. Chlorambucil is

Table 18.4 Staging of chronic lymphocytic leukaemia (CLL).

(a) Rai classification

Stage

0	Absolute lymphocytosis >15 × 10⁹/L⁺
I	As stage 0 + enlarged lymph nodes (adenopathy)
II	As stage 0 + enlarged liver and/or spleen ± adenopathy
III	As stage 0 + anaemia (Hb <10.0 g/dL)⁺ ± adenopathy ± organomegaly
IV	As stage 0 + thrombocytopenia (platelets <100 × 10⁹/L)⁺ ± adenopathy ± organomegaly

(b) International Working Party classification

Stage	Organ enlargement*	Haemoglobin† (g/dL)	Platelets† (× 10⁹/L)
A (50–60%)	0, 1 or 2 areas		
B (30%)	3, 4 or 5 areas	≥10	≥100
C (<20%)	Not considered	<10	and/or <100

*One area = lymph nodes >1 cm in neck, axillae, groins or spleen, or liver enlargement.
†Secondary causes of anaemia (e.g. iron deficiency) or autoimmune haemolytic anaemia or autoimmune thrombocytopenia must be treated before staging.
Source: (b) Binet J.L. *et al.* (1981) *Cancer* **48**, 198.

not effective in patients who are resistant to R-FC. Combination therapy with rituximab is being explored.

Monoclonal antibodies

Rituximab (anti-CD20) is valuable in combination with chemotherapy and for treatment of autoimmune cytopenias. Alemtuzumab (anti-CD52) is a monoclonal antibody that is highly effective at killing B and T lymphocytes by complement fixation. It is given intravenously or subcutaneously over several weeks either alone or with corticosteroids and is valuable in resistant and relapsed disease. It is also being tested for a potential role in killing residual leukaemia cells after R-FC treatment has been completed. It is highly immunosuppressive and antibacterial and antiviral prophylaxis is needed. Another anti-CD20 antibody of atumumab and an anti-CD23, lumiliximab are in trial.

Corticosteroids

Patients in bone marrow failure may be treated initially with prednisolone alone until there is significant recovery of the platelet, neutrophil and haemoglobin levels. The peripheral lymphocyte count initially rises as infiltrated organs shrink, but later the count falls. High dose steroid therapy is valuable in patients with 17q deletion and may be given in combination with alemtuzumab where it can be effective in reducing lymphadenopathy or splenomegaly. Corticosteroids are also indicated in autoimmune haemolytic anaemia, thrombocytopenia and red cell aplasia.

Lenalidomide is a thalidomide derivative (see p. 175) and has therapeutic activity in CLL. Initial treatment is sometimes associated with a disease 'flare' at affected tissue sites and the mechanism of action is uncertain.

Bendamustine related to alkylating and anti-purine drugs is also in trials.

Other forms of treatment

- *Radiotherapy* This is valuable in reducing the size of bulky lymph node groups that are unresponsive to chemotherapy. Radiotherapy to the spleen may be valuable in late-stage disease.
- *Combination chemotherapy* Cyclophosphamide, hydroxodaunorubicin, oncovin (vincristine) and

prednisolone (CHOP) with rituximab is sometimes used in late-stage cases.

- *Bendamustine* is both an alkylating agent and purine analogue. In trials it is combined with rituximab.
- *Ciclosporin* Red cell aplasia may respond to ciclosporin.
- *Splenectomy* This is generally reserved for those patients with immune-mediated cytopenias that do not respond to short courses of steroids or those with painful bulky enlargement of the spleen not responding to other therapy.
- *Immunoglobulin replacement* Immunoglobulin (e.g. 400 mg/kg/month by intravenous infusion) is useful for patients with hypogammaglobulinaemia and recurrent infections, especially during winter months.
- *Stem cell transplantation* This is currently an experimental approach in younger patients. Allogeneic stem cell transplantation (SCT) may be curative but has a high mortality rate.

Course of disease

Many patients in Binet stage A or Rai stage 0 or I never need therapy and this is particularly likely for those with favourable prognostic markers (Table 18.3). For those who do need treatment a typical pattern is that of a disease that is responsive to several courses of chemotherapy before the gradual onset of extensive bone marrow infiltration, bulky

disease and recurrent infection. The disease may transform into a localized high-grade lymphoma (Richter's transformation) or there may be the appearance of an increasing number of prolymphocytes that are resistant to treatment.

B-cell prolymphocytic leukaemia

Although prolymphocytic leukaemia (PLL) may initially appear similar to CLL, the diagnosis is made by the appearance of a majority of prolymphocytes in the blood. The prolymphocyte is around twice the size of a CLL lymphocyte and has a large central nucleolus (Fig. 18.6). B-cell PLL is three times more common than T-cell PLL.

PLL and CLL also differ in their clinical features. PLL typically presents with splenomegaly without lymphadenopathy and with a high and rapidly rising lymphocyte count. Anaemia is a poor prognostic feature. Treatment is difficult in PLL. Splenectomy is usually of benefit and purine nucleoside analogues, rituximab or alemtuzumab may help.

Hairy cell leukaemia

Hairy cell leukaemia (HCL) is an uncommon B-cell lymphoproliferative disease with a male : female ratio of 4 : 1 and a peak incidence at 40–60 years. Patients typically present with infections, anaemia or splenomegaly. Lymphadenopathy is very uncommon. Pancytopenia is usual at pres-

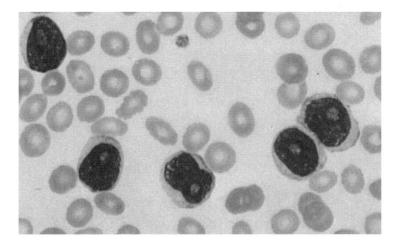

Figure 18.6 Prolymphocytic leukaemia: blood film showing prolymphocytes that have prominent central nucleoli and an abundance of pale cytoplasm.

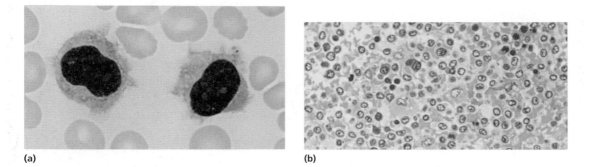

Figure 18.7 Hairy cell leukaemia: **(a)** peripheral blood film showing typical 'hairy' cells with oval nuclei and finely mottled pale grey–blue cytoplasm with an irregular edge; **(b)** bone marrow trephine.

entation and the lymphocyte count is rarely over 20×10^9/L. Monocytopenia is a distinctive feature. The blood film reveals a variable number of unusual large lymphocytes with villous cytoplasmic projections (Fig. 18.7). Immunophenotyping shows CD22, FMC7 and CD103 positivity in most cases (Table 18.2). The hairy cells stain for tartrate-resistant acid phosphatase (TRAP). The bone marrow trephine shows a characteristic appearance of mild fibrosis and a diffuse cellular infiltrate (Fig. 18.7).

There are several effective treatments for HCL and a patient can expect a long-term remission. The treatment of choice is 2-chlorodeoxyadenosine (CDA) or deoxycoformycin (DCF) and both agents achieve responses in over 90% of cases. In two-thirds of cases no relapse occurs, even after 5–10 years. HCL was one of the first diseases in which α-interferon was shown to be effective and it remains an excellent treatment. These drugs have largely replaced the need for splenectomy or combination chemotherapy. Rituximab can be combined with CDA or DCF for relapsed cases.

Lymphocytosis in non-Hodgkin lymphomas

Some cases of splenic marginal zone lymphoma show circulating monoclonal B lymphocytes with a villous cell outline and were previously termed 'splenic lymphoma with villous lymphocytes' (see p. 265).

Lymphocytosis may also be seen in other types of non-Hodgkin lymphoma (e.g. follicular, mantle cell, diffuse large B cell) and are discussed further in Chapter 20.

T-cell diseases

T-cell prolymphocytic leukaemia

This presents as B-PLL with a high white cell count but lymphadenopathy is more marked and skin lesions and serous effusions are common. Most are CD4+.

Large granular lymphocytic leukaemia

Large granular lymphocytic leukaemia (LGL-L) is characterized by the presence of circulating lymphocytes with abundant cytoplasm and large azurophilic granules (Fig. 18.8a). Such cells may be either T or natural killer (NK) cells and show variable expression of CD16, CD56 and CD57. Cytopenia, especially neutropenia, is the main clinical problem although anaemia, splenomegaly and arthropathy with positive serology for rheumatoid arthritis are also common. The mean age is 50 years. Treatment may not be needed but, if required, steroids, cyclophosphamide, ciclosporin or methotrexate may relieve the cytopenia. Granulocyte colony-stimulating factor (G-CSF) has been used in cases associated with neutropenia.

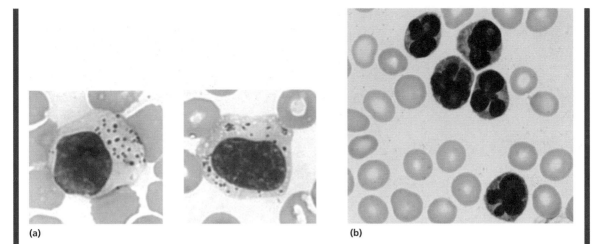

(a)   (b)

Figure 18.8 **(a)** Large granular lymphocytes in the peripheral blood. **(b)** Adult T-cell leukaemia/lymphoma. Typical convoluted lymphoid cells in peripheral blood.

Adult T-cell leukaemia/lymphoma

Adult T-cell leukaemia/lymphoma (ATLL) was the first malignancy to be associated with a human retrovirus, human T-cell leukaemia/lymphoma virus type 1 (HTLV-1). The virus is endemic in parts of Japan and the Caribbean and the disease is very rare in people who have not lived in these areas. ATLL lymphocytes have a bizarre morphology with a convoluted 'clover-leaf' nucleus and a consistent CD4+ phenotype (Fig. 18.8b).

Most subjects infected with the virus do not develop the disease. The clinical presentation is often acute and dominated by hypercalcaemia, skin lesions, hepatosplenomegaly and lymphadenopathy. Diagnosis is by morphology and serology and although combination chemotherapy may be tried the prognosis is poor.

- Chronic lymphocytic leukaemias are characterized by the accumulation of mature B or T lymphocytes in the blood.
- Individual subtypes are distinguished on the basis of morphology, immunophenotype and cytogenetics.
- Chronic lymphocytic leukaemia (CLL, B cell) represents 90% of cases and has a peak incidence between 60 and 80 years of age. There is genetic predisposition to development of the disease.
- Most cases are identified when a routine blood test is performed. As the disease progresses the patient can develop enlarged lymph nodes, splenomegaly and hepatomegaly.
- Immunosuppression is a significant problem because of hypogammaglobulinaemia and cellular immune dysfunction.
- Anaemia may also develop because of autoimmune haemolysis and bone marrow infiltration.
- Diagnosis is usually performed by immunophenotypic analysis of peripheral blood which reveals a clonal population of CD5+, CD23+ B cells.
- The best guide to prognosis is the stage of the disease. In addition, tumours that have acquired somatic mutations in the immunoglobulin genes have a relatively good prognosis.

(Continued)

SUMMARY

- ■ Treatment is usually given only when clinical symptoms start to develop. Fludarabine, cyclophosphamide and anti-CD20 monoclonal antibody usually establish disease remission but are not curative.

- ■ Less common subtypes of chronic lymphoid leukaemias include prolymphocytic leukaemia, hairy cell leukaemia and T-cell disorders.

Now visit www.wiley.com/go/essentialhaematology to test yourself on this chapter.

CHAPTER 19
Hodgkin lymphoma

Key topics

Essential Haematology, 6th Edition. © A. V. Hoffbrand and P. A. H. Moss. Published 2011 by Blackwell Publishing Ltd.

Lymphomas are a group of diseases caused by malignant lymphocytes that accumulate in lymph nodes and cause the characteristic clinical features of lymphadenopathy. Occasionally, they may spill over into blood ('leukaemic phase') or infiltrate organs outside the lymphoid tissue.

The major subdivision of lymphomas is into Hodgkin lymphoma and non-Hodgkin lymphoma and this is based on the histological presence of Reed–Sternberg (RS) cells in Hodgkin lymphoma.

History and pathogenesis

Thomas Hodgkin, curator of the anatomy museum at Guy's Hospital in London, described the disease in 1832. Dorothy Reed and Carl Sternberg were pathologists who identified the abnormal cell that defines this subtype of lymphoma in 1898. The characteristic RS cells, and the associated abnormal mononuclear cells, are neoplastic whereas the infiltrating inflammatory cells are reactive. Immunoglobulin gene rearrangement studies suggest that the RS cell is of B-lymphoid lineage and that it is often derived from a B cell with a 'crippled' immunoglobulin gene caused by the acquisition of mutations that prevent synthesis of full-length immunoglobulin. The Epstein–Barr virus (EBV) genome has been detected in over 50% of cases in Hodgkin tissue but its role in the pathogenesis is unclear.

Clinical features

The disease can present at any age but is rare in children and has a peak incidence in young adults. There is an almost 2 : 1 male predominance. The following symptoms are common.

1 Most patients present with painless, non-tender, asymmetrical, firm, discrete and rubbery enlargement of superficial lymph nodes (Fig. 19.1). The cervical nodes are involved in 60–70% of patients, axillary nodes in approximately 10–15% and inguinal nodes in 6–12%. In some cases the size of the nodes decreases and increases spontaneously. They may become matted. Typically, the disease is localized, initially to a

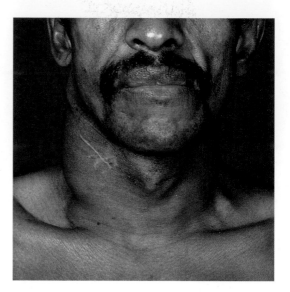

Figure 19.1 Cervical lymphadenopathy in a patient with Hodgkin lymphoma.

single peripheral lymph node region and its subsequent progression is by contiguity within the lymphatic system. Retroperitoneal nodes are also often involved but usually only diagnosed by computed tomography (CT) scan.

2 Modest splenomegaly occurs during the course of the disease in 50% of patients. The liver may also be enlarged because of liver involvement.

3 Mediastinal involvement is found in up to 10% of patients at presentation. This is a feature of the nodular sclerosing type, particularly in young women. There may be associated pleural effusions or superior vena cava obstruction.

4 Cutaneous Hodgkin lymphoma occurs as a late complication in approximately 10% of patients. Other organs (e.g. bone marrow, gastrointestinal tract, bone, lung, spinal cord or brain) may also be involved, even at presentation, but this is unusual.

5 Constitutional symptoms are prominent in patients with widespread disease. The following may be seen:
  (a) Fever occurs in approximately 30% of patients and is continuous or cyclic;
  (b) Pruritus, which is often severe, occurs in approximately 25% of cases;

(c) Alcohol-induced pain in the areas where disease is present occurs in some patients;

(d) Other constitutional symptoms include weight loss, profuse sweating (especially at night), weakness, fatigue, anorexia and cachexia. Haematological and infectious complications are discussed below.

Haematological and biochemical findings

1 Normochromic normocytic anaemia is most common. Bone marrow involvement is unusual in early disease but if it occurs bone marrow failure may develop with a leucoerythroblastic anaemia.

2 One-third of patients have a neutrophilia; eosinophilia is frequent.

3 Advanced disease is associated with lymphopenia and loss of cell-mediated immunity.

4 The platelet count is normal or increased during early disease, and reduced in later stages.

5 The erythrocyte sedimentation rate and C-reactive protein are usually raised and are useful in monitoring disease progress.

6 Serum lactate dehydrogenase is raised initially in 30–40% of cases.

Diagnosis and histological classification

The diagnosis is made by histological examination of an excised lymph node. The distinctive multinucleate polyploid RS cell is central to the diagnosis of the four classic types (Figs 19.2 and 19.3) and mononuclear Hodgkin cells are also part of the malignant clone. These cells stain with CD30 and CD15 but are usually negative for B-cell antigen expression. Inflammatory components consist of lymphocytes, neutrophils, eosinophils, plasma cells and variable fibrosis. CD68 detects infiltrating macrophages and, if strongly positive, is an unfavourable feature.

Histological classification is into four classic types and nodular lymphocyte predominant disease (Table 19.1), each of which implies a different prog-

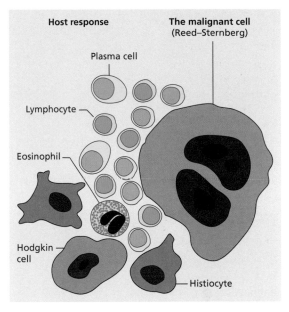

Figure 19.2 Diagrammatic representation of the different cells seen histologically in Hodgkin lymphoma.

nosis. Nodular sclerosis and mixed cellularity are most frequent. Patients with lymphocyte rich histology have the most favourable prognosis of classic Hodgkin lymphoma. Nodular lymphocyte predominant does not show RS cells and has many features of non-Hodgkin lymphoma and may be treated as such.

Clinical staging

The selection of appropriate treatment depends on accurate staging of the extent of disease (Table 19.2). Figure 19.4 shows the scheme that is used. Staging is performed by thorough clinical examination together with chest X-ray (Fig. 19.5) and CT scan to detect intrathoracic, intra-abdominal or pelvic disease (Fig. 19.6). It is also used to monitor response to therapy. Magnetic resonance imaging (MRI) scanning may be needed for particular sites (Table 19.2). Bone marrow trephine is sometimes carried out and liver biopsy may be needed in difficult cases. Positron emission tomography (PET) scanning is also useful in staging and is combined

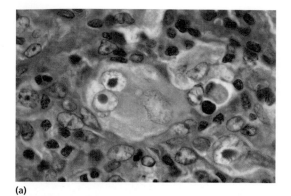

(a)

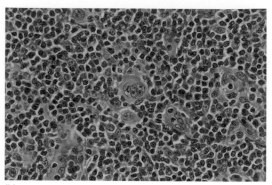

(b)

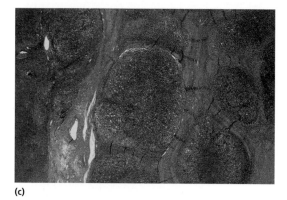

(c)

Figure 19.3 Hodgkin lymphoma: **(a)** high power view of a lymph node biopsy showing two typical multi-nucleate Reed–Sternberg cells, one with a characteristic owl eye appearance, surrounded by lymphocytes, histiocytes and an eosinophil; **(b)** mixed cellularity; and **(c)** nodular sclerosing Hodgkin lymphoma.

Table 19.1 World Health Organization (WHO) (2008) classification of Hodgkin lymphoma.	
Nodular lymphocyte-predominant (5% of cases) Reed–Sternberg cells are absent; lymphocyte predominant (LP) tumour B cells are present	
Classic Hodgkin lymphoma (95% of cases)	
Nodular sclerosis	Collagen bands extend from the node capsule to encircle nodules of abnormal tissue. A characteristic lacunar cell variant of the Reed–Sternberg cell is often found. The cellular infiltrate may be of the lymphocyte-predominant, mixed cellularity or lymphocyte-depleted type; eosinophilia is frequent
Lymphocyte rich	Scanty Reed–Sternberg cells; multiple small lymphocytes with few eosinophils and plasma cells; nodular and diffuse types
Mixed cellularity	The Reed–Sternberg cells are numerous and lymphocyte numbers are intermediate
Lymphocyte depleted	There is either a reticular pattern with dominance of Reed–Sternberg cells and sparse numbers of lymphocytes or a diffuse fibrosis pattern where the lymph node is replaced by disordered connective tissue containing few lymphocytes. Reed–Sternberg cells may also be infrequent in this latter subtype

Table 19.2 Techniques for staging of lymphoma.

Laboratory	Full blood count
	ESR
	Bone marrow aspirate and trephine (not routine)
	Liver function
	LDH
	C-reactive protein
Radiology	Chest X-ray
	CT of thorax, abdomen, chest and pelvis
	PET or PET/CT
	MRI
	Bone scan

CT, computed tomography; ESR, erythrocyte sedimentation rate; LDH, lactate dehydrogenase; MRI, magnetic resonance imaging; PET, positron emission tomography.

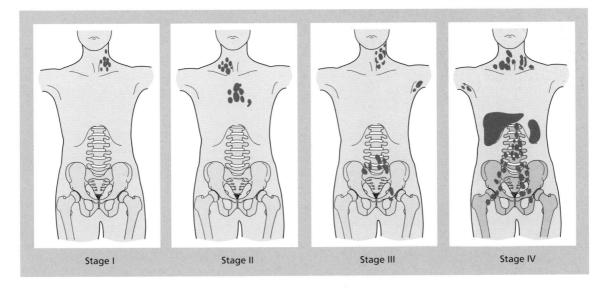

Stage I   Stage II   Stage III   Stage IV

Figure 19.4 Staging of Hodgkin lymphoma. Stage I indicates node involvement in one lymph node area. Stage II indicates disease involving two or more lymph nodal areas confined to one side of the diaphragm. Stage III indicates disease involving lymph nodes above and below the diaphragm. Splenic disease is included in stage III but this has special significance (see below). Stage IV indicates involvement outside the lymph node areas and refers to diffuse or disseminated disease in the bone marrow, liver and other extranodal sites. NB. The stage number in all cases is followed by the letter A or B indicating the absence (A) or presence (B) of one or more of the following: unexplained fever above 38°C; night sweats; or loss of more than 10% of body weight within 6 months. Localized extranodal extension from a mass of nodes does not advance the stage but is indicated by the subscript E. Thus, mediastinal disease with contiguous spread to the lung or spinal theca would be classified as I_E. As involvement of the spleen is often a prelude to widespread haematogenous spread of the disease, patients with lymph node and splenic involvement are staged as III_S. Bulky disease (widening of the mediastinum by more than one-third, or the presence of a nodal mass >10 cm in diameter) is relevant to therapy at any stage.

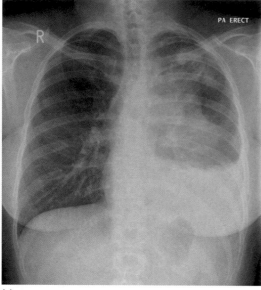

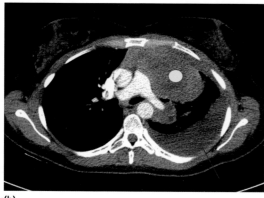

Figure 19.5 (a) Chest X-ray in Hodgkin lymphoma in 35-year-old female, revealing enlargement of left hilar lymph nodes, abnormal soft tissue projected over the upper left lung and a large left pleural effusion.
(b) Axial CT scan image with IV contrast in the same patient. Large anterior mediastinal mass (yellow circle) with left hilar enlarged nodes (red circle) and left pleural effusion (blue arrow). (Courtesy of Dr P. Wylie and Dr N. Mir.)

with CT to detect small foci of residual disease following treatment (Fig. 19.7).

Patients are also classified as A or B according to whether or not constitutional features (fever or weight loss) are present (Fig. 19.4).

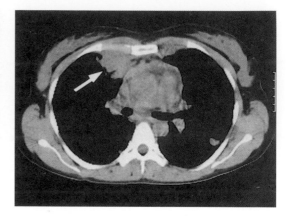

Figure 19.6 Hodgkin lymphoma (nodular sclerosing type): CT scan of chest showing anterior mediastinal mass of enlarged lymph nodes (arrowed).

Treatment

Treatment is with radiotherapy, chemotherapy or a combination of both. The choice depends primarily on the stage and whether clinically A or B (Fig. 19.4) although histological grading is an additional factor. Semen storage, if appropriate, should be carried out before therapy is begun.

Radiotherapy

Patients with stage I and IIA disease may be cured by radiotherapy alone. A dose of 4000 rad (40 Gy) is used and high-voltage radiotherapy techniques allow the treatment of all lymph node areas above or below the diaphragm by single 'upper mantle' or 'inverted Y' blocks. Radiotherapy also has a role in the treatment of bulky tumour masses such as mediastinal tumour that remains after chemotherapy or painful skeletal, nodal or soft tissue deposits.

Combined modality therapy

Concerns over late relapse and the long-term effects of radiotherapy have led to the development of regimens in which chemotherapy and radiotherapy are used together. This combination therapy allows short courses of chemotherapy to be combined with reduced levels of 'local field' radiotherapy and the most effective combinations are being assessed in clinical trials.

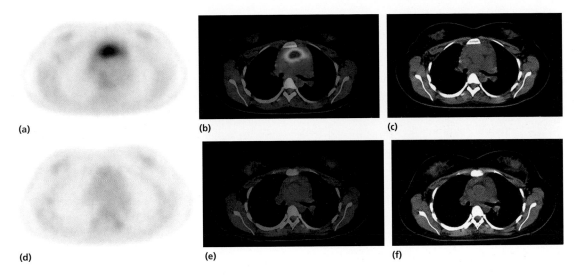

Figure 19.7 Example of the value of imaging in the management of Hodgkin lymphoma. **(a)** Axial PET, **(b)** fused PET/CT and **(c)** CT images at diagnosis demonstrate intense [^{18}]FDG uptake in an anterior mediastinal mass. Following two cycles of ABVD chemotherapy **(d)** the axial PET, **(e)** fused PET/CT and **(f)** CT images demonstrate no significant [^{18}]FDG uptake in the residual mediastinal mass, in keeping with a complete metabolic response. (Courtesy of Dr V.S. Warbey and Professor G.J.R. Cook.)

Chemotherapy

Cyclical chemotherapy is used for stage III and IV disease and also in stage I and II patients who have bulky disease, type B symptoms or have relapsed following initial radiotherapy. The combination of Adriamycin, bleomycin, vinblastine and dacarbazine (ABVD) is now most widely used. Variants such as ChlVPP (chlorambucil, vincristine, procarbazine, prednisolone) are sometimes used. It is usual to give a total of six cycles of chemotherapy or four following achievement of complete remission.

More intensive chemotherapy regimens such as escalated BEACOPP (bleomycin, etoposide, doxorubicin, cyclophosphamide, vincristine, procarbazine, prednisolone) may be useful for poor-risk disease and trials to compare these with ABVD are underway.

Assessment of response to treatment

Clinical examination and imaging (e.g. CT and PET scans) are used to assess response to treatment. Patients with Hodgkin lymphoma often show residual masses following treatment which may be because of the large degree of fibrosis present within lymph nodes. It can be difficult to assess whether or not such masses represent residual disease and the label of complete response uncertain (CRu) has been applied in these cases. PET scanning combined with CT is useful is revealing areas of active disease (Fig. 19.7). PET is now used in many centres after the first two cycles of ABVD and, if there is residual active disease, treatment is switched to more intensive chemotherapy (e.g. escalated BEACOPP). If the PET scan is negative, a further four cycles of ABVD are given.

Relapsed cases

The patient is treated with an alternative combination chemotherapy to the initial regimen and, if necessary, with radiotherapy to sites of bulky disease. If the disease remains chemosensitive, high-dose chemotherapy and autologous stem cell transplantation improve the probability of cure and are recommended for most patients below the age of 65 years. Allogeneic transplantation may also be curative in a minority of patients who fail other therapies.

Table 19.3 Hodgkin lymphoma: International Prognostic Index (Hansclever Index) for advanced disease.

Age >45 years

Male gender

Serum albumin <40 g/dL

Haemoglobin level <10.5 g/dL

Stage IV disease

Leucocytosis (white cell count $\geq 15 \times 10^9$/L)

Lymphopaenia (<0.6×10^9/L or <8% of the white cell count)

Prognosis

The prognosis depends on age, stage and histology. The International Prognostic Score (Hansclever Index) is useful for patients with advanced disease. It includes seven factors and each of these is associated with an 8% reduction in the predicted 5 year disease-free progression rate (Table 19.3). Overall, approximately 85% of patients are cured.

The late effects of Hodgkin lymphoma and its treatment

Long-term follow-up of patients has revealed a considerable burden of late disease following treatment. Secondary cancers such as lung cancer and breast cancer appear to be related to radiotherapy whereas myelodysplasia or acute myeloid leukaemia are more associated with the use of alkylating agents. Non-Hodgkin lymphomas and other cancers also occur with greater frequency than in controls. Non-malignant complications include sterility, intestinal complications, coronary artery disease and other cardiac or pulmonary complications of the mediastinal radiation or chemotherapy. These features are the main reason why less intensive treatment regimens are now being explored for this disease.

SUMMARY

- Lymphomas are a group of diseases caused by malignant lymphocytes that accumulate in lymph nodes and cause lymphadenopathy.
- The major subdivision of lymphomas is into Hodgkin lymphoma and non-Hodgkin lymphoma and this is based on the presence of Reed–Sternberg cells in Hodgkin lymphoma.
- Reed–Sternberg cells are neoplastic B cells but most cells in the lymph node are reactive inflammatory cells.
- The usual clinical presentation is with painless asymmetrical lymphadenopathy – most commonly in the neck.
- Constitutional symptoms of fever, weight loss and sweating are prominent in patients with widespread disease.
- Blood tests may show anaemia, neutrophilia and raised erythrocyte sedimentation rate (ESR) or lactic dehydrogenase (LDH).
- Diagnosis is made by histological examination of an excised lymph node and there are four subtypes of disease.
- Staging of the disease is important for determining treatment and prognosis. History, examination, blood tests, CT and PET scan are typically used.
- Treatment is with radiotherapy, chemotherapy or a combination of both. The choice depends on the stage and grade of the disease.
- The response to treatment can be monitored by CT and PET scans. Disease relapse can be treated with chemotherapy, sometimes with stem cell transplantation.
- The prognosis is excellent and over 85% of patients can expect to be cured. Late side effects of treatment are a concern.

Now visit www.wiley.com/go/essentialhaematology to test yourself on this chapter.

CHAPTER 20

Non-Hodgkin lymphoma

Key topics

Essential Haematology, 6th Edition. © A. V. Hoffbrand and P. A. H. Moss. Published 2011 by Blackwell Publishing Ltd.

Non-Hodgkin lymphomas

These are a large group of clonal lymphoid tumours, about 85% of B cell and 15% of T or NK (natural killer) cell origin (Table 20.1). Their clinical presentation and natural history are more variable than in Hodgkin lymphoma. They are characterized by an irregular pattern of spread and a significant proportion of patients develop extranodal disease. Their frequency has increased markedly over the last 50 years and with an incidence of approximately 17 in 100 000 they now represent the fifth most common malignancy in some developed countries (see Fig 11.1). The aetiology of the majority of cases of non-Hodgkin lymphomas (NHL) is unknown although infectious agents are an important cause in particular subtypes (Table 20.2). There are also considerable geographical variation (Table 20.2). The World Health Organization (WHO) classification also recognizes age (paediatric or elderly) and site of involvement (e.g. skin, central nervous system (CNS), intestine, spleen, mediastinal) as important in disease classification.

Classification

The lymphomas are classified within a group of **mature B-cell and T-cell neoplasms**, which also includes some chronic leukaemias and myeloma which are described in Chapters 18 and 21, respectively (Table 20.1). In this chapter we consider the more common lymphoma subtypes within this classification.

Cell of origin

The normal B-cell development stages are illustrated in Fig. 9.10. B-cell lymphomas tend to mimic normal B cells at different stages of development

Table 20.1 The World Health Organization (WHO) classification of mature B-cell and T-cell neoplasms (modified), which includes the non-Hodgkin lymphomas. B-cell disorders comprise 85% of cases. T cell and NK cell together comprise 15% of cases. A few very rare subtypes have been omitted.

Mature B-cell neoplasms	Mature T-cell and NK-cell neoplasms
Chronic lymphocytic leukaemia/small lymphocytic lymphoma	T-cell prolymphocytic leukaemia
B-cell prolymphocytic leukaemia	T-cell large granular lymphocytic leukaemia
Splenic marginal zone lymphoma	Adult T-cell lymphoma/leukaemia
Hairy cell leukaemia	Extranodal NK/T-cell lymphoma, nasal type
Lymphoplasmacytic lymphoma–Waldenström macroglobulinaemia	Enteropathy-associated T-cell lymphoma
Heavy chain diseases	Mycosis fungoides
Plasma cell myeloma	Sézary syndrome
Plasmacytoma	Peripheral T-cell lymphoma
Extranodal marginal zone lymphoma of mucosa-associated lymphoid tissue (MALT lymphoma)	Angioimmunoblastic T-cell lymphoma
Follicular lymphoma	Anaplastic large cell lymphoma, *ALK* positive
Mantle cell lymphoma	
Diffuse large B-cell lymphoma	
Burkitt lymphoma	

ALK, anaplastic lymphoma kinase, the gene on chromosome 2 which is overexpressed; NK, natural killer.

Table 20.2 Infections associated with haemopoietic malignancies.

Infection	Tumour
Virus	
HTLV-1	Adult T-cell leukaemia/ lymphoma
Epstein–Barr virus	Burkitt and Hodgkin lymphomas; PTLD
HHV-8	Primary effusion lymphoma; multicentric Castleman's disease
HIV-1	High-grade B-cell lymphoma, primary CNS lymphoma, Hodgkin lymphoma
Hepatitis C	Marginal zone lymphoma
Bacteria	
Helicobacter pylori	Gastric lymphoma (MALT)
Protozoa	
Malaria	Burkitt lymphoma

HHV-8, human herpes virus 8; HIV, human immunodeficiency virus; HTLV-1, human T-lymphotropic virus type 1; MALT, mucosa-associated lymphoid tissue; PTLD, post-transplant lymphoproliferative disease.

(Fig. 20.2). They can be divided into those resembling precursor (bone marrow) B cells, those resembling germinal centre (GC) cells and those post-GC cells in lymph nodes. T-cell lymphomas resemble precursor T cells in bone marrow or thymus, or peripheral mature T cells.

Low- and high-grade non-Hodgkin lymphomas

The NHL are a diverse group of diseases and vary from highly proliferative and potentially rapidly fatal diseases to some of the most indolent and well-tolerated malignancies. For many years clinicians have subdivided lymphomas into low- and high-grade disease. This approach is valuable as, in general terms, the low-grade disorders are relatively indolent, respond well to chemotherapy but are very difficult to cure whereas high-grade lymphomas are aggressive and need urgent treatment but are more often curable.

Leukaemias and lymphomas

The difference between *lymphomas*, in which lymph nodes, spleen or other solid organs are involved, and

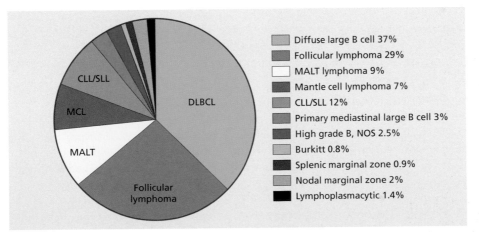

Figure 20.1 The relative frequencies of B-cell non-Hodgkin lymphomas. CLL, chronic lymphocytic lymphoma; DLBCL, diffuse large B-cell lymphoma; MALT, mucosa-associated lymphoid tissue; MCL, mantle cell lymphoma; NOS, not otherwise specified; PMLBCL, primary mediastinal large B-cell lymphoma; SLL, small lymphocytic lymphoma.

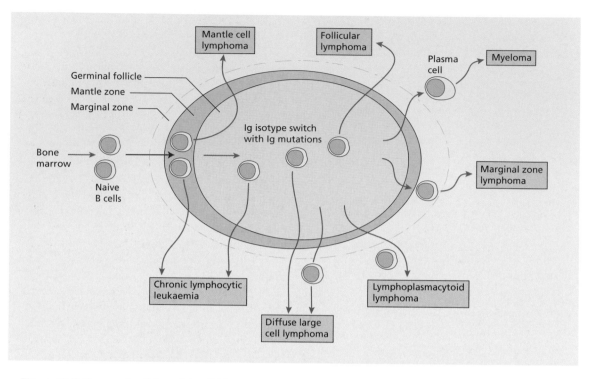

Figure 20.2 Proposed cellular origin of B-lymphoid malignancies. Normal B cells migrate from the bone marrow and enter secondary lymphoid tissue. When they encounter antigen a germinal centre is formed and B cells undergo somatic hypermutation of the immunoglobulin genes. Finally, B cells exit the lymph node as memory B cells or plasma cells. The cellular origin of the different lymphoid malignancies can be inferred from immunoglobulin gene rearrangement status and membrane phenotype. Mantle cell lymphoma and a proportion of B-cell chronic lymphocytic lymphoma (B-CLL) cases have unmutated immunoglobulin genes whereas marginal zone lymphoma, diffuse large cell lymphoma, follicle cell lymphoma, lymphoplasmacytoid lymphoma and some B-CLL cases have mutated immunoglobulin genes.

leukaemias, with predominant bone marrow and circulating tumour cells, may be blurred. A single lymphoproliferative disease (e.g. chronic lymphocytic leukaemia and small lymphocytic lymphoma) merge with each other with the identical cell genotype and immunophenotype. Lymphoma cells may circulate (e.g. in follicular, mantle cell, diffuse large B-cell lymphomas and the Sézary syndrome). B-cell acute lymphoblastic leukaemia (B-ALL) and T-ALL and the corresponding B- and T-lymphoblastic lymphomas are different manifestations of the same diseases and are usually treated in identical fashion.

Clinical features of non-Hodgkin lymphomas

1 *Superficial lymphadenopathy* The majority of patients present with asymmetric painless enlargement of lymph nodes in one or more peripheral lymph node regions.

2 *Constitutional symptoms* Fever, night sweats and weight loss occur less frequently than in Hodgkin lymphoma and their presence is usually associated with disseminated disease.

3 *Oropharyngeal involvement* In 5–10% of patients there is disease of the oropharyngeal lymphoid

structures (Waldeyer's ring) which may cause complaints of a 'sore throat' or noisy or obstructed breathing.

4 *Symptoms due to anaemia*, infections due to neutropenia or purpura with thrombocytopenia may be presenting features in patients with diffuse bone marrow disease. Cytopenias may also be autoimmune in origin or due to sequestration in the spleen. Infections may occur as a result of neutropenia or reduced cell immunity (e.g. herpes zoster).

5 *Abdominal disease* The liver and spleen are often enlarged and involvement of retroperitoneal or mesenteric nodes is frequent. The gastrointestinal tract is the most commonly involved extranodal site after the bone marrow, and patients may present with acute abdominal symptoms.

6 *Other organs* Skin, brain, testis or thyroid involvement is not infrequent. The skin is also primarily involved in two unusual, closely related T-cell lymphomas, mycosis fungoides and Sézary syndrome.

Investigations

Histology

Lymph node biopsy or trucut biopsy of lymph node or of other involved tissue (e.g. bone marrow or extranodal tissue) is the definitive investigation (Figs 20.3 and 20.4). Morphological examination is assisted by immunophenotypic and, in some cases, genetic analysis (Table 20.3). For B-cell lymphomas, expression of either κ or λ light chains confirms clonality and distinguishes the disease from a reactive node (Fig. 20.5). A fine needle aspiration may be performed to exclude another cause of lymphadenopathy (e.g. tuberculosis, carcinoma) but is not useful in establishing a diagnosis of lymphoma.

Laboratory investigations

1 In advanced disease with marrow involvement there may be anaemia, neutropenia or thrombocytopenia (especially if the spleen is enlarged or there are leucoerythroblastic features).

Figure 20.3 Non-Hodgkin lymphoma: histological sections of lymph nodes showing: **(a)** a diffuse pattern of involvement in lymphocytic lymphoma with the normal architecture totally replaced by neoplastic lymphocytic cells; **(b)** a follicular or nodular pattern in follicular lymphoma – the 'follicles' or 'nodules' of neoplastic cells compress surrounding tissue and lack a mantle of small lymphocytes.

(a)

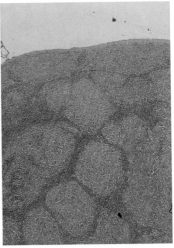

(b)

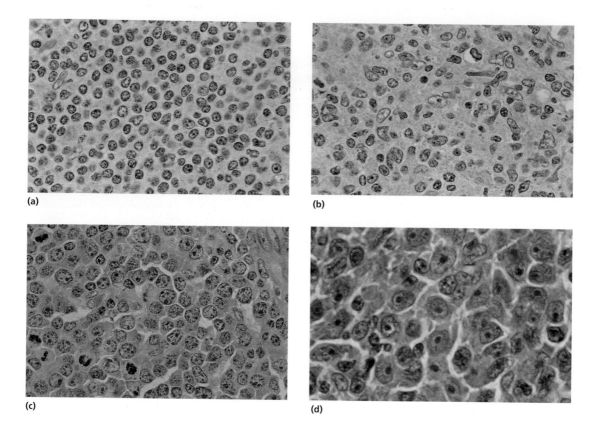

Figure 20.4 Non-Hodgkin lymphoma: high power view of lymph node biopsies: **(a)** Lymphocytic lymphoma showing predominantly small lymphocytes with round nuclei containing densely clumped heterochromatin. **(b)** Mantle cell lymphoma: showing characteristic deformed pattern of small lymphocytes with angular nuclei ('centrocytes'). **(c)** Diffuse large B-cell lymphoma: the neoplastic cells are much larger than normal lymphocytes and have a round nucleus with prominent nucleoli, many of which are adjacent to the nuclear membrane ('centroblasts'). A number of mitotic figures are seen. **(d)** Diffuse large B-cell lymphoma showing large neoplastic cells with a single prominent nucleolus and abundant dark-staining cytoplasm (previously termed immunoblasts).

2 Lymphoma cells (e.g. mantle zone cells, 'cleaved follicular lymphoma' or 'blast' cells) may be found in the peripheral blood in some patients (Fig. 20.6).

3 HIV should be tested for in all patients.

4 Trephine biopsy of marrow is valuable (Fig. 20.7). Paradoxically, bone marrow involvement is found more frequently in low-grade malignant lymphomas.

5 The serum lactate dehydrogenase (LDH) level is raised in more rapidly proliferating and extensive disease and is used as a prognostic marker (Table 20.4). Elevation of serum uric acid may occur.

6 Immunoglobulin electrophoresis may reveal a paraprotein.

Cytogenetics

The various subtypes of NHL are associated with characteristic chromosomal translocations which are of diagnostic and prognostic value (Table 20.3). Particularly characteristic translocations are t(14; 18) in follicular lymphoma, t(11; 14) in mantle cell lymphoma, t(8; 14) in Burkitt lymphoma and t(2; 5) in anaplastic large cell lymphoma.

In B-cell lymphomas the immunoglobulin genes are clonally rearranged whereas in T-cell

Table 20.3 Characteristic immunophenotype and cytogenetics of B-cell lymphomas.

Lymphoma	Surface immunoglobulin	CD5	CD10	CD20	CD23	BCL-2	BCL-6	Cyclin D₁	Typical cytogenetics
CLL/lymphocytic lymphoma	Weak	+	−	+	+	+	−	−	13q14, 17p or 11q deletions; trisomy 12
Lymphoplasmacytic	+/−	−	−	+	−	+	−	−	No specific findings
MALT lymphoma	+	−	−	+	+/−	+	−	−	t(1; 14)
Follicular lymphoma	+	−	+	+	+/−	+	+	−	t(14; 18)
Mantle cell lymphoma	+	+	−	+	−	+	−	+	t(11; 14)
Diffuse large cell lymphoma	+/−	−	+/−	+	−	+/−	+/−	−	t(3; 14) t(14; 18)
Burkitt lymphoma	+	−	+	+	−	−	+	−	t(8; 14) t(2; 8) t(8; 22)

CLL, chronic lymphocytic leukaemia; MALT, mucosa-associated lymphoid tissue.
More detailed cytogenetics are given in Table 11.1.

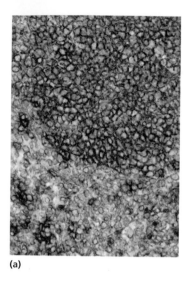

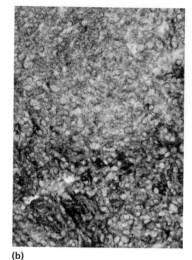

(a)

(b)

Figure 20.5 Non-Hodgkin lymphoma: lymph node stained by immunoperoxidase shows **(a)** brown ring staining for κ in the malignant lymphoid nodule, and **(b)** no labelling for λ confirming the monoclonal origin of the lymphoma.

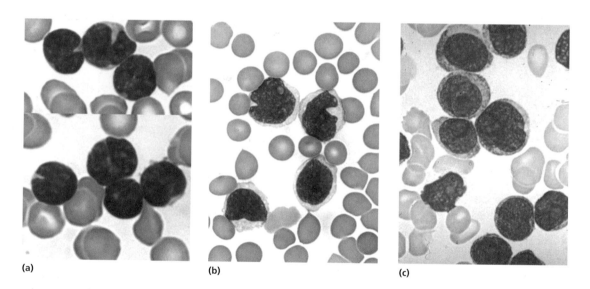

(a)

(b)

(c)

Figure 20.6 Blood involvement by malignant lymphoma: **(a)** small cleaved lymphoid cells in follicle centre cell lymphoma; **(b)** mantle cell lymphoma; **(c)** large B-cell lymphoma.

lymphomas there is clonal rearrangement of the T-cell receptor genes (see Chapter 11). These tests may be carried out on biopsy tissue. DNA microarray patterns of gene expression have been shown to give valuable diagnostic information (Fig. 20.8) but are not used in routine clinical practice.

Staging

The staging system (Cotswold modification of Ann Arbor) is the same as that described for Hodgkin lymphoma but is less clearly related to prognosis than histological type. Staging procedures usually

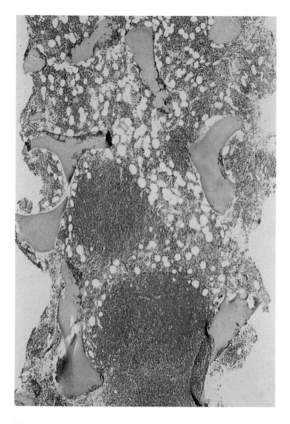

Figure 20.7 Iliac crest trephine biopsy in lymphocytic lymphoma. Prominent nodules of lymphoid tissue are seen in the intertrabecular space and paratrabecular areas.

Table 20.4 International prognostic index for high-grade lymphoma.

	Good	Bad
Age	<60 years	>60 years
Performance status	0 or 1	>2
Stage (see p. 247)	I or II	III or IV
Number of extranodal sites	0 or 1	>2
Serum LDH	Normal	Raised

LDH, lactate dehydrogenase.

include chest X-ray and computed tomography (CT) scanning (Fig. 20.9). Positron-emission tomography (PET) may detect disease not seen on CT scan and is used to follow treatment response (Fig. 20.10). Bone marrow aspiration and trephine are also performed for diagnosis and staging and HIV testing is needed.

Specific subtypes of non-Hodgkin lymphoma

Low-grade non-Hodgkin lymphoma

Small lymphocytic lymphoma

This term is used for cases with the same morphology, immunophenotype and cytogenetics as chronic lymphocytic lymphoma (CLL), less than $5 \times 10^9/L$ peripheral blood B cells and no cytopenias due to bone marrow involvement. Most of the patients are elderly and often no treatment is required ('watch and wait').

Lymphoplasmacytoid lymphoma (Waldenström's macroglobulinaemia)

This is an uncommon condition, seen most frequently in men over 50 years of age. When, as usually is the case, the disease produces a monoclonal IgM paraprotein, lymphoplasmacytoid lymphoma (LPL) may be termed Waldenström's macroglobulinaemia. The cell of origin appears to be a post-germinal centre B cell with the characteristics of an IgM-bearing memory B cell. The disease usually presents with an insidious onset, often with fatigue and weight loss. Hyperviscosity syndrome (see Fig. 21.13) is a common complication as IgM paraprotein (a pentamer) increases blood viscosity more than equivalent concentrations of IgG or IgA. Visual upset is frequent and the retina may show a variety of changes such as engorged veins, haemorrhages, exudates and a blurred disc (see Fig. 21.13). If the macroglobulin is a cryoglobulin, features of cryoprecipitation, such as Raynaud's phenomenon, may be present. LPL may also be diagnosed by chance in symptomless patients.

Anaemia, at least partly caused by an increased plasma volume, is usually a significant problem and a bleeding tendency may result from macroglobulin interference with coagulation factors and platelet function. Neurological symptoms, neuropathy, dyspnoea and heart failure may be presenting symptoms. Moderate lymphadenopathy and enlargement of the liver and spleen are frequently seen.

Diagnosis is made by the finding of a monoclonal serum IgM together with bone marrow or lymph node infiltration with lymphoplasmacytoid cells (Fig. 20.11). The erythrocyte sedimentation rate (ESR) is raised and there may be a peripheral blood lymphocytosis.

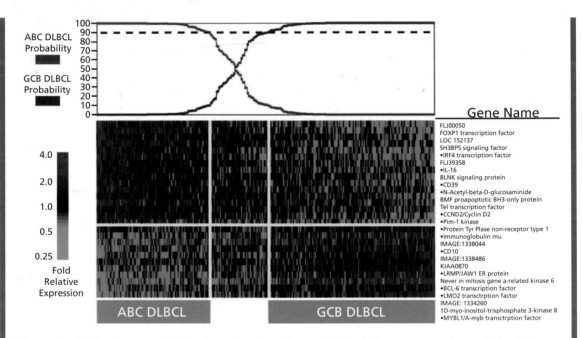

Figure 20.8 DNA microarray of diffuse large B-cell lymphoma (DLCL) which uses expression analysis of 27 genes to divide cases into those with a typical activated B cell (ABC) or germinal centre B cell (GCB) pattern (Wright *et al.*, 2003).

Figure 20.9 Non-Hodgkin lymphoma. **(a)** Computed tomography (CT) colonography examination performed for weight loss and abdominal pain in a 86-year-old female showing enlarged para-aortic (yellow arrow) and mesenteric lymph nodes (blue circle). Histology revealed diffuse large B-cell non-Hodgkin lymphoma. (Courtesy of Dr P. Wylie.) **(b)** CT scan of the abdomen: enlarged retroperitoneal and mesenteric nodes from a man causing the 'floating aorta' (arrowed) appearance. (Courtesy of Professor A. Dixon and Dr R.E. Marcus.) **(c)** Magnetic resonance imaging (MRI) scan of the chest showing large mediastinal lymph nodes (white and arrowed) adjacent to the great vessels (black). **(d)** MRI T$_2$-weighted midline saggital image of a lumbosacral spine showing compression of the dural sac by an extradural mass. A, spinal cord; B, extradural mass; C, roots of corda equina. (Courtesy of Dr A. Valentine.) **(e)** Positron emission tomography (PET) body scan of a 59-year-old woman with high-grade non-Hodgkin lymphoma. (i) The first scan showed no evidence of disease prior to allogeneic transplant. Normal physiological uptake is seen in the brain and bladder. Two months post-transplant the patient relapsed clinically with a mass on the anterior chest wall. (ii) The PET scan showed evidence of widespread relapse in nodal (para-aortic and iliac nodes) and extranodal sites including the lung and bone. The uptake in bone is clearly demonstated in the left humerus and femur (arrowed). This scan illustrates how well PET can detect both nodal and extranodal disease and allows whole body assessment at a single scanning session. (Courtesy of Dr S.F. Barrington.)

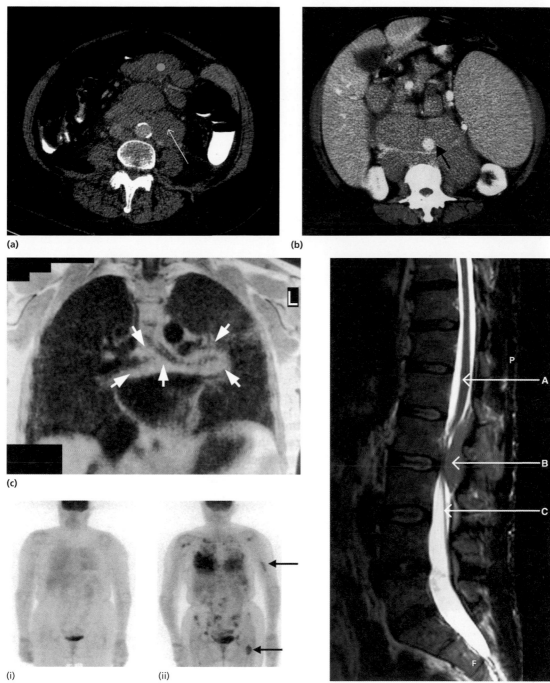

(a)

(b)

(c)

(d)

(i)   (ii)

(e)

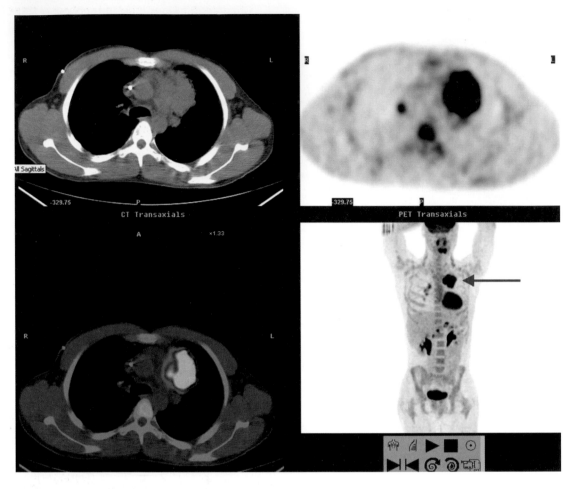

Figure 20.10 Non-Hodgkin lymphoma. PET/CT scan of male aged 26 years. Red arrow shows the level at which transaxial section is performed. Upper right-hand panel showing FDG uptake in anterior mediastinal mass and right hilar node. Upper left-hand panel shows corresponding CT section, bottom left-hand panel shows the CT and PET fused image of the corresponding section. Bottom right-hand panel, coronal section showing FDG uptake in mediastinal mass and right hilar node. There is also FDG uptake in the thyroid, heart, bowel, kidneys and bladder. (Courtesy of the Department of Nuclear Medicine, University College, London.)

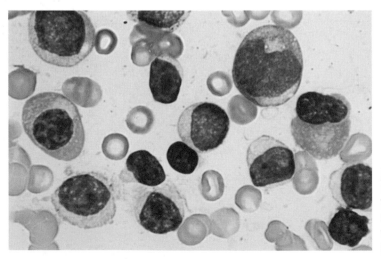

Figure 20.11 Lymphoplasmacytoid lymphoma associated with Waldenström's macroglobulin-aemia. Bone marrow shows cells with features of lymphocytes and plasma cells.

Treatment

No treatment is required for patients without symptoms, but treatment should be started if there is significant organomegaly, anaemia, thrombocytopenia, neuropathy, amyloidosis or hyperviscosity. Rituximab, a humanized monoclonal antibody to CD20 (Fig. 20.12), is used, generally in combination with cyclophosphamide, fludarabine or other purine analogue, bendamustine or bortezomib (but is omitted if there is hyperviscosity). Combination chemotherapy as for follicular or large cell diffuse B lymphoma may be needed in late stages. Autologous or allogeneic stem cell transplantation (SCT) is considered for advanced disease. Erythropoictin or regular transfusions may be required for chronic anaemia.

Acute hyperviscosity syndrome is treated with repeated plasmapheresis. As IgM is mainly intravascular, plasmapheresis is more effective than with IgG or IgA paraproteins when much of the protein is extravascular and so rapidly replenishes the plasma compartment.

Marginal zone lymphomas

Marginal zone lymphomas are low-grade lymphomas that arise from the marginal zone of B-cell germinal follicles. It is thought that lymphoid hyperplasia initially occurs in response to antigen or inflammation and then cells acquire secondary genetic damage that leads to lymphoma. They are classified according the anatomical site at which they arise, such as the spleen, mucosa (MALT) or lymph node (nodal). Mucosa-associated lymphoid tissue (MALT) lymphomas usually arise in the stomach (Fig. 20.13) or thyroid. Gastric MALT lymphoma is the most common form and is preceded by *Helicobacter pylori* infection. In the early stages it may respond to antibiotic therapy aimed at eliminating *H. pylori*.

Splenic marginal zone lymphoma usually presents as splenomegaly and may be associated with circulating 'villous' lymphocytes. Splenectomy is useful for symptomatic patients.

If chemotherapy is needed for marginal zone lymphoma it is usually based on regimens used in

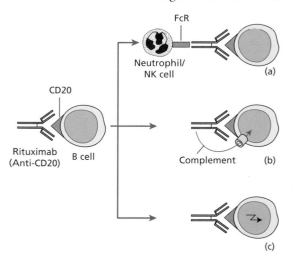

Figure 20.12 The potential mechanisms of action of rituximab. Rituximab binds to CD20 on the surface of B cells. It can elicit a number of effector mechanisms including: **(a)** antibody dependent cell-mediated cytotoxicity; **(b)** complement mediated lysis of tumour cells; and **(c)** direct apoptosis of the target cell.

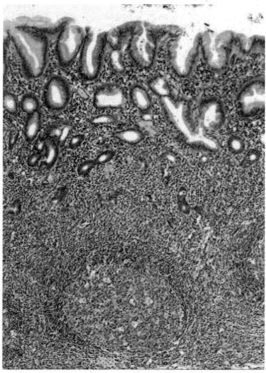

Figure 20.13 Gastric mucosa-associated lymphoid tissue (MALT) lymphoma: the tumour cells surround reactive follicles and infiltrate the mucosa. The follicle has a 'starry sky' appearance. (Courtesy of Professor P. Isaacson.)

other low-grade lymphomas such as follicular lymphoma. Radiotherapy and rituximab are also used.

Follicular lymphoma

This represents around 25% of NHL with a median age of onset of 60 years. It is associated with the t(14; 18) translocation in the great majority of cases (Figs 20.14 and 20.15). The translocation leads to constitutive expression of the *BCL-2* gene with increased survival of cells because of reduced apoptosis.

Patients are likely to be middle-aged or elderly and their disease is often characterized by a benign course for many years. The median survival from diagnosis is approximately 10 years. The histological appearances are graded as I–III according to the relative proportion of centrocytes and centroblasts, Grade IIIb patients, who are treated according to diffuse large B-cell lymphoma (DLBCL) guidelines (see below), having the worst prognosis. Bone marrow involvement is frequent.

Presentation is usually with painless lymphadenopathy, often widespread, and the majority of patients will have stage III or IV disease. Relatively benign types may present rarely as polyps in the duodenum, in the skin, or in children. However, sudden transformation may occur at a rate of about 3% a year to aggressive diffuse tumours which are

sometimes associated with a leukaemic phase. Around 10% of patients have initially localized (Stage 1) disease and may achieve cure with radiotherapy alone. Those with disseminated (Stage II–IV) disease are generally not treated in the absence of symptoms ('watch and wait') but treatment is introduced when complications occur. At the current time, chemotherapy is not a curative option. Therapy is usually based on monthly courses of rituximab, in combination with cyclophosphamide, vincristine and prednisolone (R-CVP), or rituximab with bendamustine or chlorambucil. These regimens can provide clinical responses in up to 90% of patients and usually achieve a remission of several years. Rituximab infusions can also be given as maintenance therapy, and are typically administered every 2–6 months as the antibody has a long half-life in the circulation.

Disease relapse for stage II–IV disease is almost inevitable and is usually treated initially with similar chemotherapy regimens followed by rituximab maintenance. Over time the disease becomes increasingly difficult to control and more intensive chemotherapy or radiolabelled antibody therapy (anti-CD20) may be considered. Autologous SCT may be valuable in patients with a history of at least one relapse and allogeneic SCT using reduced intensity protocols offers the prospect of cure for some patients.

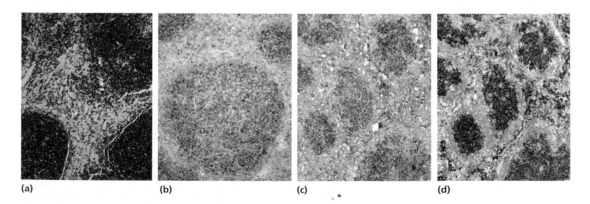

(a)   (b)   (c)   (d)

Figure 20.14 Follicular lymphoma: immunostain. **(a)** The neoplastic cells are diffusely positive for B-cell markers (CD20). **(b)** Immunostain: the neoplastic cells are diffusely positive for CD10, a germinal centre marker, and are located in the follicular and interfollicular areas. **(c)** The neoplastic cells are positive for BCL-6, a germinal centre marker. **(d)** Immunostain: the neoplastic cells are positive for BCL-2.

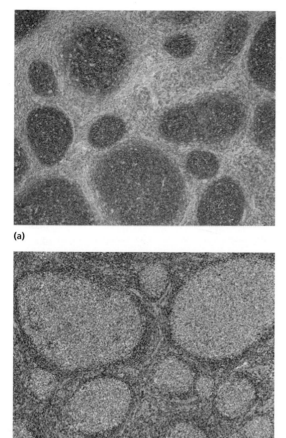

(a)

(b)

Figure 20.15 Follicular lymphoma: immunostain.
(a) CD20 expressed in tumour cells. **(b)** CD3 is
confined to reactive T cells.

Mantle cell lymphoma

Mantle cell lymphoma is derived from pre-germinal
centre cells localized in the primary follicles or in
the mantle region of secondary follicles. It has a
characteristic phenotype of CD19⁺ and CD5⁺ (like
CLL) but in contrast to CLL is CD22⁺ and CD23⁻.
A specific t(11; 14) translocation juxtaposes the
cyclin D1 gene to the immunoglobulin heavy-chain
gene, and leads to increased expression of cyclin D1.
Presence of this translocation is required for diagnosis. Clinical presentation is typically with lymphadenopathy and often there is bone marrow

infiltration. The cells have characteristically angular
nuclei in histological sections (Fig. 20.4) and often
circulate in the blood (Fig. 20.6).

Current treatment regimens include:

1 R-CHOP
2 Intensive combinations such as R-Hyper-
CVAD
3 Cytosine arabinoside, rituximab and autologous
SCT and
4 Purine analogues with or without cyclophosphamide and rituximab.

The roles of bortezomid and lenalidomide are being
investigated. Allogeneic SCT may also be considered in some patients. The prognosis is usually poor
and overall survival is 4–6 years, although 15% of
patients show an indolent course similar to CLL.

Heavy-chain diseases

These are rare disorders in which neoplastic cells
secrete only incomplete 'immunoglobulin' heavy
chains (γ, α or μ). The most common is α chain
disease which occurs in the Mediterranean area and
starts as a malabsorption syndrome which may
progress to systemic lymphoma.

High-grade non-Hodgkin lymphoma

Diffuse large B-cell lymphomas (DLBCL)

DLBCL are a heterogeneous group of disorders rep-
resenting the classic 'high-grade' lymphomas. As
such they typically present with rapidly progressive
lymphadenopathy associated with a fast rate of cellular proliferation. Progressive infiltration may
affect the bone marrow, gastrointestinal tract, brain
(Fig. 20.16), spinal cord, the kidneys or other
organs.

A variety of clinical and laboratory findings are
relevant to the outcome of therapy. According to
the International Prognostic Index these include
age, performance status, stage, number of extranodal sites and serum LDH (Table 20.4). Bulky
disease (major mass >5 cm in diameter) and prior
history of low-grade disease or AIDS are also associated with a poorer prognosis. There are a variety of
histological patterns including centroblastic, immu-

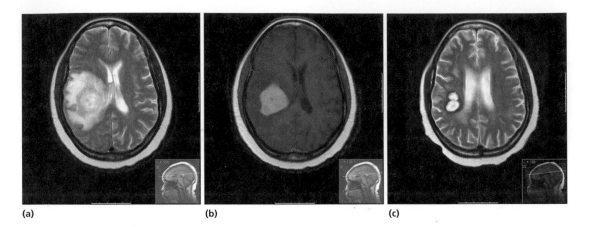

(a)   (b)   (c)

Figure 20.16 AIDS, cerebral lymphoma; MRI. **(a)** T2 weighted magnetic resonance brain scan showing heterogeneous mass and adjacent oedema in right inferior frontoparietal region. There is compression of the right lateral ventricle and displacement of midline structures. Biopsy showed diffuse large B-cell lymphoma. **(b)** The mass enhances after intravenous gadolinium injection. **(c)** Enhanced image after chemotherapy showing regression of the mass. (Courtesy of the Department of Radiology, Royal Free Hospital, London.)

noblastic, anaplastic (Fig. 20.4). The most common cytogenetic changes involve the *BCL-6* gene at chromosome 3q27; and translocation of the *BCL-2* gene, occurs in 20%.

The mainstay of treatment is rituximab in combination with the CHOP chemotherapy regimen (cyclophosphomide, hyroxodaunorubicin, vincristine (Oncovin) and prednisolone) and these are given in 2- or 3-weekly cycles, typically for six to eight courses. Granulocyte colony-stimulating factor (G-CSF) injections are often used to support the neutrophil count. For localized disease, combined radiotherapy and chemotherapy (e.g. three courses of R-CHOP) may be optimal. Prophylactic therapy to prevent CNS disease, such as intrathecal or high-dose systemic methotrexate, should be considered for patients with high-risk disease, particularly those with bone marrow involvement. The response to treatment should be monitored by repeat CT or PET-CT scans midway through chemotherapy and then following completion. For patients who relapse, high-dose chemotherapy with drug regimens such as ESHAP (etoposide, cytosine arabinoside, methylprednisolone and cisplatin) or R-ICE (rituximab, ifosfamide, carboplatin and etoposide) can be effective. In those patients who respond to these treatments, autologous SCT is

often used. Reduced intensity allogeneic SCT has also been shown to be effective For those with primary refractory or chemoresistant disease the outlook is poor. Overall long-term survival is approximately 65%.

Burkitt lymphoma

Burkitt lymphoma occurs in endemic or sporadic forms. Endemic (African) Burkitt lymphoma is seen in areas with chronic malaria exposure and is associated with Epstein–Barr virus (EBV) infection. In virtually all cases the *MYC* oncogene is overexpressed because it is translocated to an immunoglobulin gene, usually the heavy-chain locus t(8; 14) (see Fig. 11.11). As a result, expression of the *MYC* gene is deregulated and the gene is expressed in parts of the cell cycle during which it should normally be switched off.

Typically the patient, usually a child, presents with massive lymphadenopathy, often of the jaw (Fig. 20.17), which is initially very responsive to chemotherapy although long-term cure is uncommon. Sporadic Burkitt lymphoma may occur anywhere in the world and EBV infection is seen in 20% of cases. There is an increased incidence in HIV infection. The histological picture is distinctive

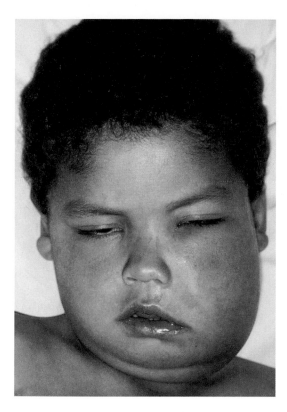

Figure 20.17 Burkitt lymphoma: characteristic facial swelling caused by extensive tumour involvement of the mandible and surrounding soft tissues.

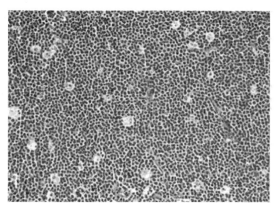

Figure 20.18 Burkitt lymphoma: histological section of lymph node showing sheets of lymphoblasts and 'starry sky' tingible body macrophages.

with a very high proliferative index of over 95% (Fig. 20.18). The prognosis is excellent with the introduction of chemotherapy regimens which include high-doses of methotrexate, cytosine arabinoside and cyclophosphamide, e.g. CODOX-M/IVAC (which includes doxorubicin, ifosphamide and etoposide). Intrathecal chemotherapy is also given. DA-Epoch, an infusional regimen using similar agents, has also proved effective.

Primary central nervous system lymphoma

These are rare tumours, more common in older patients and those with HIV infection. Patients are treated with high-dose methotrexate (with high-dose cytosine arabinoside) followed by whole brain radiotherapy. Long-term cognitive dysfunction is an issue.

Lymphoblastic lymphomas

Lymphoblastic lymphomas (B or T cell) occur mainly in children and young adults and these conditions merge clinically and morphologically with ALL. They are treated using similar protocols.

T-cell lymphomas

Peripheral T-cell lymphomas that present with lymphadenopathy rather than extranodal disease are a heterogeneous group of rare tumours and are usually of CD4$^+$ phenotype. Several variants of T-cell lymphomas are recognized.

Peripheral T-cell non-Hodgkin lymphoma, unspecified

These derive from post-thymic T cells at various stages of differentiation. They are treated with combined chemotherapy (e.g. CHOP). The prognosis is poor.

Autografting for patients with chemosensitive disease is often performed.

Angioimmunoblastic lymphadenopathy

Angioimmunoblastic lymphadenopathy usually occurs in elderly patients with lymphadenopathy, hepatosplenomegaly, skin rashes and a polyclonal increase in serum IgG. Patients are treated with chemotherapy or other agents such as thalidomide or ciclosporin.

Mycosis fungoides

Mycosis fungoides is a chronic cutaneous T-cell lymphoma that presents with severe pruritus and psoriasis-like lesions (Fig. 20.19). Ultimately, deeper organs are affected, particularly lymph nodes, spleen, liver and bone marrow.

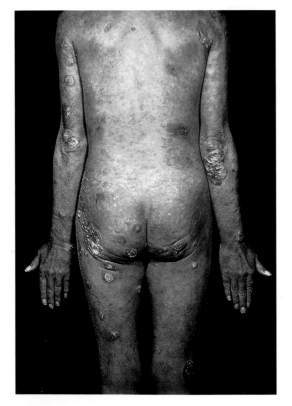

Figure 20.19 Mycosis fungoides.

Sézary syndrome

In Sézary syndrome there is dermatitis, erythroderma, generalized lymphadenopathy and circulating T-lymphoma cells. The cells are usually CD4$^+$ and have a folded or cerebriform nuclear chromatin. Initial treatment of these conditions is by local irradiation, topical chemotherapy or photochemotherapy with psoralen and ultraviolet light (PUVA). Chemotherapy (e.g. CHOP) may be needed but is rarely effective for long.

Adult T-cell leukaemia/lymphoma

This is associated with human T-cell leukaemia/lymphoma virus type 1 (HTLV-1) infection (see Chapter 18).

Enteropathy-associated T-cell lymphomas

Enteropathy-associated T-cell lymphomas are associated with coeliac disease and have a very poor response to treatment. Trials using high-dose methotrexate and autografts are in progress.

Anaplastic large cell lymphoma

Anaplastic large cell lymphoma is particularly common in children and is usually of T-cell phenotype. The disease is CD30$^+$ and usually associated with the t(2; 5) (p23; q35) translocation. This leads to overexpression of anaplastic lymphoma kinase (ALK). It has an aggressive course characterized by systemic symptoms and extranodal involvement. ALK– cases occur and have a worse prognosis. ALK+ large B-cell lymphoma is also described.

Histiocytic and dendritic cell neoplasms

These are rare tumours including dendritic and macrophage-derived sarcomas which may be localized or disseminated. They usually present as tumours at extranodal sites, especially the intestinal tract, skin and soft tissues. Systemic symptoms are present. The outlook is poor except for those with small localized tumours who may do well. Langerhans' cell histiocytosis, a clonal disease of histiocytes, is discussed on page 122.

SUMMARY

- Non-Hodgkin lymphomas are a large group of clonal lymphoid tumours. Approximately 85% are of B-cell origin and 15% derive from T or NK cells.
- Their clinical presentation and natural history are more variable than Hodgkin lymphoma and can vary from very indolent disease through to rapidly progressive subtypes that need urgent treatment.
- For many years clinicians have divided lymphomas into low-grade and high-grade disease. This is useful as low-grade disorders are typically slowly progressive, respond well to chemotherapy but are very difficult to cure, whereas high-grade lymphomas are aggressive and need urgent treatment but are more often curable.
- Investigation is with lymph node biopsy, blood tests and radiology. Immunohistochemistry of the lymph node is valuable and cytogenetic analysis is performed in many cases.
- Clinical staging is performed as for Hodgkin lymphoma.
- Some of the more common subtypes include:

  Small lymphocytic lymphoma is the lymphoma equivalent of chronic lymphocytic leukaemia.

  Lymphoplasmacytic lymphoma usually produces an IgM paraprotein, when it is also known as Waldenström's macroglobulinaemia, and often leads to anaemia and hyperviscosity.

  Marginal zone lymphomas arise from marginal zone B cells of lymphoid follicles and can occur in many organs, usually as a result of chronic antigenic stimulation.

  Follicular lymphoma represents 25% of all NHL and is associated with the t(14; 18) translocation. Treatment usually achieves disease remission but the only curative option is allogeneic stem cell transplantation.

  Mantle cell lymphoma is associated with increased expression of the cyclin D1 gene and has clinical features of an 'intermediate grade' lymphoma.

  Diffuse large B-cell lymphoma is a common subtype and is an aggressive disease which needs urgent treatment. It shares features with acute leukaemia and the majority of cases are cured.

  Burkitt lymphoma is one of the most highly proliferative subtypes of any tumour. Endemic cases in Africa are associated with EBV infection. Treatment is with aggressive chemotherapy regimens.

  T-cell lymphomas are less common but include *mycosis fungoides, peripheral T-cell lymphomas* and *anaplastic large cell lymphoma.*

- Treatments for NHL are based on a variety of chemotherapy regimens. Anti-CD20 antibodies are used in most cases of B-cell lymphomas and have markedly improved the outlook.

Now visit www.wiley.com/go/essentialhaematology to test yourself on this chapter.

CHAPTER 21
Multiple myeloma and related disorders

Key topics

Paraproteinaemia

This is the presence of a monoclonal immunoglobulin band in the serum. Normally, serum immunoglobulins are polyclonal and represent the combined output from millions of different plasma cells. A monoclonal band (M-protein), or *paraprotein*, reflects the synthesis of immunoglobulin from a single clone of plasma cells. This may occur as a primary neoplastic disease or secondary to an underlying benign or neoplastic disease affecting the immune system (Table 21.1).

Multiple myeloma

Multiple myeloma (myelomatosis) is a neoplastic disease characterized by plasma cell accumulation in the bone marrow, the presence of monoclonal protein in the serum and/or urine and, in symptomatic patients, related tissue damage. Ninety-eight per cent of cases occur over the age of 40 years with a peak incidence in the seventh decade. The term asymptomatic (smouldering) multiple myeloma is used for cases with similar laboratory findings but no organ or tissue damage. Retrospective analysis of serum samples has shown that almost all cases of myeloma develop from a pre-existing monoclonal gammopathy of undetermined significance (MGUS; see below). Other plasma cell neoplasms are listed in Table 21.2.

The myeloma cell is a post-germinal centre plasma cell that has undergone immunoglobulin class switching and somatic hypermutation and secretes the paraprotein that is present in serum. Immunoglobulin heavy and light chain genes are clonally rearranged. Plasma cells naturally home to the bone marrow and this characteristic is retained by the tumour cell. The aetiology of the disease is unknown but it is more common in certain racial groups such as black individuals. Tumour cells accumulate complex genetic changes but dysregulated or increased expression of cyclin D (see p. 278) is believed to be an early unifying event.

Diagnosis

Symptomatic myeloma is diagnosed if there is:

1 Monoclonal protein in serum and/or urine (Fig. 21.1)
2 Increased clonal plasma cells in the bone marrow (Fig. 21.2) and
3 Related organ or tissue impairment.

A useful acronym for tissue damage is CRAB (hypercalaemia, renal impairment, anaemia, bone

---

Table 21.1 Diseases associated with monoclonal immunoglobulins.

Neoplastic
Multiple myeloma
Solitary plasmacytoma
Monoclonal gammopathy of undetermined significance (MGUS)
Waldenström macroglobulinaemia
Non-Hodgkin lymphoma
Chronic lymphocytic leukaemia
Primary amyloidosis
Heavy-chain disease

Benign
Chronic cold haemagglutinin disease
Transient (e.g. with infections)
HIV infection
Gaucher's disease

Table 21.2 Plasma cell neoplasms (WHO, 2008).

Monoclonal gammopathy of undetermined significance (MGUS)

Plasma cell myeloma
Variants:
  Asymptomatic (smouldering) myeloma
  Non-secretory myeloma
  Plasma cell leukaemia

Plasmacytoma
Solitary plasmacytoma of bone
Extraosseous (extramedullary) plasmacytoma

Immunoglobulin deposition diseases
Primary amyloidosis
Systemic light and heavy chain deposition diseases

Osteosclerotic myeloma (POEMS syndrome)

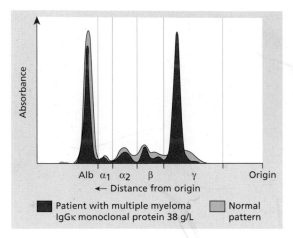

Figure 21.1 Serum protein electrophoresis in multiple myeloma showing an abnormal paraprotein in the γ-globulin region with reduced levels of background β- and γ-globulins.

disease). Also, amyloid, hyperviscosity and recurrent infection may also be present.

Asymptomatic (smouldering) myeloma is diagnosed if there is an M protein in serum at myeloma levels (>30 g/L) and/or 10% or more of clonal plasma cells in the marrow but no related organ or tissue impairment (e.g. CRAB or myeloma-related symptoms).

Clinical features

1 Bone pain (especially backache) resulting from vertebral collapse and pathological fractures (Fig. 21.3a,b).
2 Features of anaemia, e.g. lethargy, weakness, dyspnoea, pallor, tachycardia.
3 Recurrent infections: related to deficient antibody production, abnormal cell-mediated immunity and neutropenia.

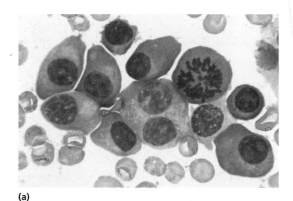

(a)

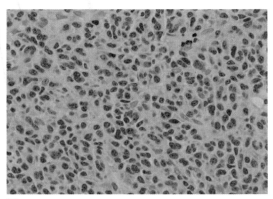

(b)

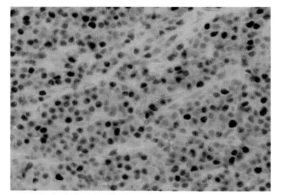

(c)

Figure 21.2 (a) The bone marrow in multiple myeloma showing large numbers of plasma cells, with many abnormal forms. **(b)** Low power view showing sheets of plasma cells replacing normal haemopoietic tissue. **(c)** Immunohistochemical staining of the bone marrow in myeloma with antibody to CD138 revealing extensive numbers of plasma cells.

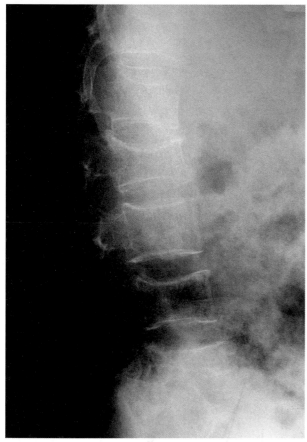

(a)

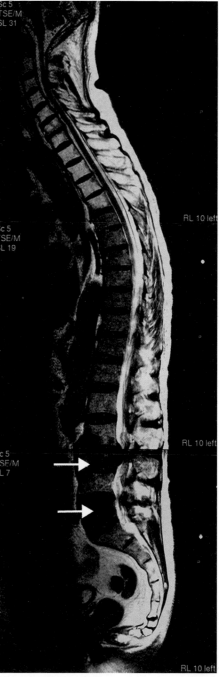

(b)

Figure 21.3 (a) Multiple myeloma: X-ray of lumbar spine showing severe demineralization with partial collapse of L_3. **(b)** Magnetic resonance imaging (MRI) of spine: T_2-weighted study. There is infiltration and destruction of L_3 and L_5 with bulging of the posterior part of the body of L_3 into the spinal canal compressing the corda equina (arrowed). Radiotherapy has caused a marrow signal change in vertebrae C_2–D_4 because of replacement of normal red marrow by fat (bright white signal). (Courtesy of Dr A. Platts.)

4 Features of renal failure and/or hypercalcaemia: polydipsia, polyuria, anorexia, vomiting, constipation and mental disturbance.

5 Abnormal bleeding tendency: myeloma protein may interfere with platelet function and coagulation factors; thrombocytopenia occurs in advanced disease.

6 Amyloidosis occurs in 5% with features such as macroglossia, carpal tunnel syndrome and diarrhoea.

7 In approximately 2% of cases there is a hyperviscosity syndrome with purpura, haemorrhages, visual failure, central nervous system (CNS) symptoms, neuropathies and heart failure.

Laboratory findings include the following:

1 **Presence of a paraprotein** Serum and urine should be screened by immunoglobulin electrophoresis. The paraprotein is immunoglobulin G (IgG) in 60% of cases, IgA in 20% and light chain only in almost all the rest. Less than 1%

have IgD or IgE paraprotein and a similar number are non-secretory.

2 **Elevated serum immunoglobulin-free light chains** Immunoglobulin-free light chains (FLC) are κ or λ light chain proteins, synthesized by plasma cells that have not been paired with heavy chain (Fig. 21.4). They are normally made in small quantities and filtered from the serum into the kidney but can be measured in serum. Free light chains are produced by almost all malignant plasma cells and so the *serum free light chain* assay is useful in diagnosis and monitoring of myeloma and other forms of malignant paraproteinaemia. Typically in myeloma there is an increase in either the κ or λ serum free light chain value. The normal κ:λ serum free light chain ratio of 0.6 (range 0.26–1.65) is also skewed with an excess of either κ or λ chains. Light chain assays have largely replaced the need for analysis of urine paraproteinaemia.

3 Normal serum immunoglobulin levels (IgG, IgA and IgM) are reduced, a feature known as

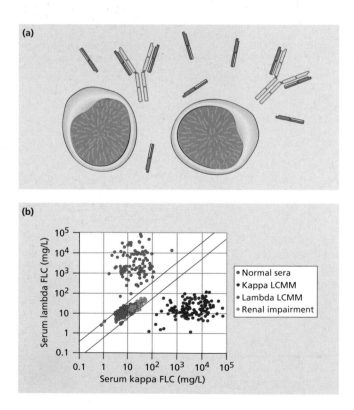

Figure 21.4 The value of serum immunoglobulin-free light chain (FLC) measurement in multiple myeloma. **(a)** Serum free light chains are immunoglobulin light chains that are synthesized by plasma cells but not paired with heavy chains before they are released into the blood. Low levels are found in normal individuals and these are increased in patients with myeloma. **(b)** Profile of serum free light chains in healthy controls, patients with renal impairment and those with κ or λ light chain multiple myeloma (LCMM). As light chains are normally filtered by the kidney, their levels rise in patients with renal impairment although the κ:λ ratio remains normal. (From Hutchison C. (2008) *BMC Nephrology* 9, 11–19; Bradwell A.R. (2003) *Lancet* 361, 489–91.)

immune paresis. The urine contains free light chains, ***Bence-Jones protein***, in two-thirds of cases. Rare cases of myeloma are non-secretory and therefore not associated with a paraprotein or Bence-Jones proteinuria although some will still show a disturbed free light chain ratio in the serum.

4 There is usually a normochromic, normocytic or macrocytic anaemia. Rouleaux formation is marked in most cases (Fig. 21.5). Neutropenia and thrombocytopenia occur in advanced disease. Abnormal plasma cells appear in the blood film in 15% of patients and can be detected by sensitive flow cytometry in over 50%.

5 High erythrocyte sedimentation rate (ESR).

6 Increased plasma cells in the bone marrow (usually >20%) often with abnormal forms (Fig. 21.2). The characteristic **immunophenotype** of malignant plasma cells is CD38^{high}CD138^{high} and CD45^{low}. Anti-CD138 is used to measure the number of plasma cells in the marrow biopsy (Fig. 21.2). Interleukin 6 is a potent growth factor for myeloma cells and is often active by an autocrine mechanism (secreted by, and acting on, the same cell).

7 Radiological investigation of the skeleton reveals bone lesions such as osteolytic areas without evidence of surrounding osteoblastic reaction or sclerosis in 60% of patients (Fig. 21.6) or generalized osteoporosis in 20% (Fig. 21.3). Twenty per cent have no bone lesions. In addition, pathological fractures or vertebral collapse (Fig. 21.3b) are common. The osteolytic lesions are caused by osteoclast activation resulting from high serum levels of RANKL (receptor activator of nuclear factor-κB (NF-κB) ligand), produced by plasma cells and bone marrow stroma, which binds to activatory RANK receptors on the osteoclast surface.

8 Serum calcium elevation occurs in 45% of patients. Typically, the serum alkaline phos-

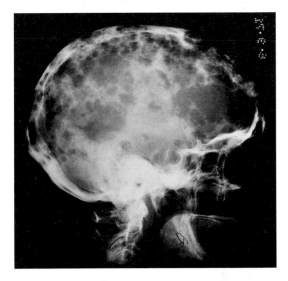

Figure 21.6 Skull X-ray in multiple myeloma showing many 'punched-out' lesions.

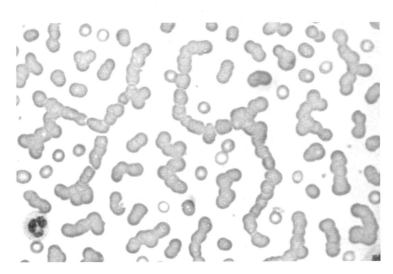

Figure 21.5 The peripheral blood film in multiple myeloma showing Rouleaux formations.

phatase is normal (except following pathological fractures).

9 The serum creatinine is raised in 20% of cases. Proteinaceous deposits from heavy light chain proteinuria, hypercalcaemia, uric acid, amyloid and pyelonephritis may all contribute to renal failure (Fig. 21.7).

10 A low serum albumin occurs with advanced disease.

11 Serum β_2-microglobulin is often raised and is a useful indicator of prognosis. Levels less than 3.5 mg/L imply a relatively good prognosis, above 5.5 mg/L bad.

12 Cytogenetic analysis shows that approximately half the tumours have an increased number of chromosomes (*hyperdiploid*) whereas non-hyperdiploid cases have a high incidence of translocations involving the immunoglobulin heavy-chain gene (*IGH*). The D-cyclin genes, D_1, D_2 or D_3, are often involved in the translocations. Monoallelic loss of 13q is frequent in both categories and all these genetic abnormalities may also be seen in MGUS (see p. 282).

Treatment

This may be divided into specific and supportive (Fig. 21.8).

Specific

At the current time the disease remains incurable except for those very few, mostly younger, patients who may be cured by allogeneic stem cell transplantation (SCT). For all other patients the major treatment decision is between the use of *intensive therapy* (mostly for patients aged less than 65–70 years) and *non-intensive therapy* for older patients.

Intensive therapy involves the combination of 4–6 courses of chemotherapy to reduce the tumour burden usually followed by stem cell collection and autologous SCT after high-dose chemotherapy. Repeated intravenous or oral chemotherapy cycles use drugs such as cyclophosphamide, dexamethasone and thalidomide (CDT), lenalidomide, dexamethasone, Adriamycin or the proteasome inhibitor, bortezomib. After several courses of treatment, when the number of tumour cells has been markedly reduced, peripheral blood stem cells are usually collected after mobilization using a combination of chemotherapy and granulocyte colony-stimulating factor (G-CSF). High-dose melphalan, with or without radiotherapy, is the typical conditioning regimen for autologous SCT. Two consecutive SCT procedures are used in some centres. Maintenance treatment after autologous SCT with thalidomide, lenalidomide, bortezomib and other drugs is under trial as are protocols that omit SCT altogether.

Although *allogeneic transplantation* may cure the disease it carries a high procedure-related mortality and patients frequently relapse after the procedure.

Non-intensive therapy In elderly patients courses of the oral alkylating agent melphalan usually in combination with prednisolone, thalidomide or bortezomib are effective in reducing the tumour burden. Typically, paraprotein levels gradually fall, bone lesions show improvement and blood counts may improve. Cyclophosphamide is also effective and simple to use as a single agent. However, after a variable number of courses a 'plateau phase' is reached in which the paraprotein level stops falling. At this point treatment is stopped and the patient is seen at regular intervals in the outpatient clinic. After a variable period of time, often around 18 months, the disease 'escapes' from plateau with rising paraprotein and worsening symptoms. Further chemotherapy may be given although the disease becomes increasingly difficult to control.

Notes on specific drugs used in myeloma

Thalidomide is useful in first-line therapy and also in the management of relapsed disease. Its precise mechanism of action is unknown and it has a number of side-effects such as sedation, constipation, neuropathy and thrombosis (Table 21.3). The addition of dexamethasone increases the response rate but venous thrombosis becomes a major concern. Prophylactic anticoagulation with heparin, warfarin or aspirin is needed when thalidomide is used in induction regimens.

Lenalidomide is an analogue of thalidomide and is highly active in the management of myeloma. It is widely used for relapsed disease and is being

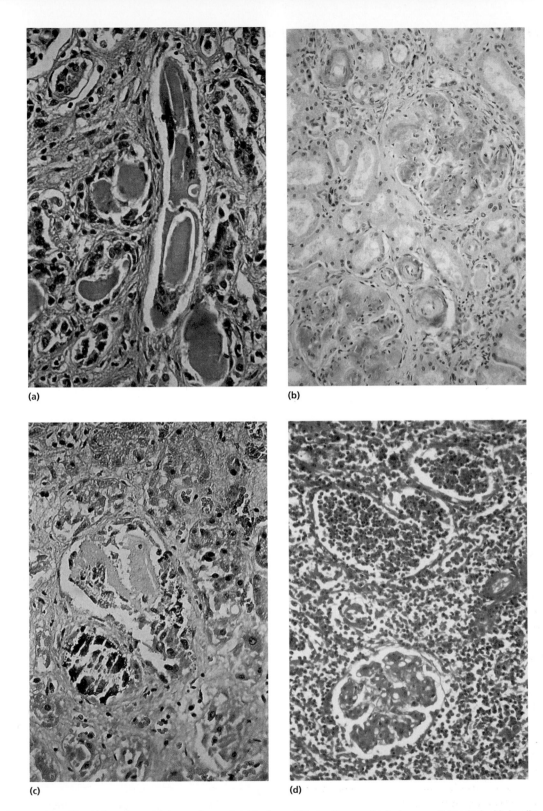

Figure 21.7 The kidney in multiple myeloma. **(a)** Myeloma kidney: the renal tubules are distended with hyaline protein (precipitated light chains or Bence-Jones protein). Giant cells are prominent in the surrounding cellular reaction. **(b)** Amyloid deposition: both glomeruli and several of the small blood vessels contain an amorphous pink-staining deposit characteristic of amyloid (Congo red stain). **(c)** Nephrocalcinosis: calcium deposition (dark 'fractured' material) in the renal parenchyma. **(d)** Pyelonephritis: destruction of renal parenchyma and infiltration by acute inflammatory cells.

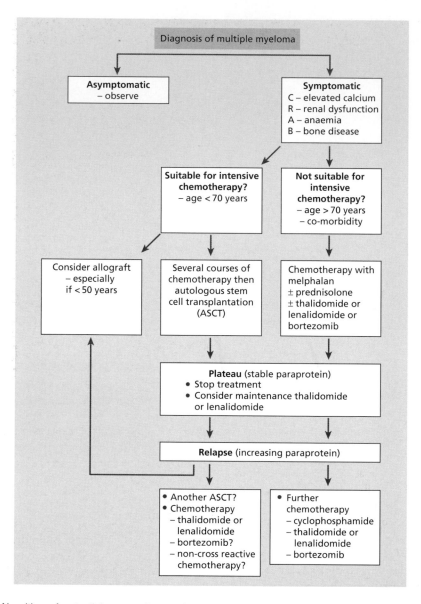

Figure 21.8 Algorithm of potential approaches to the management of multiple myeloma.

assessed as first-line therapy. It is associated with myelosuppression and increased risk of thrombosis, but causes less neuropathy than thalidomide (Table 21.3). *Pomalidomide* is the most recent addition to this class of drugs.

Bortezomib (Velcade®) inhibits the cellular pro-teasome and NF-κB activation and is very valuable in the treatment of myeloma. Already proven in refractory disease, it is now being assessed in earlier phases of treatment. Its main side-effect is neuropathy.

Radiotherapy is highly effective in treating the symptoms of myeloma. It may be used for areas of bone pain or spinal cord compression.

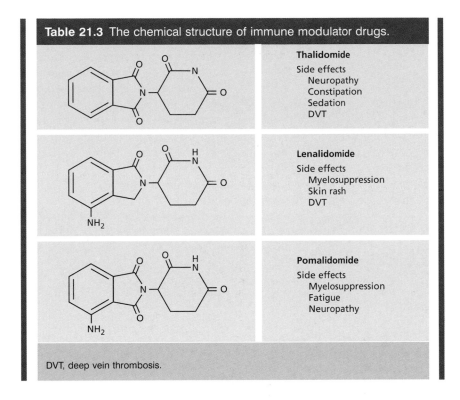

Table 21.3 The chemical structure of immune modulator drugs.

Thalidomide
Side effects
  Neuropathy
  Constipation
  Sedation
  DVT

Lenalidomide
Side effects
  Myelosuppression
  Skin rash
  DVT

Pomalidomide
Side effects
  Myelosuppression
  Fatigue
  Neuropathy

DVT, deep vein thrombosis.

Support care

Renal failure Rehydrate and treat the underlying cause (e.g. hypercalcaemia, hyperuricaemia). Dialysis is generally well tolerated. It is important that all patients with myeloma drink at least 3 L of fluid each day throughout the course of their disease.

Bone disease and hypercalcaemia Bisphosphonates such as pamidronate, clodronate or zoledronic acid are effective in reducing the progression of bone disease and may also improve overall survival. Acute hypercalcaemia is treated with rehydration with isotonic saline, a diuretic and corticosteroids followed by a biphosphonate.

Compression paraplegia Use decompression laminectomy or irradiation; corticosteroid therapy may help.

Anaemia Transfusion or erythropoietin are used.

Bleeding Bleeding caused by paraprotein interference with coagulation and hyperviscosity syndrome may be treated by repeated plasmapheresis.

Infections Rapid treatment of any infection is essential. Prophylactic infusions of immunoglobulin concentrates together with oral broad-spectrum antibiotics and antifungal agents may be needed for recurrent infections.

Prognosis

An international prognostic index has been used based on serum β_2-microglobulin (β_2M) and albumin levels. Patients with serum β_2M >5.5 mg/L and an albumin <35 g/L have a poor survival as do those with frequent circulating plasma cells. Overall, the median survival with non-intensive chemotherapy is 3–4 years and this is improved by approximately 1–2 years with autologous transplantation.

Other plasma cell tumours

Solitary plasmacytoma

These are isolated plasma cell tumours, usually of bone or soft tissue (e.g. the mucosa of the upper respiratory and gastrointestinal tracts or the skin).

The associated paraprotein disappears following radiotherapy to the primary lesion.

Plasma cell leukaemia

This rare disease is characterized by a high number of circulating malignant plasma cells. The clinical features tend to be a combination of those found in acute leukaemia (pancytopenia and organomegaly) with features of myeloma (hypercalcaemia, renal involvement and bone disease). Treatment is with supportive care and systemic chemotherapy but prognosis is poor.

Heavy-chain disease

These are now classified with non-Hodgkin lymphoma (see p. 267).

Monoclonal gammopathy of undetermined significance

Transient or persistent paraproteins can occur in many other conditions as well as in multiple myeloma (Table 21.1). A serum paraprotein may be sometimes be detected without any evidence of myeloma or other underlying disease and is termed *monoclonal gammopathy of undetermined significance (MGUS)*. It is increasingly common with age, being present in 1% of persons older than 50 years and 3% of those over 70 years. There are no clinical complications and the proportion of plasma cells in the marrow is normal (<4%) or only slightly raised (<10%) (Table 21.4). The concentration of monoclonal immunoglobulin in serum is less than 30 g/L and other serum immunoglobulins are not depressed. The κ or λ light chain is increased in serum in one-third of patients; the greater the imbalance, the more the risk of transformation. No treatment is needed but patients with MGUS develop overt myeloma or lymphoma at a rate of approximately 1% each year and so are usually followed up regularly in the outpatient clinic. The survival of patients with MGUS is reduced compared with control populations and this effect increases with duration of follow-up and age (Fig. 21.9).

Amyloidosis

The amyloidoses are a heterogeneous group of disorders characterized by the extracellular deposition of protein in an abnormal fibrillar form (Table 21.5). Amyloidosis may be hereditary or acquired and deposits may be focal, localized or systemic in distribution. The amyloid is made from different amyloid fibril precursor proteins in each type of disease. Except for intracerebral amyloid plaques, all amyloid deposits contain a non-fibrillary glycoprotein amyloid P which is derived from a normal serum precursor structurally related to C-reactive protein (CRP). The classic diagnostic histological test is red–green birefringence after staining with Congo red and viewing under polarized light (Fig. 21.10).

Table 21.4 Features of benign and malignant paraproteinaemia.

	Benign	Malignant
Bence-Jones proteinuria	Absent	May be present
Serum paraprotein concentration	Usually <30 g/L and stationary	Usually >30 g/L and rising
Serum free light chain ratio	Normal	Abnormal
Immuneparesis (hypogammaglobulinaemia)	Absent	Present
Underlying lymphoproliferative disease or myeloma	Absent	Present
Bone lesions	Absent	Present
Plasma cells in marrow	<10%	>10%

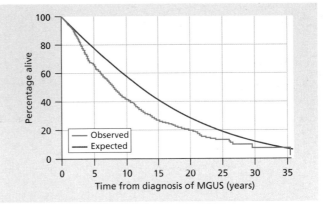

Figure 21.9 Survival of patients with monoclonal gammopathy of undetermined significance (MGUS) (n = 1384) is reduced compared to the control population; median 8.1 *vs.* 11.8 years, respectively ($p < 0.001$). (Reproduced from Kyle R.A. *et al.* (2009) *Haematologica* **94**: 1714.)

Table 21.5 Classification of amyloidosis: types, structure and organ involvement.

Type	Chemical nature	Organs involved
Systemic AL amyloidosis Associated with myeloma, Waldenström's macroglobulinaemia or MGUS May also occur on its own as primary amyloidosis (associated with an occult plasma cell proliferation) May also occur in localized form with local 'immunocyte' proliferation	Immunoglobulin light chains (AL)	Tongue Skin Heart Nerves Connective tissue Kidneys Liver Spleen
Reactive systemic AA amyloidosis Rheumatoid arthritis, tuberculosis, bronchiectasis, chronic osteomyelitis, inflammatory bowel disease, Hodgkin lymphoma, carcinomas, familial Mediterranean fever	Protein A (AA)	Liver Spleen Kidneys Bone marrow
Familial amyloidosis	e.g. Transthyretin abnormalities	Nerves Heart Eyes
Localized amyloidosis Central nervous system Endocrine Senile	β-Amyloid protein Peptic hormones Various	Alzheimer's disease Endocrine tumours Heart, brain, joints, prostate, etc.

AA, AL, these are defined by their chemical nature as in the table; MGUS, monoclonal gammopathy of undetermined significance.

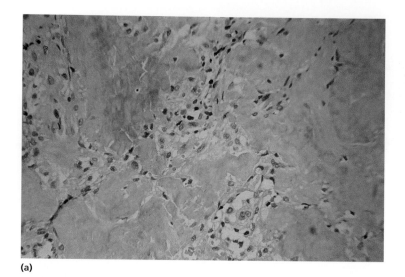

(a)

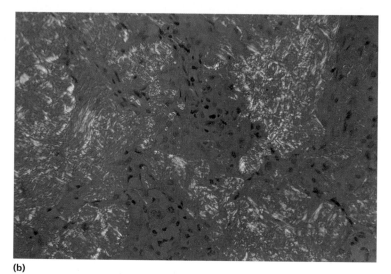

(b)

Figure 21.10 Amyloidosis:
(a) Congo red staining and
(b) blue–green birefringence
under polarized light.

Systemic AL amyloidosis

Systemic amyloid light chain (AL) amyloid disease is caused by deposition of monoclonal light chains produced from a clonal plasma cell proliferation. The level of paraprotein may be very low and is not always detectable in serum or urine but the serum free light chain ratio is usually abnormal (Fig. 21.4). The clinical features are caused by involvement of the heart, tongue (Fig. 21.11), peripheral nerves and kidneys (Fig. 21.7), and the patient may present with heart failure, macroglossia, peripheral neu-ropathy, carpal tunnel syndrome or renal failure. A serum amyloid P (SAP) scan (Fig. 21.12) is used to determine the extent and severity of disease. Treatment is with chemotherapy similar to that used in myeloma, possibly with autologous SCT, which may improve prognosis.

Hyperviscosity syndrome

The most common cause is polycythaemia (see p. 204). Hyperviscosity may also occur in patients

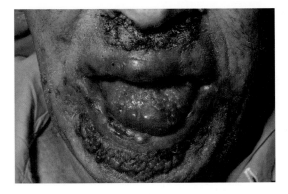

Figure 21.11 Multiple myeloma: the tongue and lips are enlarged because of nodular and waxy deposits of amyloid.

with myeloma or Waldenström's macroglobulinaemia or in patients with chronic myeloid or acute leukaemias associated with very high white cell counts.

The clinical features of the hyperviscosity syndrome include visual disturbances, lethargy, confusion, muscle weakness, nervous system symptoms and signs, and congestive heart failure. The retina may show a variety of changes: engorged veins, haemorrhages, exudates and a blurred disc (Fig. 21.13).

Emergency treatment varies with the cause: venesection or isovolaemic exchange with a plasma substitute for red cells in a polycythaemic patient;

Figure 21.12 Serial anterior whole body ^{123}I-labelled serum amyloid P component (SAP) scans of a 52-year-old woman who presented with renal failure resulting from systemic AL amyloidosis. **(a)** The initial scan demonstrates a large amyloid load with hepatic, splenic, renal and bone marrow deposits. The underlying plasma cell dyscrasia responded to high-dose melphalan followed by autologous stem cell rescue. **(b)** Follow-up SAP scintigraphy 3 years after chemotherapy showed greatly reduced uptake of tracer indicating substantial regression of her amyloid deposits. (Courtesy of Professor P.N. Hawkins, National Amyloidosis Centre, Royal Free Hospital, London.)

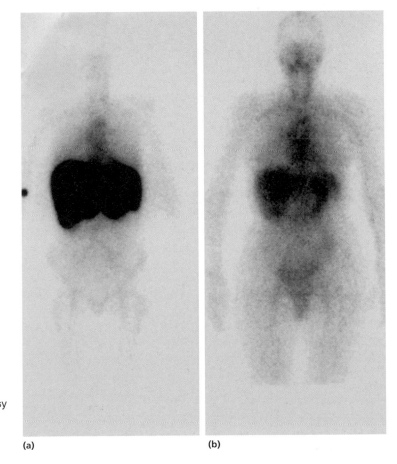

(a)   (b)

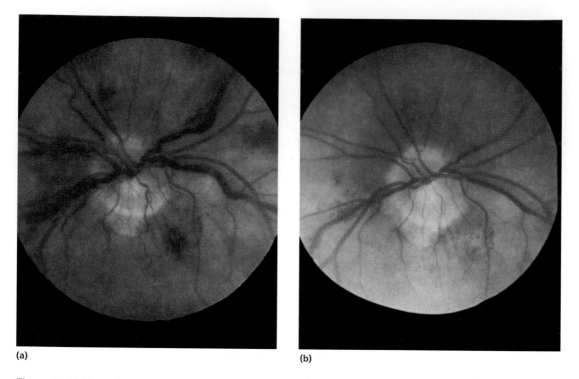

(a) (b)

Figure 21.13 Hyperviscosity syndrome in Waldenström's macroglobulinaemia. **(a)** The retina before plasmapheresis shows distension of retinal vessels, particularly the veins which show bulging and constriction (the 'linked sausage' effect) and areas of haemorrhage; **(b)** following plasmapheresis the vessels have returned to normal and the areas of haemorrhage have cleared.

plasmapheresis in myeloma, Waldenström's disease or hyperfibrinogenaemia; and leucopheresis or chemotherapy in leukaemias associated with high white cell counts. The long-term treatment depends on control of the primary disease with specific therapy.

SUMMARY

- The term *paraproteinaemia* refers to the presence of a monoclonal immunoglobulin band in serum and reflects the synthesis of immunoglobulin from a single clone of plasma cells.
- Multiple myeloma (myelomatosis) is a tumour of plasma cells that accumulate in the bone marrow, release a paraprotein and cause tissue damage. The disease has a peak incidence in the seventh decade.
- Almost all cases of myeloma develop from a pre-existing *monoclonal gammopathy of undetermined significance (MGUS)* in which there is low level paraprotein and no evidence of tissue damage. Approximately 1% of cases progress to myeloma each year.
- A useful reminder for the spectrum of tissue damage in myeloma is *CRAB* – hyper**c**alaemia, **r**enal impairment, **a**naemia, **b**one disease.

- In patients younger than 70 years, myeloma is usually treated by intensive chemotherapy followed by an autologous stem cell transplant using stem cells harvested from the patient.
- In older patients chemotherapy alone is used. However, in both age groups the disease is virtually never cured. New drugs such as thalidomide, bortezomib and lenalidomide are improving the outlook for patients and average survival is now 4–5 years.
- A *plasmacytoma* is a localized mass of malignant plasma cells and is usually treated with radiotherapy. Many cases progress to myeloma.

- *Amyloidoses* are caused by extracellular deposition of protein in an abnormal fibrillar form. Systemic AL amyloid disease is caused by monoclonal light chains produced from a clonal plasma cell proliferation and may cause heart failure, macroglossia, peripheral neuropathy or renal failure.
- *Hyperviscosity syndrome* may occur in paraproteinaemia or in patients with very high red or white cell counts. Clinical features include visual disturbances, confusion and heart failure. Venesection, plasma exchange or chemotherapy may be required.

Now visit www.wiley.com/go/essentialhaematology to test yourself on this chapter.

CHAPTER 22

Aplastic anaemia and bone marrow failure

Key topics

Essential Haematology, 6th Edition. © A. V. Hoffbrand and P. A. H. Moss. Published 2011 by Blackwell Publishing Ltd.

Pancytopenia

Pancytopenia is a reduction in the blood count of all the major cell lines – red cells, white cells and platelets. It has several causes (Table 22.1) which can be broadly divided into decreased bone marrow production or increased peripheral destruction.

Aplastic anaemia

Aplastic (hypoplastic) anaemia is defined as pancytopenia resulting from aplasia of the bone marrow. It is classified into primary (congenital or acquired) or secondary types (Table 22.2).

Pathogenesis

The underlying defect in all cases appears to be a substantial reduction in the number of haemopoietic pluripotential stem cells, and a fault in the remaining stem cells or an immune reaction against them, which makes them unable to divide and differentiate sufficiently to populate the bone marrow (Fig. 22.1). A primary fault in the marrow microenvironment has also been suggested but the success of stem cell transplantation (SCT) shows this can only be a rare cause because normal donor stem cells are usually able to thrive in the recipient's marrow cavity.

Congenital

The Fanconi type has an autosomal recessive pattern of inheritance and is often associated with growth retardation and congenital defects of the skeleton (e.g. microcephaly, absent radii or thumbs), of the renal tract (e.g. pelvic or horseshoe kidney) (Fig. 22.2) or skin (areas of hyper- and hypopigmentation); sometimes there is mental retardation. The syndrome is genetically heterogeneous with 13 different genes involved, A, B, C, D1, D2, E, F, G, I, J, L, M and N in different families. The encoded proteins cooperate in a common cellular pathway which results in ubiquitination of FANCD2, which protects cells against genetic damage.

Table 22.1 Causes of pancytopenia.

Decreased bone marrow function
Aplasia
Acute leukaemia, myelodysplasia, myeloma
Infiltration with lymphoma, solid tumours, tuberculosis
Megaloblastic anaemia
Paroxysmal nocturnal haemoglobinuria
Myelofibrosis
Haemophagocytic syndrome

Increased peripheral destruction
Splenomegaly

Table 22.2 Causes of aplastic anaemia.

Primary	Secondary
Congenital (Fanconi and non-Fanconi types)	**Ionizing radiation**: Accidental exposure (radiotherapy, radioactive isotopes, nuclear power stations)
Idiopathic acquired	**Chemicals**: Benzene, organophosphates and other organic solvents, DDT and other pesticides, organochlorines, recreational drugs (ecstasy) **Drugs**: Those that regularly cause marrow depression (e.g. busulfan, melphalan, cyclophosphamide, anthracyclines, nitrosoureas). Those that occasionally or rarely cause marrow depression (e.g. chloramphenicol, sulphonamides, gold, anti-inflammatory, antithyroid, psychotropic, anticonvulsant/antidepressant drugs) **Viruses**: Viral hepatitis (non-A, non-B, non-C, in most cases), EBV

EBV, Epstein–Barr virus.

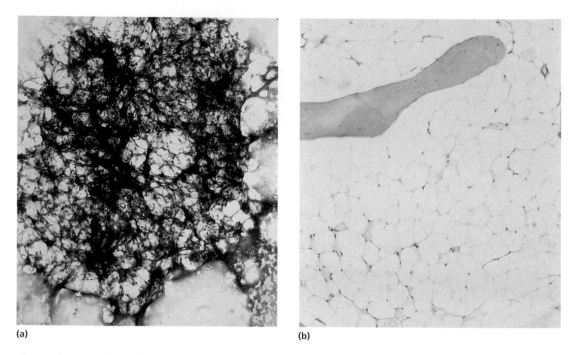

(a) (b)

Figure 22.1 Aplastic anaemia: low power views of bone marrow show severe reduction of haemopoietic cells with an increase in fat spaces. **(a)** Aspirated fragment. **(b)** Trephine biopsy.

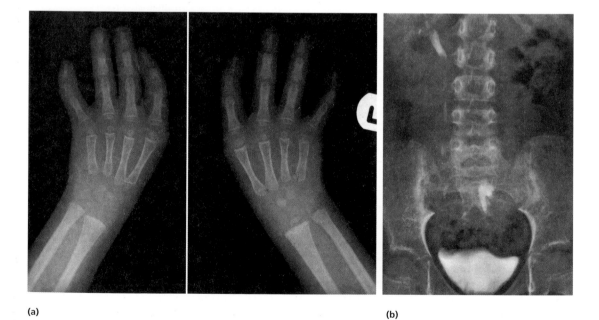

(a) (b)

Figure 22.2 **(a)** X-rays showing absent thumbs in a patient with Fanconi's anaemia (FA). **(b)** Intravenous pyelogram in a patient with FA showing a normal right kidney but a left kidney abnormally placed in the pelvis.

Cells from patients with Fanconi's anaemia (FA) show an abnormally high frequency of spontaneous chromosomal breakage and the diagnostic test is elevated breakage after incubation of peripheral blood lymphocytes with the DNA cross-linking agent diepoxybutane (DEB test).

The usual age of presentation of FA is 5–10 years. Approximately 10% of patients develop acute myeloid leukaemia. Treatment is usually with androgens and/or SCT. The blood count usually improves with androgens but side-effects, especially in children, are distressing (virilization and liver abnormalities); remission rarely lasts more than 2 years. SCT may cure the patient. Because of the sensitivity of the patient's cells to DNA damage, conditioning regimens are mild.

Dyskeratosis congenita (DC) is a rare sex-linked disorder with nail and skin atrophy, aplastic anaemia and a high risk of cancer. It is associated with mutations in the *DKC1* (dyskerin) or *TERC* (telomerase reverse transcriptase RNA template) genes which are both involved in the maintenance of telomere length.

Other inherited bone marrow failure syndromes include Diamond–Blackfan anaemia (DBA), (see p. 294), Shwachman–Diamond syndrome (SDS), (see p. 295), severe congenital neutropenia (see p. 119), amegakaryocytic thrombocytopenia (see p. 333) and thrombocytopenia with absent radii (see p. 333). In DC, DBA and SDS there are defects in ribosomal biosynthesis and function (Fig. 22.3).

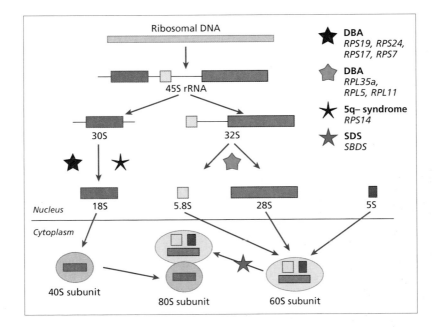

Figure 22.3 Schematic showing scheme of rRNA processing in human cells and the points at which this is possibly disrupted in the different bone marrow failure syndromes. The ribosomal RNAs (rRNAs) are transcribed by RNA polymerase I as a single precursor transcript (45S rRNA). The 45S rRNA is then processed to 18S, 5.8S and 28S rRNAs. The 18S is a component of the 40S ribosomal subunit. The 5.8S and 28S together with 5S (synthesized independently) are components of the 60S ribosomal subunit. The 40S and 60S subunits are assembled to form the 80S ribosomes. The processing steps affected in Diamond–Blackfan anaemia (due to heterozygous mutations in *RPS19, RPS17, RPS24, RPS7, RPL35a, RPL5, RPL11*), 5q-syndrome (haploinsufficiency of *RPS14*) and Shwachman–Diamond syndrome (biallelic mutations in *SBDS*) are indicated by the different coloured stars. DBA, Diamond Blackfan anaemia; SDS, Shwachman–Diamond syndrome; S, sedimentation coefficient.

Idiopathic acquired

This is the most common type of aplastic anaemia, accounting for at least two-thirds of acquired cases. In most cases haemopoetic tissue is the target of an immune process dominated by oligoclonal expression of cytotoxic T cells which secrete γ-interferon and tumour necrosis factor. In approximately one-third of cases short telomeres are found in leucocytes, especially in those with a prolonged clinical course. Mutations in the telomere repair complex have been described but their relevance is unclear. The favourable responses to antilymphocyte globulin (ALG) and ciclosporin support the concept that autoimmune T-cell mediated damage, possibly against functionally and structurally altered stem cells, is important.

Secondary

This is often caused by direct damage to the haemopoietic marrow by radiation or cytotoxic drugs. The antimetabolite drugs (e.g. methotrexate) and mitotic inhibitors (e.g. daunorubicin) cause only temporary aplasia but the alkylating agents, particularly busulfan, may cause chronic aplasia closely resembling the chronic idiopathic disease. Some individuals develop aplastic anaemia as a rare idiosyncratic side-effect of drugs such as chloramphenicol or gold which are not known to be cytotoxic (Table 22.2). They may also develop the disease, during or within a few months of, viral hepatitis (rarely hepatitis A, B or C, but more frequently non-A, non-B, non-C). Because the incidence of marrow toxicity is particularly high for chloramphenicol, this drug should be reserved for treatment of those infections that are life-threatening and for which it is the optimum antibiotic (e.g. typhoid). Chemicals such as benzene may be implicated and rarely aplastic anaemia may be the presenting feature of acute lymphoblastic or myeloid leukaemia, especially in childhood. Myelodysplasia (see Chapter 16) may also present with a hypoplastic marrow.

Clinical features

The onset is at any age with a peak incidence around 30 years and a slight male predominance; it can be insidious or acute with symptoms and signs resulting from anaemia, neutropenia or thrombocytopenia. Infections, particularly of the mouth and throat, are common and generalized infections are frequently life-threatening. Bruising, bleeding gums, epistaxes and menorrhagia are the most frequent haemorrhagic manifestations and the usual presenting features, often with symptoms of anaemia. The lymph nodes, liver and spleen are not enlarged.

Laboratory findings

1 Anaemia is normochromic, normocytic or macrocytic (mean cell volume often 95–110 fL). The reticulocyte count is usually extremely low in relation to the degree of anaemia.
2 Leucopenia. There is a selective fall in granulocytes, usually but not always to below 1.5×10^9/L. In severe cases, the lymphocyte count is also low. The neutrophils appear normal.
3 Thrombocytopenia is always present and, in severe cases, is less than 20×10^9/L.
4 There are no abnormal cells in the peripheral blood.
5 The bone marrow shows hypoplasia, with loss of haemopoietic tissue and replacement by fat which comprises over 75% of the marrow. Trephine biopsy is essential and may show patchy cellular areas in a hypocellular background (Fig. 22.1b). The main cells present are lymphocytes and plasma cells; megakaryocytes in particular are severely reduced or absent.

Severe cases show neutrophils $<0.5 \times 10^9$/L (very severe $<0.2 \times 10^9$/L), platelets $<20 \times 10^9$/L, reticulocytes $<20 \times 10^9$/L and marrow cellularity $<25\%$.

Diagnosis

The disease must be distinguished from other causes of pancytopenia (Table 22.1) and this is not usually difficult provided an adequate bone marrow sample is obtained. Cytogenetic analysis should be performed. Paroxysmal nocturnal haemoglobinuria (PNH) must be excluded by flow-cytometry testing of red cells for CD55 and CD59. In older patients, hypoplastic myelodysplasia may show similar appearances. Qualitative abnormalities of the cells and clonal cytogenetic changes suggest myelodysplasia rather than aplastic anaemia. Some patients diagnosed as having aplastic anaemia develop PNH, myelodysplasia or acute myeloid leukaemia in subsequent years. This may occur even in patients who have responded well to immunosuppressive therapy.

Treatment

General

The cause, if known, is removed (e.g. radiation or drug therapy is discontinued). Initial management consists largely of supportive care with blood transfusions, platelet concentrates and treatment and prevention of infection. All blood products should be leucodepleted to reduce the risk of alloimmunisation and irradiated to prevent grafting of live donor lymphocytes. In severely thrombocytopenic (platelet count $<10 \times 10^9/L$) and neutropenic patients (neutrophils $<0.5 \times 10^9/L$), management is similar to the supportive care of patients receiving intensive chemotherapy with reverse barrier isolation. An antifibrinolytic agent (e.g. tranexamic acid) may be used in patients with severe prolonged thrombocytopenia. Oral antifungal agents and oral antibiotics are used prophylactically in some units to reduce the incidence of infection.

Specific

This must be tailored to the severity of the illness as well as the age of the patient and potential sibling stem cell donors. Severity is assessed by the reticulocyte, neutrophil and platelet counts and degree of marrow hypoplasia. Severe cases have a high mortality in the first 6–12 months unless they respond to specific therapy. Less severe cases may have an acute transient course or a chronic course with ultimate recovery, although the platelet count often remains subnormal for many years. Relapses, sometimes severe and occasionally fatal, may also occur and rarely the disease transforms into myelodysplasia, acute leukaemia or PNH (see Chapter 6).

The following 'specific' treatments are used with varying success.

1 *Antilymphocyte or antithymocyte globulin* (ALG or ATG) This is prepared in animals (e.g.

horse or rabbit) and is of benefit in approximately 50–60% of acquired cases. It is usually given with corticosteroids which reduce the side-effects of ALG including the serum sickness of fever, rash and joint pains which may occur approximately 7 days after administration. Corticosteroids should not be used alone as they increase the risk of infection. Typically, if there is no response to ALG after 4 months a second course may be tried, prepared from another species. Overall, up to 80% of patients respond to combined ALG.

2 *Ciclosporin* This is an effective agent which appears particularly valuable in combination with ALG and steroids.

3 *Alemtuzumab* (Anti-CD52) This has proved effective in about 50% of pateint in small studies and is usually used after ATG has failed.

4 *Androgens* These are beneficial in some patients with FA and acquired aplastic anaemia although an overall improved survival in acquired aplastic anaemia has not been proven. Danazol, nandrolone, oxymetholone have all been tried but side-effects are marked including virilization, salt retention and liver damage with cholestatic jaundice or rarely hepatocellular carcinoma. A response if any occurs is seen as a rise in haemoglobin level with neutrophils and platelets unchanged. If there is no response in 4–6 months, androgens should be stopped. If there is a response the drug should be withdrawn gradually.

5 *Stem cell transplantation* Allogeneic transplantation offers the chance of permanent cure. For aplastic anaemia conditioning is with cyclophosphamide without irradiation but with ciclosporin, which reduces the risks of graft failure and (with methotrexate) of graft-versus-host disease. The relative role of SCT versus immunosuppressive therapy in individual patients with aplastic anaemia is under constant review. In general terms, SCT is favoured in younger patients with severe aplastic anaemia and a human leucocyte antigen (HLA) matching sibling donor. Cure rates of up to 80% are obtained. However, non-myeloablative transplants (see p. 301) are used in selected patients over the age of 40 years. SCT using unrelated volunteer donors and mismatched family members is achieving a survival ratio over 50% in patients with severe aplastic anaemia. In older subjects and those with less severe disease, immunosuppression is usually tried first.

6 *Haemopoietic growth factors* Granulocyte colony-stimulating factor (G-CSF) may produce minor responses but does not lead to sustained improvement. Other growth factors have not proved helpful.

Red cell aplasia

Chronic

This is a rare syndrome characterized by anaemia with normal leucocytes and platelets and grossly reduced or absent erythroblasts in the marrow (Fig. 22.3). The congenital form is known as Diamond–Blackfan syndrome (Table 22.3) and is inherited as a recessive condition. It is associated with a varying number of somatic disorders (e.g. of the face or heart). Mutation of a gene on chromosome 19 or other genes that encode ribosomal proteins underlies most cases (Fig. 22.3). Corticosteriods are the first line of treatment and SCT may be curative. Androgens may also produce improvement but side-effects on growth can be severe.

The acquired chronic form can occur without any obvious associated disease or precipitating factor (idiopathic), or may be seen with autoimmune diseases (especially systemic lupus erythematosus), with a thymoma, lymphoma or chronic lymphocytic leukaemia (CLL). Red cell aplasia from anti-erythropoietin antibodies has been rarely described in patients with chronic renal failure receiving recombinant erythropoietin. In some cases, immunosuppression with corticosteroids, ciclosporin, azathioprine or ALG is helpful. Thymectomy may help in those with a thymoma, and treatment of the underlying disease may help cases secondary to lymphoma or CLL. Monoclonal

Table 22.3 Classification of pure red cell aplasia.

Acute, transient	Chronic congenital	Chronic acquired
Parvovirus infection Drugs (e.g. azathioprine, co-trimoxazole) Idiopathic in infancy and childhood	Diamond–Blackfan syndrome	Idiopathic Associated with thymoma, systemic lupus erythematosus, rheumatoid arthritis, lymphoma, chronic lymphocytic leukaemia, T-large granular lymphocytosis, myelodysplasia, viral infection, drugs

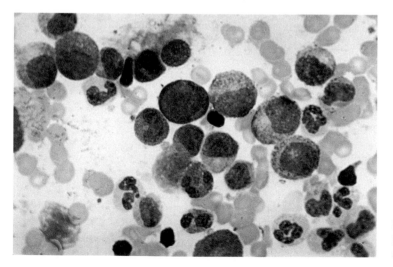

Figure 22.4 The bone marrow in primary red cell aplasia. There is selective loss of erythropoiesis.

antibodies (e.g. Campath (anti-CD52) or rituximab (anti-CD20)) are being increasingly used in treatment of refractory acquired red cell aplasia and other autoimmune cytopenias.

If regular blood transfusions are needed, iron chelation therapy will also be necessary. SCT has been carried out in some severe cases.

Transient

Parvovirus B19 infects red cell precursors via the P antigen and causes a transient (5–10 days) red cell aplasia with the rapid onset of severe anaemia in patients with pre-existing shortened red cell survival (e.g. sickle cell disease or hereditary spherocytosis; Fig. 22.4). Transient red cell aplasia with anaemia may also occur in association with drug therapy (Table 22.3), and in normal infants or children, often with a history of a viral infection in the preceding 3 months.

Shwachman–Diamond syndrome

This is a rare autosomal recessive syndrome characterized by varying degrees of cytopenia, especially neutropenia with a propensity to transform to myelodysplasia or acute myeloid leukaemia. Exocrine pancreatic dysfunction is an invariable feature while skeletal abnormalities, hepatic impairment and short stature are frequent. The gene SBDS, involved in ribosome synthesis, shows mutations (Fig. 22.3).

Congenital dyserythropoietic anaemia

Congenital dyserythropoietic anaemias (CDAs) are a group of hereditary refractory anaemias characterized by ineffective erythropoiesis and erythroblast multinuclearity. The patient may be jaundiced with bone marrow expansion. The white cell and platelet counts are normal. The reticulocyte count is low for the degree of anaemia, despite increased marrow cellularity. The anaemia is of variable severity and is usually first noted in infancy or childhood. Iron overload may develop and splenomegaly is common. The CDAs have been classified into four types based on the degree to which megaloblastic changes, giant erythroblasts and dyserythropoietic changes are

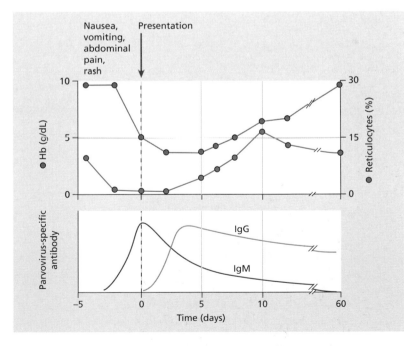

Figure 22.5 Parvovirus infection: flow chart showing transient fall in haemoglobin and reticulocytes in a patient with hereditary spherocytosis.

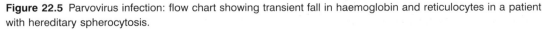

present. CDA1 is associated with somatic abnormalities. It is caused by mutation of the gene *CDAN1* or chromosome 15q15 active during the S phase of the cell cycle. Type II is known as HEMPAS, hereditary erythroblast multinuclearity with a positive acidified serum lysis test, with some sera but not the patient's serum. The basic lesion in HEMPAS is a mutation of the gene *SEC23B* at 20q coding for a protein involved in synthesis of endoplasmic reticulum derived vesicles destined for the Golgi compartment. α-Interferon has induced remission in some cases.

SUMMARY

- Aplastic anaemia presents as pancytopenia (subnormal haemoglobin, neutrophils and platelets) associated with a hypoplastic bone marrow.
- Aplastic anaemia may be congenital (Fanconi) or acquired (idiopathic or due to drugs, viral infection or toxins).
- Fanconi anaemia is autosomal recessive, associated with congenital skeletal, skin or renal abnormalities. It is caused by inherited mutations of genes involved in DNA repair.
- Acquired aplastic anaemia is treated with immunosuppressive drugs (e.g. antilymphocyte globulin, ciclosporin or by stem cell transplantation.

- Red cell aplasia causes anaemia with normal white cell and platelet counts. It may be transient, usually caused by parvovirus infection, or chronic. This may be congenital (Diamond–Blackfan) or acquired associated with, e.g. systemic lupus erythematosus, lymphoma or chronic lymphocytic leukaemia.
- Congenital dyserythropoietic anaemias are a group of rare inherited disorders of erythropoiesis.

Now visit www.wiley.com/go/essentialhaematology to test yourself on this chapter.

CHAPTER 23
Stem cell transplantation

Key topics

Essential Haematology, 6th Edition. © A. V. Hoffbrand and P. A. H. Moss. Published 2011 by Blackwell Publishing Ltd.

Principles of stem cell transplantation

Stem cell transplantation (SCT) involves eliminating a patient's haemopoietic and immune system by chemotherapy and/or radiotherapy and replacing it with stem cells either from another individual or with a previously harvested portion of the patient's own haemopoietic stem cells (Fig. 23.1). The term encompasses **bone marrow transplantation** (BMT), in which stem cells are collected from bone marrow, **peripheral blood stem cell** (PBSC) **transplantation** and umbilical cord stem cell transplantation.

SCT may be **syngeneic** (from an identical twin), **allogeneic** (from another person) or **autologous** (from the patient's own stem cells) (Table 23.1).

The principal diseases for which SCT is performed are listed in Table 23.2. However, the exact role of SCT in the management of each disease is complex and depends on factors such as disease severity and subtype, remission status, age and, for allogeneic transplantation, availability of a donor.

Collection of stem cells

Stem cells can be collected from the peripheral blood, bone marrow or umbilical cord blood.

Peripheral blood stem cell collection

PBSCs are taken using a cell-separator machine connected to the patient or donor via peripheral cannulae (Fig. 23.2). Blood is taken through one cannula and pumped around the machine where mononuclear cells are collected by centrifugation before the red cells are returned to the patient. This continuous process may take a few hours before enough mononuclear cells are collected.

Peripheral blood normally contains too few haemopoietic stem cells to allow collection of sufficient numbers for transplantation. Chemotherapy and growth factors can each increase the number by around 10–100 times. Chemotherapy is used in patients undergoing autologous stem cell collection but not in healthy donors. PBSCs are usually collected during the recovery phase from a cycle of chemotherapy (e.g. $1.5\,g/m^2$ cyclophosphamide). In

Table 23.1 Stem cell transplantation: potential donors.

HLA-matching sibling	Allogeneic
Unrelated HLA-matching volunteer	
Umbilical cord blood	
Identical twin	Syngeneic
Self	Autologous

HLA, human leucocyte antigen.

Table 23.2 Stem cell transplantation: indications.

Allogeneic (or syngeneic)	Autologous
Acute lymphoblastic or myeloid leukaemia. Other malignant disorders of the marrow (e.g. chronic myeloid leukaemia, myelodysplasia, multiple myeloma, lymphoma, severe aplastic anaemia including Fanconi's anaemia)	Hodgkin lymphoma and non-Hodgkin lymphoma, multiple myeloma, AML, primary amyloidosis
Inherited disorders: thalassaemia major, sickle cell anaemia, immune deficiencies, inborn errors of metabolism in the haemopoietic and mesenchymal system (e.g. osteopetrosis) Other acquired severe marrow diseases (e.g. paroxysmal nocturnal haemoglobinuria, red cell aplasia, myelofibrosis)	

AML, acute myeloid leukaemia.

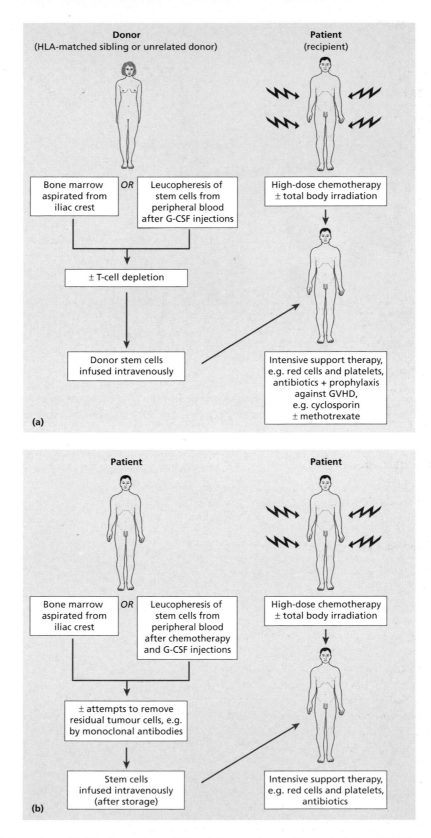

Figure 23.1 Procedures for **(a)** allogeneic, and **(b)** autologous stem cell transplantation. G-CSF, granulocyte colony-stimulating factor; GVHD, graft-versus-host disease; HLA, human leucocyte antigen. For non-myeloblative (reduced intensity) allogeneic SCT, lower doses of chemotherapy with or without radiotherapy are used.

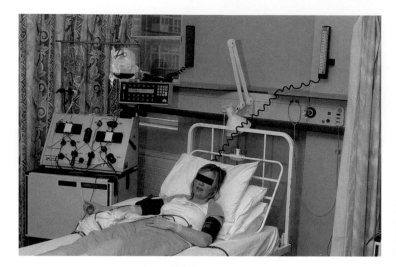

Figure 23.2 Peripheral blood stem cell (PBSC) collection: a donor undergoing collection of PBSCs on a cell separator.

future it is possible that stem cell populations may also be expanded *in vitro*.

Granulocyte colony-stimulating factor (G-CSF) is given to patients or donors as a course of injections (typically 10 μg/kg/day for 4–6 days) until the white cell count starts to rise. PBSC collections are then taken and, depending on the efficiency of stem cell mobilization, repeated collections may be needed for up to 3 days. The adequacy of the collection may be assessed by:

1 CD34$^+$ cell count. Generally >2.0 × 10^6/kg are needed for transplantation.
2 *In vitro* colony assays, particularly granulocyte–macrophage colony-forming unit (CFU-GM) (see p. 3), of which 1–5 × 10^5/kg would be considered adequate for transplantation.

Bone marrow collection

The donor is given a general anaesthetic and 500–1200 mL marrow is harvested from the pelvis. The marrow is anticoagulated and a mononuclear cell count is taken to assess the yield, which should be approximately 2–4 × 10^8 nucleated cells/kg body weight of the recipient.

Umbilical cord blood

Fetal blood is a rich source of haemopoietic stem cells which may be collected from cord blood.

Because of the relatively small numbers of stem cells collected from a single cord, they are most useful for children who do not have a fully matching sibling or unrelated donor. Less stringent human leucocyte antigen (HLA) matching is needed. Double cord donations may be needed to obtain sufficient stem cells for adult recipients.

Stem cell processing

After collection the stem cell harvest can be processed with removal of red cells and concentration of the mononuclear cells. Autologous collections may be 'purged' by chemotherapy or antibodies in an attempt to remove residual malignant cells. Allogeneic collections may be treated with antibodies to remove T cells to reduce graft-versus-host disease (GVHD). CD34$^+$ stem cells may be selected from both types of harvest (Fig. 23.3).

Conditioning

Prior to infusion of haemopoietic stem cells patients receive chemotherapy, sometimes in combination with total body irradiation (TBI; Fig. 23.1) in a procedure called ***conditioning***. This is designed to eradicate the patient's haemopoietic and immune system and, if present, malignancy. In addition, in the setting of allogeneic SCT, by suppressing the host immune system it helps to prevent rejection of

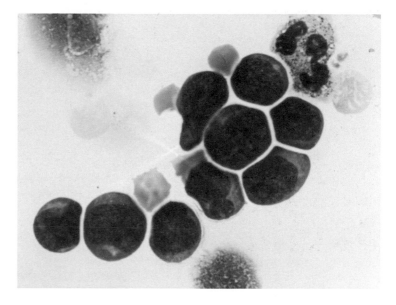

Figure 23.3 Peripheral blood stem cell collection: enriched CD34⁺ cells stained by May–Grünwald-Giemsa stain. The cells have the appearance of small- and medium-sized lymphocytes.

the 'foreign' stem cells. An important development that has occurred in SCT is a major shift from **myeloablative** regimens to **non-myeloablative** conditioning.

Myeloablative conditioning regimens irreversibly destroy the haemopoietic function of the bone marrow with high doses of chemotherapy or radiotherapy. TBI is usually used in patients with malignant disease and is administered as a single dose or in smaller doses over several days (*fractionated*). The most commonly used chemotherapy drug is cyclophosphamide but busulfan, melphalan, cytosine arabinoside, etoposide or nitrosoureas are given in some protocols. At least 36 hours are allowed for the elimination of the drugs from the circulation following the last dose of chemotherapy before donor stem cells are infused. Conditioning therapy is often complicated by mucositis and patients sometimes need parenteral nutrition. Trials are taking place in which monoclonal antibodies directed against specific antigens such as CD45 are attached to toxins or radioactive isotopes in an attempt to selectively target white cells as an aid to conditioning.

Non-myeloablative conditioning regimens have been developed to reduce the morbidity and mortality of allogeneic transplantation and do not completely destroy the host bone marrow. These can include agents such as fludarabine, low-dose irradiation, antilymphocyte globulin or other antibodies that delete T cells, and low doses of busulfan or cyclophosphamide. The aim in these 'mini- or reduced-intensity-transplants' is to use enough immunosuppression to allow donor stem cells to engraft without completely eradicating host marrow stem cells. Donor leucocyte infusions (DLI) are commonly used at a late stage in order to encourage complete donor engraftment. Such regimens extend the age range and increase the treatment indications for allogeneic transplantation.

Post-transplant engraftment and immunity

After a period of typically 1–3 weeks of severe pancytopenia, the first signs of successful engraftment are monocytes and neutrophils in the blood with a subsequent increase in platelet count (Fig. 23.4). A reticulocytosis also begins and natural killer (NK) cells are among the earliest donor-derived lymphocytes to appear. G-CSF may be used to reduce the period of neutropenia. Engraftment is usually quicker following PBSC transplantation than BMT.

The marrow cellularity gradually returns to normal but the marrow reserve remains impaired

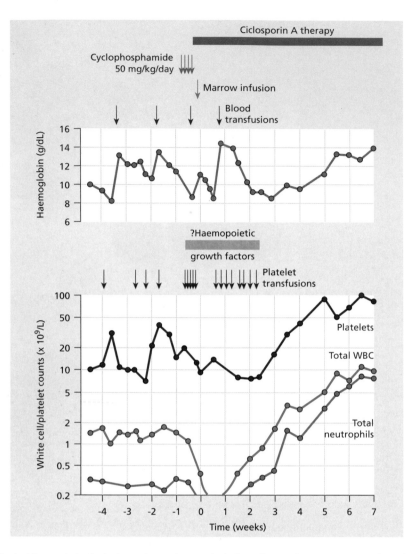

Figure 23.4 Typical haematological chart of a patient undergoing allogeneic marrow transplantation for aplastic anaemia. WBC, white blood cells.

for 1–2 years. There is profound immunodeficiency for 3–12 months with a low level of CD4 helper cells and a raised CD8:CD4 ratio for 6 months or more. Immune recovery is quicker after autologous and syngeneic SCT than following allogeneic SCT. The patient's blood group changes to that of the donor and antigen-specific immunity becomes that of the donor after approximately 60 days.

Autologous stem cell transplantation

This allows the delivery of a high dose of chemotherapy, with or without radiotherapy, which otherwise would result in prolonged bone marrow aplasia. Stem cells are harvested and stored before the treatment is given and are then reinfused to 'rescue' the patient from the myeloablative effects of the treatment (Fig. 23.1). A limitation of the procedure is that tumour cells contaminating the stem cell harvest may be reintroduced into the patient. Nevertheless, autografting has a major role in the treatment of haematological diseases such as lymphoma and myeloma. The major problem associated with autografting is recurrence of the original disease. GVHD is not an issue. Procedure-related mortality is generally well below 5%.

Allogeneic stem cell transplantation

In this procedure, stem cells harvested from another person are infused into the patient. The procedure has a significant morbidity and mortality and one of the major reasons is the immunological incompatibility between donor and patient despite HLA matching. This may manifest as immunodeficiency, GVHD or graft failure. Paradoxically, there is also a graft-versus-leukaemia (GVL) effect which probably underlies much of the success of the procedure.

The human leucocyte antigen system

Allografting would be impossible without the ability to perform HLA typing. The short arm of chromosome 6 contains a cluster of genes known as the major histocompatibility complex (MHC) or the HLA region (Fig. 23.5a). Genes in this region encode the HLA antigens and many other molecules including complement components, tumour necrosis factor (TNF) and proteins associated with antigen processing. HLA proteins are divided into two types: class I and II (Table 23.3). Their role is to bind intracellular peptides and 'present' these to T lymphocytes for antigen recognition (see Chapter 9). Class I molecules (HLA-A, -B and -C) present antigen to $CD8^+$ T cells and class II molecules (HLA-DR, -DQ and -DP) present to $CD4^+$ T cells (Fig. 23.5b).

Class I antigens are present on most nucleated cells and on the cell surface they are associated with β_2-microglobulin. Class II antigens have a more restricted tissue distribution and comprise α and β

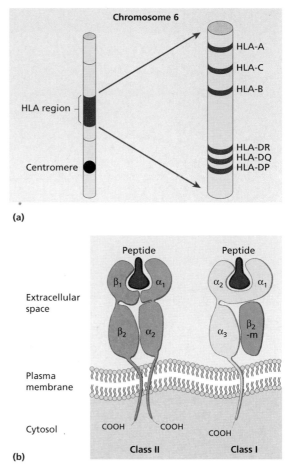

Figure 23.5 **(a)** The human leucocyte antigen (HLA) complex. **(b)** HLA class I and II molecules showing protein domains and bound peptide.

chains, both encoded by genes in the HLA region. The inheritance of the four loci (HLA-A, -B, -C and -DR) is closely linked, one set of loci is inherited from each parent so that there is approximately a one in four chance of two siblings having identical HLA antigens (Fig. 23.6a). Crossing-over of genes during meiosis accounts for occasional unexpected disparities. The inheritance is independent of sex or blood group.

Table 23.3 The human leucocyte antigens (HLA).

	Class I	Class II
Antigens	HLA-A, -B, -C	HLA-DR, -DP, -DQ
Distribution	All nucleated cells, platelets	B lymphocytes Monocytes Macrophages Activated T cells
Structure	Large polypeptide chain (MHC coded) and a β_2-microglobulin	Two polypeptide chains (α and β) both MHC coded
Interacts with	CD8 lymphocytes	CD4 lymphocytes

MHC, major histocompatibility complex.

Human leucocyte antigen and transplantation

The natural role of HLA molecules is in directing T-lymphocyte responses and the greater the HLA mismatch the more severe is the immune response between transplanted cells. HLA typing is critical in donor selection for allogeneic SCT.

Minor histocompatibility antigens are peptides that are presented by HLA molecules and are able to act as antigens in SCT either because (e.g. HA-1, HA-2) they are polymorphic in the population or because they are encoded on the Y chromosome and therefore represent novel antigens when a female immune system engrafts in a male. They are likely to be important antigens in GVHD and the GVL reaction (see below).

HLA typing may be carried out by serological or molecular techniques. Serological testing involves the use of antibodies that are specific for individual HLA alleles or small families of alleles. Positivity may be detected by direct binding of a labelled antibody or by the use of complement to kill target cells that bind antibody (the two-stage lymphocytotoxicity test).

Molecular testing is performed with DNA primers or probes that react with polymorphic sequence motifs present within the nucleotide sequence of the *HLA* allele.

The nomenclature for *HLA* alleles is now standardized. A single antigenic specificity (gene) defined by serological typing (e.g. *HLA-A*) can be divided into different alleles by DNA sequencing. Each allele is given in numerical designation. The gene name is followed by an asterisk. The first two subsequent digits indicate the allele group. The third and fourth digits list subtypes. Subsequent digits indicate minor differences in non-coding regions. As an example, alleles at the *HLA-A* loci are written as *HLA-A*01:01* to *HLA-A*80:01*. The type often corresponds to the serological antigen carried by the alleles (e.g. HLA-A2 for the *HLA-A*02:01* to *HLA-A*02:30* alleles). The nomenclature for the class II genes is similar but complicated by the fact that there may be more than one *HLA-DRB* gene on each chromosome (Fig. 23.6b).

When searching for an unrelated donor the aim is to match HLA alleles between recipient and donor and this is then called a 10/10 match based on A, B, C, DRB1 and DQB1 matching. An exception is when a donor with only a single HLA haplotype match, usually a parent or sibling, is used in a ***haploidentical SCT***. Such transplants usually require a stem cell graft that is heavily depleted of T cells in order to limit the development of GVHD. There are over 14 million volunteer donors on international registries and the chance of identifying a matched unrelated donor for a patient lacking an HLA identical sibling (depending on the ethnic group) is usually greater than 50%.

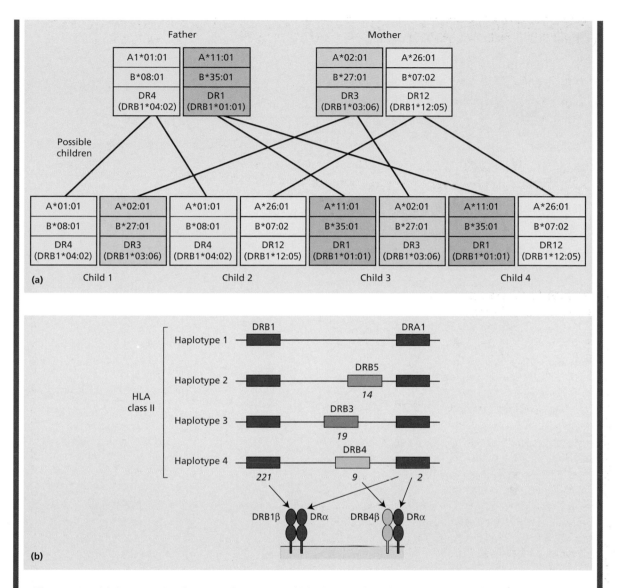

Figure 23.6 (a) An example of the possible pattern of inheritance of the A, B and DR (*DRB1*) series alleles of the human leucocyte antigen (HLA) complex. **(b)** Molecular genetics of the HLA class II gene complex. There are four major haplotypes of major histocompatibility complex (MHC) class II genes in the population and each individual may have up to two (one on each chromosome). The *DRA1* gene codes for the DRα protein and the *DRB1*, *DRB3*, *DRB4* and *DRB5* genes encode DRβ chains. Expression from the *DRB1* gene is higher than from the other genes. The number of alleles at each gene is shown underneath the gene in italics. Alleles at each locus have a standard nomenclature (e.g. the alleles at the *DRB1* gene are termed *DRB1*01:01* to *DRB1*16:08*). It is now known that the DR51, DR52 and DR53 antigens, which are defined by serological testing, are encoded from the *DRB5*, *DRB4* and *DRB3* genes, respectively.

Chimerism analysis

Following allogeneic SCT, the recipient's blood shows the presence of both donor and recipient cells (chimerism). This can be by fluorescence *in situ* hybridization (FISH) analysis of the proportion of Y chromosome containing cells if there is a sex mismatch or by DNA analysis techniques.

Complications (Table 23.4)

Graft-versus-host disease

This is caused by donor-derived immune cells, particularly T lymphocytes, reacting against recipient tissues. Its incidence is increased with increasing age of donor and recipient and if there is any degree of HLA mismatch between them. GVHD prophylaxis is usually given as ciclosporin (intravenously or orally or tacrolimus for 6–12 months) and methotrexate (three or four injections). An alternative is to remove T cells from the donor stem cell infusion. In addition, anti-T-cell antibodies may be given to the patient.

In **acute GVHD**, usually occurring in the first 100 days, the skin, gastrointestinal tract or liver are affected (Table 23.5). The skin rash typically affects the face, palms, soles and ears but may in severe cases affect the whole body (Fig. 23.7). Diarrhoea may lead to fluid and electrolyte depletion. Typically, bilirubin and alkaline phosphatase are raised but the other hepatic enzymes are relatively normal. Acute GVHD is usually treated by high doses of corticosteroids which are effective in the majority of cases.

In **chronic GVHD**, which usually occurs after 100 days and may evolve from acute GVHD,

these tissues are involved but also the joints and other serosal surfaces, the oral mucosa and lacrimal glands. Features of scleroderma, Sjögren's syndrome and lichen planus may develop. The immune system is impaired (including hyposplenism) with risk of

Table 23.4 Complications of stem cell transplantation.

Early (usually <100 days)	Late (usually >100 days)
Infections, especially bacterial, fungal, herpes simplex virus, CMV	Infections, especially varicella-zoster, capsulate bacteria
Haemorrhage	Chronic pattern GVHD (arthritis, malabsorption, hepatitis, scleroderma, sicca syndrome, lichen planus, pulmonary disease, serous effusions)
Acute pattern GVHD (skin, liver, gut)	Chronic pulmonary disease
Graft failure	Autoimmune disorders
Haemorrhagic cystitis	Cataract
Interstitial pneumonitis	Infertility
Others: veno-occlusive disease, cardiac failure	Second malignancies

CMV, cytomegalovirus; GVHD, graft-versus-host disease.

Table 23.5 Acute pattern graft-versus-host disease: clinical staging (Seattle system).

Stage	Skin	Liver (bilirubin, μmol/L)	Gut (diarrhoea, L/day)
I	Rash <25%	20–35	0.5–1.0
II	Rash 25–50%	35–80	1.0–1.5
III	Erythroderma	80–150	1.5–2.5
IV	Bullae, desquamation	>150	>2.5; severe pain, ileus

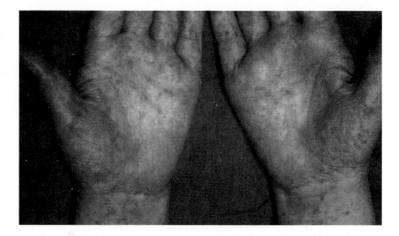

Figure 23.7 Widespread erythematous skin rash in acute graft-versus-host disease following bone marrow transplantation.

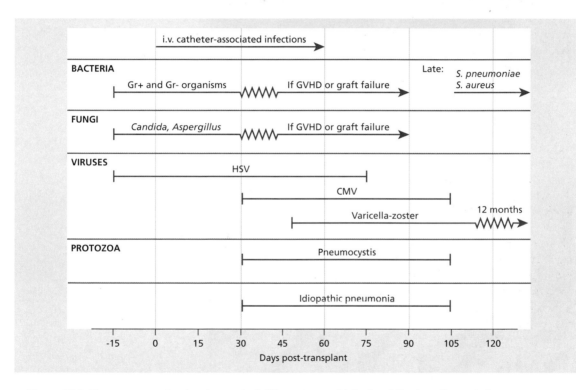

Figure 23.8 Time sequence for development of different types of infection following allogeneic bone marrow transplantation. CMV, cytomegalovirus; Gr+, Gr–, Gram-positive or -negative; GVHD, graft-versus-host disease; HSV, herpes simplex virus.

infection. Malabsorption and pulmonary abnormalities are frequent. Drugs such as ciclosporin, corticosteroids, mycophenolate mofetil or thalidomide are used although response may be poor.

Infections

In the early post-transplant period, bacterial or fungal infections are frequent (Fig. 23.8). These may be reduced by barrier nursing, the use of skin and mouth antiseptics and treatment in units with high efficiency particulate (HEPAR) air filtration. Prophylactic therapy with aciclovir, antifungal agents and oral antibiotics is often added. If a fever or other evidence of an infection occurs, broad-spectrum intravenous antibiotics are commenced immediately after blood cultures and other appropriate microbiological specimens have been taken. Failure of response to antibacterial agents is usually an indication to commence systemic antifungal therapy with amphotericin B, caspofungin or voriconazole (see p. 171). Fungal infections, especially *Candida* and *Aspergillus* species (Fig. 23.9), are a particular problem because of the prolonged neutropenia.

Viral infections, particularly with the herpes group of viruses, are frequent with herpes simplex, cytomegalovirus (CMV) and varicella zoster virus

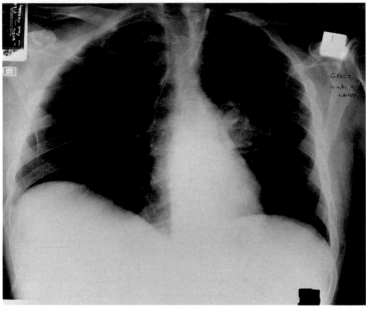

(a)

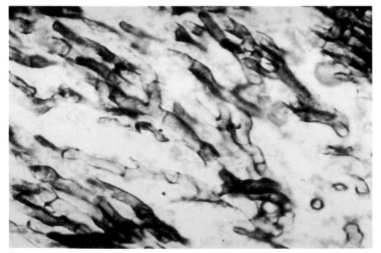

(b)

Figure 23.9 (a) Chest radiograph showing an aspergilloma in a patient following stem cell transplantation. **(b)** Cytology of sputum illustrates the branching septate hyphae of *Aspergillus* (methenamine silver stain).

(VZV) occurring at different peak intervals (Fig. 23.8).

CMV presents a particular threat and is associated with a potentially fatal interstitial pneumonitis as well as with hepatitis and falling blood counts. The infection may be caused by reactivation of CMV in the recipient or a new infection transmitted by the donor. In CMV-seronegative patients with CMV-seronegative donors, CMV-negative blood products or leucodepleted blood must be given. Aciclovir may be useful in prophylaxis. Most centres screen patients regularly for evidence of CMV reactivation following allogeneic transplantation using polymerase chain reaction (PCR) or antibody-based tests. If these tests become positive, ganciclovir may suppress the virus before disease occurs. Ganciclovir, valganciclovir and foscarnet may be used for established CMV infection.

VZV infection is also frequent post-SCT but occurs later with a median onset at 4–5 months. Rarely, disseminated VZV infection occurs. Intravenous aciclovir is indicated. Epstein–Barr virus (EBV) infections and EBV-associated lymphoproliferative disease are less frequent after SCT than after solid organ transplants.

Pneumocystis carinii is another cause of pneumonitis that may be prevented by prophylactic co-trimoxazole or pentamidine inhalations.

Interstitial pneumonitis

This is one of the most frequent causes of death post-SCT (Fig. 23.10). CMV is a frequent agent

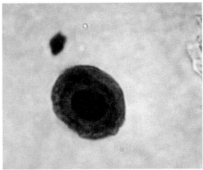

(b)

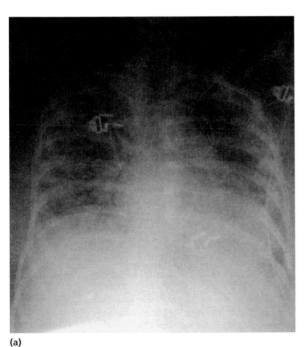

(a)

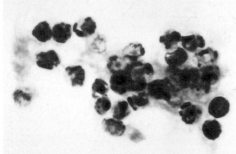

(c)

Figure 23.10 (a) Chest radiograph showing interstitial pneumonitis following bone marrow transplantation. Widespread diffuse mottling can be seen. The patient had received total body irradiation and had grade III graft-versus-host disease. No infective cause of the pneumonitis was identified. Possible causes include pneumocystis, cytomegalovirus (CMV), herpes zoster, fungal infection or a combination of these. **(b)** Sputum cytology: intranuclear CMV inclusion body in a pulmonary cell. Papanicolaou stain. **(c)** *Pneumocystis carinii* in bronchial washings, Gram–Weigert stain.

but other herpes viruses and *P. carinii* account for other cases; in most cases, no cause other than the previous radiation and chemotherapy can be implicated. Bronchoalveolar lavage or open lung biopsy may be needed to establish the diagnosis.

Blood product support

Platelet concentrates are given to maintain a count of 10×10^9/L or more. Platelets and blood transfusions given in the post-transplant period must be irradiated prior to administration in order to kill any lymphocytes that might cause GVHD.

Other complications of allogeneic transplantation

Graft failure

The risk of graft failure is increased if the patient has aplastic anaemia or if T-cell depletion of donor marrow is used as GVHD prophylaxis. This suggests that donor T cells are needed to overcome host resistance to engraftment of stem cells.

Haemorrhagic cystitis

This is usually caused by the cyclophosphamide metabolite acrolein. Mesna is given in an attempt to prevent this. Certain viruses (e.g. adenovirus or polyomavirus) may also cause this complication.

Other complications

These include veno-occlusive disease of the liver (manifest as jaundice, hepatomegaly and ascites or weight gain) and cardiac failure as a result of the conditioning regimen (especially high doses of cyclophosphamide) and previous chemotherapy on the heart. Haemolysis because of ABO incompatibility between donor and recipient may cause problems in the first weeks. Microangiopathic haemolytic anaemia may also occur.

Late complications

Relapse of the original disease (e.g. acute or chronic leukaemia) may occur. Bacterial infections are frequent, especially with encapsulated organisms affecting the respiratory tract. Oral penicillin is given prophylactically to reduce this risk. VZV and fungal infections are also frequent. The use of prophylactic co-trimoxazole and oral aciclovir for 3–6 months reduces the risk of *Pneumocystis* and herpes infections, respectively.

Delayed pulmonary complications include restrictive pneumonitis and bronchiolitis obliterans. Endocrine complications include hypothyroidism, growth failure in children, impaired sexual development and infertility. These endocrine problems are more marked if TBI has been used. Clinically apparent autoimmune disorders are infrequent and include myasthenia, rheumatoid arthritis, anaemia, thrombocytopenia or neutropenia. Autoantibodies are frequently detected in the absence of symptoms. Second malignancies (especially non-Hodgkin lymphoma) occur with a six- or sevenfold incidence compared with controls. CNS complications include neuropathies and eye problems caused by chronic GVHD (sicca syndrome) or cataracts.

Graft-versus-leukaemia effect and donor leucocyte infusions

After allogeneic transplantation the donor immune system helps to eradicate the patient's leukaemia, a phenomenon known as the **graft-versus-leukaemia** effect. Evidence includes the decreased relapse rate in patients with GVHD, the increased relapse rate in identical twins and, most convincingly, the ability of **donor leucocyte infusions** to cure relapsed leukaemia in some patients. Graft-versus-lymphoma and graft-versus-myeloma effects also exist. The principle of DLI is that peripheral blood mononuclear cells are collected from the original allograft donor and directly infused into the patient at the time of leukaemia relapse (Fig. 23.11).

There is a large difference in the outcome of different diseases treated by DLI. Chronic myeloid leukaemia (CML) is most sensitive whereas acute lymphoblastic leukaemia rarely responds. In CML the response to DLI is better in cases of early relapse. PCR is used to monitor serial blood

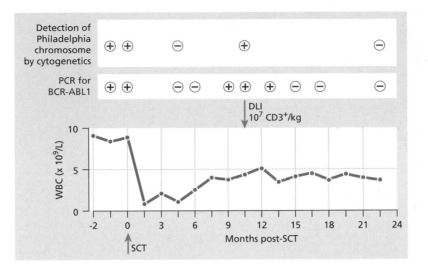

Figure 23.11 Donor leucocyte infusions. Example of donor leucocyte infusion (DLI) in the treatment of chronic myeloid leukaemia (CML) which relapsed following allogeneic stem cell transplantation (SCT). Polymerase chain reaction (PCR) analysis of the blood for the BCR-ABL1 transcript shows that there was transient loss of the transcript but molecular and cytogenetic relapse occurred at 10 months. One infusion of donor leucocytes led to re-establishment of a durable complete remission.

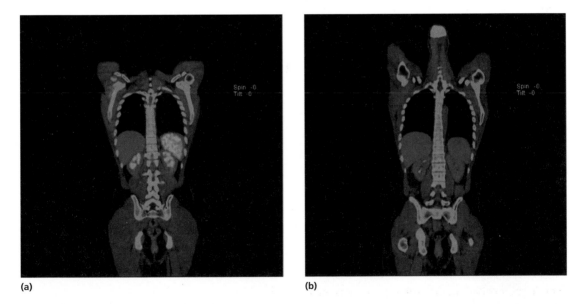

(a) (b)

Figure 23.12 Example of disease control following administration of a donor leucocyte infusion (DLI) after stem cell transplantation. **(a)** A PET scan revealed residual disease activity in a patient at 6 months following allogeneic transplantation for non-Hodgkin lymphoma. The bright signals reflect the metabolic activity of malignant cells in the spleen and axillary lymph nodes. Donor leucocyte infusion was then given and after 3 months a repeat PET scan **(b)** revealed no evidence of residual disease. (Image with kind permission of Professor Nigel Russell.)

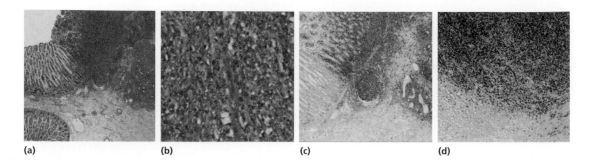

(a) (b) (c) (d)

Figure 23.13 Post-transplantation lymphoproliferative diseases: 17-year-old male 5 months after renal transplantation had small bowel perforation caused by diffuse large B-cell lymphoma. **(a)** Low-power view of lymphoid mass invading small bowel. **(b)** High-power view of lymphoid mass. **(c)** Immunostaining for CD20. **(d)** EBV-ISH (*in situ* hybridization) stain showing the tumour cells are positive for Epstein–Barr virus (EBV). (Courtesy of Professor P. Amrolia and Dr N. Sebire.)

samples for evidence of recurrence of the *BCR-ABL1* transcript before karyotypic or clinical relapse occurs (Fig. 23.11). DLI can then be used in cases of molecular relapse. The response to DLI may take several weeks but usually results in a permanent cure. The mechanism is unclear but a T-cell-mediated alloreactive immune response is likely to be a major component. Positron emission tomography (PET) scans are now being used to detect the presence of residual disease and can be used to guide both the requirement for DLI and also determining the disease response (Fig. 23.12).

Post-transplant lymphoproliferative diseases

These are polyclonal or monoclonal lymphoid proliferations that occur in recipients of stem cell or more frequently solid organ allografts, as a result of the intensive immunosupression. They may be EBV driven and are usually of B-cell origin. There is often involvement of bowel, lung or bone marrow (Fig. 23.13). Treatment is by reduction of immunosupression (if feasible), anti-CD20 (rituximab) and, if appropriate, chemotherapy or cytotoxic T cells engineered to kill the EBV+ tumour cells.

SUMMARY

- Stem cell transplantation (SCT) involves replacing the haemopoietic and immune systems by stem cells from either the same subject (autologous) or another individual (allogeneic). The donor stem cells can be harvested from bone marrow, peripheral blood or umbilical cord.
- Autologous SCT is most frequently performed for lymphomas or myeloma.
- For allogeneic SCT the recipient's own haemopoietic and immune systems are eliminated by chemotherapy, radiotherapy and monoclonal antibodies.

- Allogeneic SCT requires a tissue (HLA) matching sibling or unrelated donor. The human leukocyte antigens (HLA) are coded for by genes on chromosome 6. They are extremely polymorphic and are involved in presentation of antigens to T lymphocytes.
- Allogeneic SCT is indicated in selected cases of acute leukaemia, other malignant bone marrow diseases, and severe acquired or genetic marrow diseases (e.g. aplastic anaemia, thalassaemia major). Reduced intensity conditioning SCT may be preferred in older subjects.

- Donor leucocyte infusions may be given to cure relapse of leukaemia post-allogeneic SCT, by a 'graft-versus-leukaemia' effect.
- Early complications of allogeneic SCT include graft-versus-host disease (which may be acute or chronic), infections, graft failure and veno-occlusive disease. Long-term complications include damage to many different organs (e.g. skin, heart, lungs and liver) and post-transplant lymphoproliferative disease.

Now visit www.wiley.com/go/essentialhaematology to test yourself on this chapter.

CHAPTER 24

Platelets, blood coagulation and haemostasis

Key topics

Essential Haematology, 6th Edition. © A. V. Hoffbrand and P. A. H. Moss. Published 2011 by Blackwell Publishing Ltd.

The normal haemostatic response to vascular damage depends on a closely linked interaction between the blood vessel wall, circulating platelets and blood coagulation factors (Fig. 24.1).

An efficient and rapid mechanism for stopping bleeding from sites of blood vessel injury is clearly essential for survival. Nevertheless, such a response needs to be tightly controlled to prevent extensive clots developing and to break down such clots once damage is repaired. The haemostatic system thus represents a delicate balance between procoagulant and anticoagulant mechanisms allied to a process for fibrinolysis. The five major components involved are platelets, coagulation factors, coagulation inhibitors, fibrinolysis and blood vessels. These are described later in the haemostatic response section on p. 324.

Components of the haemostatic response

Platelets

Platelet production

Platelets are produced in the bone marrow by fragmentation of the cytoplasm of megakaryocytes, one of the largest cells in the body. The precursor of the megakaryocyte – the megakaryoblast – arises by a process of differentiation from the haemopoietic stem cell (see Fig. 1.2). The megakaryocyte matures by endomitotic synchronous replication (i.e. DNA replication in the absence of nuclear or cytoplasmic division) enlarging the cytoplasmic volume as the number of nuclear lobes increase in multiples of

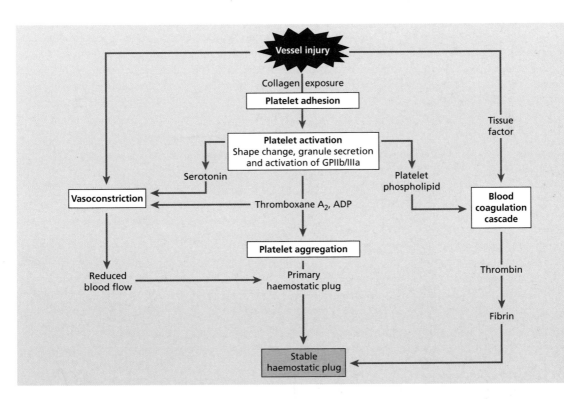

Figure 24.1 The involvement of blood vessels, platelets and blood coagulation in haemostasis. ADP, adenosine diphosphate.

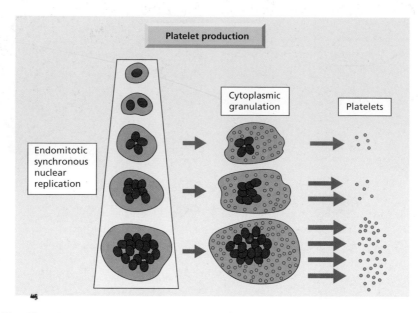

Figure 24.2 Simplified diagram to illustrate platelet production from megakaryocytes.

two (Fig. 24.2). Very early on invaginations of plasma membrane are seen, called the demarcation membrane, which evolves through the development of the megakaryocyte into a highly branched network. At a variable stage in development, most commonly at the eight nucleus stage, the cytoplasm becomes granular. Mature megakaryocytes are extremely large, with an eccentric placed single lobulated nucleus and a low nuclear:cytoplasmic ratio (Fig. 24.3). Platelets form by fragmentation from the tips of cytoplasmic extensions of megakaryocyte cytoplasm, each megakaryocyte giving rise approximately to 1000–5000 platelets (Fig. 24.3c). The time interval from differentiation of the human stem cell to the production of platelets averages 10 days.

Thrombopoietin is the major regulator of platelet production and is constitutively produced by the liver and kidneys. Thrombopoietin increases the number and rate of maturation of megakaryocytes via c-MPL receptor. Platelet levels start to rise 6 days after the start of therapy and remain high for 7–10 days. Although thrombopoietin itself is not available for clinical use, thrombomimetic agents which bind to c-MPL are now used clinically to increase the platelet count (see p. 336). Platelets also have

c-MPL receptors for thrombopoietin and remove it from the circulation. Therefore, levels are high in thrombocytopenia as a result of marrow aplasia but low in patients with raised platelet counts.

The normal platelet count is approximately $250 \times 10^9/L$ (range $150–400 \times 10^9/L$) and the normal platelet lifespan is 7–10 days. This is determined by the ratio of the apoptotic BAX and anti-apoptotic BCL-2 proteins in the cell. Up to one-third of the marrow output of platelets may be trapped at any one time in the normal spleen but this rises to 90% in cases of massive splenomegaly (see Fig. 25.9).

Platelet structure

Platelets are extremely small and discoid, $3.0 \times 0.5\,\mu m$ in diameter, with a mean volume of 7–11 fL. The ultrastructure of platelets is represented in Figure 24.4. The glycoproteins of the surface coat are particularly important in the platelet reactions of adhesion and aggregation which are the initial events leading to platelet plug formation during haemostasis. Adhesion to collagen is facilitated by glycoprotein Ia (GPIa). Glycoproteins Ib (defective in Bernard–Soulier syndrome) and IIb/IIIa (also called αIIb and β3) (defective in

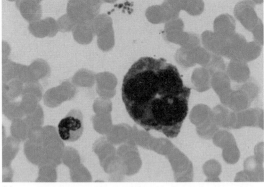

(a)

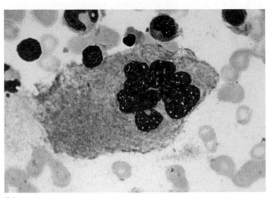

(b)

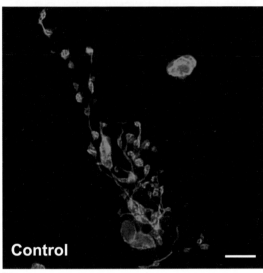

Control

(c)

Figure 24.3 Megakaryocytes: **(a)** immature form with basophilic cytoplasm; **(b)** mature form with many nuclear lobes and pronounced granulation of the cytoplasm. **(c)** Megakaryocyte in culture, stained for α-tubulin (green). Proplatelets can be seen budding from the tips of megakaryocyte cytoplasm. (From Pecci A. et al. (2009) *Thrombosis and Haemostasis* **109**, 90–96, with permission; with thanks to Professor Pecci for Fig. 24.3c.)

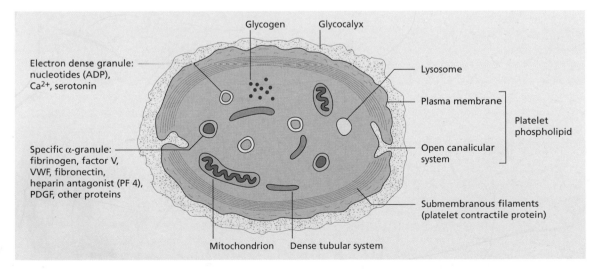

Figure 24.4 The ultrastructure of platelets. ADP, adenosine diphosphate; PDGF, platelet-derived growth factor; PF, platelet factor; VWF, von Willebrand factor.

Glanzmann's thrombasthenia) are important in the attachment of platelets to von Willebrand factor (VWF) and hence to vascular subendothelium (Fig. 24.5) where signalling interactions occur (Fig. 24.6). The binding site for IIb/IIIa is also the receptor for fibrinogen which is important in platelet–platelet aggregation.

The plasma membrane invaginates into the platelet interior to form an open membrane (canalicular) system which provides a large reactive surface to which the plasma coagulation proteins may be selectively absorbed. The membrane phospholipids (previously known as platelet factor 3) are of particular importance in the conversion of coagulation factor X to Xa and prothrombin (factor II) to thrombin (factor IIa) (Fig. 24.7).

The platelet contains three types of storage granules: dense, α and lysosomes (Fig. 24.4). The more frequent specific α granules contain clotting factors, VWF, platelet-derived growth factor (PDGF) and other proteins. Dense granules are less common and contain adenosine diphosphate (ADP), adenosine triphosphate (ATP), serotonin and calcium. Lysosomes contain hydrolytic enzymes. Platelets are also rich in signalling and cytoskeletal proteins which support the rapid switch from quiescent to activation that follows vessel damage. During the

release reaction described below, the contents of the granules are discharged into the open canalicular system.

Platelet antigens

Several platelet surface proteins have been found to be important antigens in platelet-specific autoimmunity and they have been termed human platelet antigens (HPA). In most cases, two different alleles exist, termed a or b alleles (e.g. HPA-1a). Platelets also express ABO and human leucocyte antigen (HLA) class I but not class II antigens.

Platelet function

The main function of platelets is the formation of mechanical plugs during the normal haemostatic response to vascular injury. In the absence of platelets, spontaneous leakage of blood through small vessels may occur. Platelet function falls into three: **adhesion, aggregation** and **release reactions. There is also amplification**. The immobilization of platelets at the sites of vascular injury requires specific platelet–vessel wall (adhesion) and platelet–platelet (aggregation) interactions, both partly mediated through VWF which is discussed next.

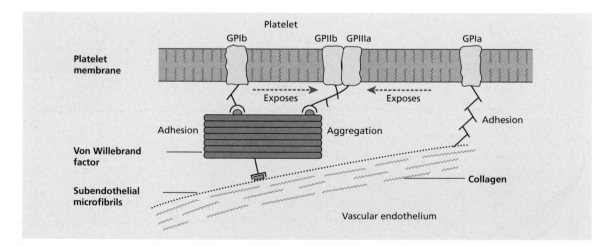

Figure 24.5 Platelet adhesion. The binding of glycoprotein (GP) Ib (which consists of four proteins: GPIbα, GPIbβ, GPIX, GPV) to von Willebrand factor leads to adhesion to the subendothelium and also exposes the GPIIb/IIIa ($\alpha_{IIb}\beta_3$ integrin) binding sites to fibrinogen and von Willebrand factor leading to platelet aggregation. The GPIa site permits direct adhesion to collagen and also explores the GPIIb/IIIa binding site.

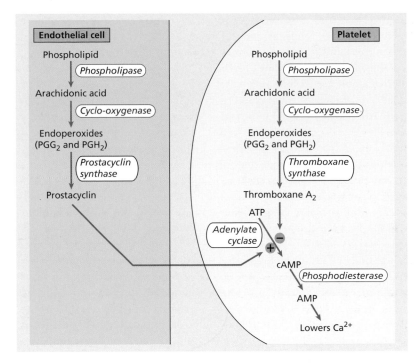

Figure 24.6 The synthesis of prostacyclin and thromboxane A_2. The opposing effects of these agents are mediated by changes in the concentration of cyclic adenosine monophosphate (cAMP) in platelets via stimulation or inhibition of the enzyme adenylate cyclase. cAMP controls the concentration of free calcium ions in the platelet which are important in the processes that cause adhesion and aggregation. High levels of cAMP lead to low free calcium ion concentrations and prevent aggregation and adhesion. ATP, adenosine triphosphate; Ca, calcium; PG, prostaglandin (G_2 and H_2).

Von Willebrand factor

VWF is involved in shear dependent platelet adhesion to the vessel wall (see p. 318) and to other platelets (aggregation) (Fig. 24.5). It also carries factor VIII. It is a large cysteine-rich glycoprotein, with multimers made up on average of 2–50 dimeric subunits, with a molecular weight (MW) range of $0.8–20 \times 10^6$. VWF is encoded by a gene on chromosome 12 and is synthesized both in endothelial cells and megakaryocytes, and stored in Weibel–Palade bodies and platelet α granules, respectively.

Plasma VWF is almost entirely derived from endothelial cells, with two distinct pathways of secretion. The majority is continuously secreted and a minority is stored in Weibel–Palade bodies. The stored VWF can raise the plasma levels when released under the influence of several secretagogues, such as stress, exercise, adrenaline and infusion of desmopressin (1-diamino-8-D-arginine vasopressin; DDAVP). The VWF released from Weibel–Palade bodies is in the form of large and ultra large multimers, the most adhesive and reactive form of VWF. They are in turn cleaved in plasma to smaller multimers and monomeric VWF by the specific plasma metalloprotease, ADAMTS13 (see Fig. 25.7).

Platelet aggregation

This is characterized by cross-linking of platelets through active GPIIb/IIIa receptors with fibrinogen bridges. A resting platelet has about 50–80 000 GPIIb/IIIa receptors, which do not bind fibrinogen, VWF or other ligands. Stimulation of a platelet leads to an increase in GPIIb/IIIa molecules, enabling platelet cross-linking with fibrinogen bridges.

Platelet release reaction and amplification

Primary activation by various agonists induces intracellular signalling, leading to the release of α granule contents. These have an important role in platelet aggregate formation and stabilization and, in addition, the ADP released from dense granules has a major positive feedback role in promoting platelet activation.

Thromboxane A_2 (TXA2) is the second of the two major platelet positive feedback loops important in secondary amplification of platelet activation to form a stable platelet aggregate. It is formed *de novo* upon activation of cytosolic phospholipase A_2 (PL_{A2}) (Fig. 24.6). TXA2 is a labile substance and lowers platelet cyclic adenosine monophosphate (cAMP) levels and initiates the release reaction (Fig. 24.6). TXA2 not only potentiates platelet aggregation, but also has powerful vasoconstrictive activity. The release reaction is inhibited by substances that increase the level of platelet cAMP. One such substance is prostacyclin (PGI_2) which is synthesized by vascular endothelial cells. It is a potent inhibitor of platelet aggregation and prevents their deposition on normal vascular endothelium.

Platelet procoagulant activity

After platelet aggregation and release, the exposed membrane phospholipid (platelet factor 3) is available for two reactions in the coagulation cascade. Both phospholipid-mediated reactions are calcium-ion dependent. The first (tenase) involves factors IXa, VIIIa and X in the formation of factor Xa (Fig. 24.7). The second (prothrombinase) results in the formation of thrombin from the interaction of factors Xa, Va and prothrombin (II). The phospholipid surface forms an ideal template for the crucial concentration and orientation of these proteins.

Growth factor

PDGF found in the α granules of platelets stimulates vascular smooth muscle cells to multiply and this may hasten vascular healing following injury.

Natural inhibitors of platelet function

Nitric oxide (NO) is constitutively released from endothelial cells (Fig. 24.8) and also from macrophages and platelets. It has a short half-life of 3–5 s.

It inhibits platelet activation and promotes vasodilatation. Prostacyclin synthesized by endothelial cells also inhibits platelet function (Fig. 24.8) and causes vasodilatation by raising cyclic guanosine monophosphate (GMP) levels. An ectonucleotidase (CD39) acts as an ADPase and helps prevent platelet aggregation in the intact vessel wall.

Blood coagulation

The coagulation cascade

Blood coagulation involves a biological amplification system in which relatively few initiation substances sequentially activate by proteolysis a cascade of circulating precursor proteins (the coagulation factor enzymes) which culminates in the generation of thrombin; this, in turn, converts soluble plasma fibrinogen into fibrin (Fig. 24.7). Fibrin enmeshes the platelet aggregates at the sites of vascular injury and converts the unstable primary platelet plugs to firm, definitive and stable haemostatic plugs. A list of the coagulation factors appears in Table 24.1. The operation of this enzyme cascade requires local concentration of circulating coagulation factors at the site of injury.

Surface-mediated reactions occur on exposed collagen, platelet phospholipid and tissue factor. With the exception of fibrinogen, which is the fibrin clot subunit, the coagulation factors are either enzyme precursors or cofactors (Table 24.1). All the enzymes, except factor XIII, are serine proteases (i.e. their ability to hydrolyse peptide bonds depends upon the amino acid serine at their active centre; Fig. 24.9). The scale of amplification achieved in this system is dramatic, (e.g. 1 mol of activated factor XI through sequential activation of factors IX, X and prothrombin may generate up to 2×10^8 mol of fibrin).

Coagulation *in vivo*

The generation of thrombin *in vivo* is a complex network of amplification and negative feedback loops to ensure a localized and limited production. The generation of thombin is dependent on three enzyme complexes, each consisting of protease, cofactor, phospholipids (PL) and calcium. They are

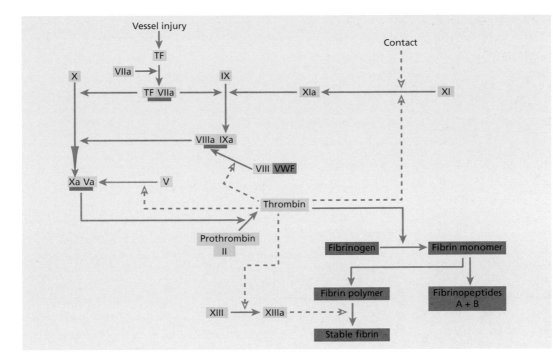

Figure 24.7 The pathway of blood coagulation initiated by tissue factor (TF) on the cell surface. When plasma comes into contact with TF, factor VII binds to TF. The complex of TF and activated VII (VIIa) activates X and IX. TF pathway inhibitor (TFPI) is an important inhibitor of TF/VIIa. The VIIIa–IXa complex greatly amplifies Xa production from X. The generation of thrombin from prothrombin by the action of Xa–Va complex leads to fibrin formation. Thrombin also activates XI (dashed line), V and XIII. Thrombin cleaves VIII from its carrier von Willebrand factor (VWF), greatly increasing the formation of VIIIa–IXa and hence of Xa–Va. Pale green, serine proteases; yellow, cofactors.

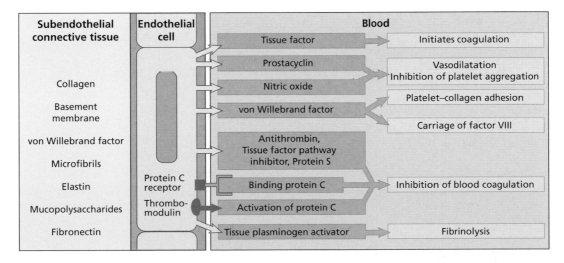

Figure 24.8 The endothelial cell forms a barrier between platelets and plasma clotting factors and the subendothelial connective tissues. Endothelial cells produce substances that can initiate coagulation, cause vasodilatation, inhibit platelet aggregation or haemostasis, or activate fibrinolysis.

Table 24.1 The coagulation factors.

Factor number	Descriptive name	Active form
I	Fibrinogen	Fibrin subunit
II	Prothrombin	Serine protease
III	Tissue factor	Receptor/cofactor*
V	Labile factor	Cofactor
VII	Proconvertin	Serine protease
VIII	Antihaemophilic factor	Cofactor
IX	Christmas factor	Serine protease
X	Stuart–Prower factor	Serine protease
XI	Plasma thromboplastin antecedent	Serine protease
XII	Hageman (contact) factor	Serine protease
XIII	Fibrin-stabilizing factor Prekallikrein (Fletcher factor) HMWK (Fitzgerald factor)	Transglutaminase Serine protease Cofactor*

HMWK, high molecular weight kininogen.
* Active without proteolytic modification.

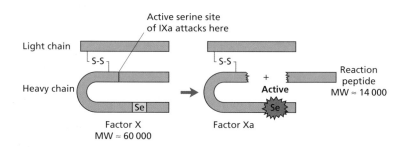

Figure 24.9 Serine (Se) protease activity. This example shows the activation of the serine site of factor X by factor IX.

extrinsic Xase (VIIa, TF, PL, Ca^{2+}), intrinsic Xase (IXa, VIIIa, PL, Ca^{2+}) generating FXa and pro-thrombinase complex (Xa, Va, PL, Ca^{2+}) generating thrombin. The generation of thrombin following vascular injury occurs in two waves of very different magnitude with different functions. During the initiation phase small amounts are generated (picomolar concentrations) which prepares the coagulation cascade for the second larger thrombin burst in the amplification when micromolar concentrations are produced, i.e. a million-fold higher concentration than produced during the initiation phase.

Initiation

Coagulation is initiated by the interaction of the membrane bound tissue factor (TF), exposed and activated by an enzyme protein disulphide isomerase after vascular injury, with plasma factor VIIa. TF is the sole initiator of thrombin generation and fibrin formation. It is expressed on fibroblasts of the adventitia and small muscle of the vessel wall and in the blood stream on microparticles, and on other non-vascular cells. One to two per cent of the total factor VII circulates in the activated form, but does not express proteolytic activity unless bound to TF. The factor VIIa-tissue factor (extrinsic factor Xase) complex activates both factor IX and factor X. The factor Xa, in the absence of its cofactor, forms small amounts of thrombin from prothrombin. This is insufficient to initiate significant fibrin polymerization. Amplification is needed and this is discussed next.

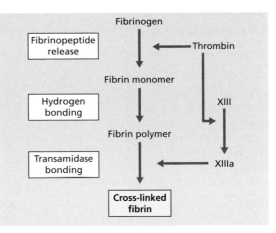

Figure 24.10 The formation and stabilization of fibrin.

Amplification

The initiation pathway or extrinsic Xase is rapidly inactivated by tissue factor pathway inhibitor (TFPI) which forms a quaternary complex with VIIa, TF and Xa. Thrombin generation is now dependent on the traditional intrinsic pathway. Factor VIII and V are converted to VIIIa and Va by the small amounts of thrombin generated during initiation. In this amplification phase the intrinsic Xase formed by IXa and VIIIa on phospholipid surface in the presence of Ca^{2+} activates sufficient Xa which then in combination with Va, PL and Ca^{2+} forms the prothrombinase complex and results in the explosive generation of thrombin which acts on fibrinogen to form the fibrin clot.

Factor XI does not seem to have a role in the physiological initiation of coagulation. It has a supplementary role in the activation of factor IX (see above) and may be important at major sites of trauma or at operations and potentially causes excess bleeding in factor XI deficient individuals.

Thrombin hydrolyses fibrinogen, releasing fibrinopeptides A and B to form fibrin monomers (Fig. 24.10). Fibrin monomers link spontaneously by hydrogen bonds to form a loose insoluble fibrin polymer. Factor XIII is also activated by thrombin together with calcium. Activated factor XIII stabilizes the fibrin polymers with the formation of covalent bond cross-links.

Fibrinogen has a MW of 340 000 and consists of two identical subunits, each containing three dissimilar polypeptide chains (α, β and γ) which are linked by disulphide bonds. After cleavage by thrombin of small fibrinopeptides A and B from the α and β chains, fibrin monomer consists of three paired α, β and γ chains which rapidly polymerise.

Some of the properties of the coagulation factors are listed in Table 24.2. The activity of factors II, VII, IX and X is dependent upon vitamin K which is responsible for carboxylation of a number of terminal glutamic acid residues on each of these molecules (see Fig. 26.8).

Although factor VIII and V cofactors are not protease enzymes, they circulate in a precursor form that requires limited cleavage by thrombin for expression of full cofactor activity.

Endothelial cells

The endothelial cell has an active role in the maintenance of vascular integrity. This cell provides the basement membrane that normally separates collagen, elastin and fibronectin of the subendothelial connective tissue from the circulating blood (Fig. 24.8). Loss or damage to the endothelium results in both haemorrhage and activation of the

Table 24.2 The coagulation factors.

Factor	Plasma half-life (h)	Plasma concentration (mg/L)	Comments
II	65	100	Prothrombin group: vitamin K needed for synthesis; require Ca^{2+} for activation
VII	5	0.5	
IX	25	5	
X	40	10	
I	90	3000	Thrombin interacts with them; increase in inflammation, pregnancy, oral contraceptives
V	15	10	
VIII	10	0.1	
XI	45	5	
XIII	200	30	

haemostatic mechanism. The endothelial cell also has a potent inhibitory influence on the haemostatic response, largely through the synthesis of prostaglandin, NO, and the ectonucleotidase CD39 which have vasodilatatory properties and inhibit platelet aggregation.

Synthesis of tissue factor that initiates haemostasis only occurs in endothelial cells following activation and its natural inhibitor, TFPI, is also synthesized. Endothelial synthesis of prostacyclin, VWF, plasminogen activator, antithrombin and thrombomodulin, the surface protein responsible for activation of protein C, provides agents that are vital to both platelet reactions and blood coagulation (Fig. 24.8).

Haemostatic response (Fig. 24.1)

Vasoconstriction

Immediate vasoconstriction of the injured vessel and reflex constriction of adjacent small arteries and arterioles is responsible for an initial slowing of blood flow to the area of injury. When there is widespread damage this vascular reaction prevents exsanguination. The reduced blood flow allows contact activation of platelets and coagulation factors. The vasoactive amines and TXA2 liberated from platelets (Fig. 24.6), and the fibrinopeptides liberated during fibrin formation (Fig. 24.10), also have vasoconstrictive activity.

Platelet reactions and primary haemostatic plug formation

Following a break in the endothelial lining, there is an initial adherence of platelets (via GP1a and GP1b receptors) to exposed connective tissue, mediated (GP1b) by VWF. Under conditions of high shear stress (e.g. arterioles) the exposed subendothelial matrix is initially coated with VWF. Collagen exposure and thrombin generated through activation of tissue factor produced at the site of injury cause the adherent platelets to release their granule contents and also activate platelet prostaglandin synthesis leading to the formation of TXA2. Released ADP causes platelets to swell and aggregate. Platelet rolling in the direction of blood flow over exposed VWF with activation of GPIIb/IIIa receptors results in firmer binding. Additional platelets from the circulating blood are drawn to the area of injury. This continuing platelet aggregation promotes the growth of the haemostatic plug which soon covers the exposed connective tissue. The unstable primary haemostatic plug produced by these platelet reactions in the first minute or so following injury is usually sufficient to provide temporary control of bleeding. The highly localized enhancement of platelet activation by ADP and TXA2 results in a platelet mass large enough to plug the area of endothelial injury. It seems likely that prostacyclin, produced by endothelial and smooth muscle cells in the vessel wall adjacent to the area of damage, is important in limiting the extent of the initial platelet plug.

Stabilization of the platelet plug by fibrin

Definitive haemostasis is achieved when fibrin formed by blood coagulation is added to the platelet mass and by platelet-induced clot retraction/compaction.

Following vascular injury, the formation of extrinsic Xase (VIIa, TF, PL and Ca^{2+}) initiates the coagulation cascade. Platelet aggregation and release reactions accelerate the coagulation process by providing abundant membrane phospholipid. Thrombin generated at the injury site converts soluble plasma fibrinogen into fibrin, potentiates platelet aggregation and secretion and also activates factor XI and XIII and cofactors V and VIII. The fibrin component of the haemostatic plug increases as the fused platelets completely degranulate and autolyse and after a few hours the entire haemostatic plug is transformed into a solid mass of cross-linked fibrin (Fig. 24.10). Clot retraction occurs which is mediated by GPIIb/IIIa receptors which link the cytoplasmic actin filaments to surface bound fibrin polymers. Nevertheless, because of incorporation of plasminogen and TPA (see p. 326), this plug begins to autodigest during the same time frame.

Physiological limitation of blood coagulation

Unchecked, blood coagulation would lead to dangerous occlusion of blood vessels (thrombosis) if the protective mechanisms of coagulation factor inhibitors, blood flow and fibrinolysis were not in operation.

Coagulation factor inhibitors

It is important that the effect of thrombin is limited to the site of injury. The first inhibitor to act is TFPI which is synthesized in endothelial cells and is present in plasma and platelets and accumulates at the site of injury caused by local platelet activation. This inhibits Xa and VIIa and tissue factor to limit the main *in vivo* pathway by forming the quaternary complex. There is direct inactivation of thrombin and other serine protease factors by other circulating inhibitors of which antithrombin is the most potent. It inactivates serine proteases (see Fig. 27.6). Heparin potentiates its action markedly. Another protein, heparin cofactor II, also inhibits thrombin. α_2-Macroglobulins, α_2-antiplasmin, C_1 esterase inhibitor and α_1-antitrypsin also exert inhibitory effects on circulating serine proteases.

Protein C and protein S

These are inhibitors of coagulation cofactors V and VIII. Thrombin binds to an endothelial cell surface receptor, thrombomodulin. The resulting complex activates the vitamin K-dependent serine protease protein C which is able to destroy activated factors V and VIII, thus preventing further thrombin generation. The action of protein C is enhanced by another vitamin K-dependent protein, S, which binds protein C to the platelet surface (Fig. 24.11). An endothelial protein C receptor localizes protein C to the endothelial surface, promoting protein C activation by the thrombin–thrombomodulin complex (Fig. 24.11). In addition, activated protein C enhances fibrinolysis (Fig. 24.11).

As with other serine proteases, activated protein C is subject to inactivation by serum protease inactivators (serpins), e.g. antithrombin.

Blood flow

At the periphery of a damaged area of tissue, blood flow rapidly achieves dilution and dispersal of activated factors before fibrin formation has occurred. Activated factors are destroyed by liver parenchymal cells and particulate matter is removed by liver Kupffer cells and other reticuloendothelial cells.

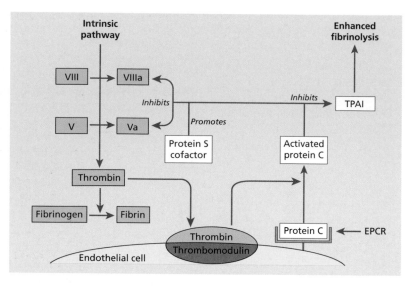

Figure 24.11 Activation and action of protein C by thrombin which has bound to thrombomodulin on the endothelial cell surface. Protein S is a cofactor that facilitates binding of activated protein C to the platelet surface. The inactivation of factors Va and VIIIa results in the inhibition of blood coagulation. The inactivation of tissue plasminogen activator inhibitor (TPAI) enhances fibrinolysis. EPCR, endothelial protein C receptor.

Fibrinolysis

Fibrinolysis (like coagulation) is a normal haemostatic response to vascular injury. Plasminogen, a β-globulin proenzyme in blood and tissue fluid, is converted to the serine protease plasmin by activators either from the vessel wall (intrinsic activation) or from the tissues (extrinsic activation) (Fig. 24.12). The most important route follows the release of TPA from endothelial cells. TPA is a serine protease that binds to fibrin. This enhances its capacity to convert thrombus-bound plasminogen into plasmin. This fibrin dependence of TPA action strongly localizes plasmin generation by TPA to the fibrin clot. Release of TPA occurs after such stimuli as trauma, exercise or emotional stress. Activated protein C stimulates fibrinolysis by destroying plasma inhibitors of TPA (Fig. 24.11). However, thrombin inhibits fibrinolysis by activating thrombin-activated fibrinolysis inhibitor (TAFI) which prevents plasminogen from binding to fibrin clot.

Plasmin generation at the site of injury limits the extent of the evolving thrombus. The split products of fibrinolysis are also competitive

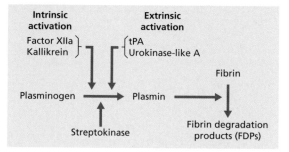

Figure 24.12 The fibrinolytic system. tPA, tissue plasminogen activator.

inhibitors of thrombin and fibrin polymerization. Normally, α_2-antiplasmin inhibits any local free plasmin.

Fibrinolytic agents are widely used in clinical practice (see p. 377). Therapeutic recombinant TPA has been synthesized using recombinant DNA technology. The bacterial agent streptokinase is a peptide produced by haemolytic streptococci and forms a complex with plasminogen, which converts other plasminogen molecules to plasmin. Urokinase is a TPA initially isolated from human urine.

Plasmin is capable of digesting fibrinogen, fibrin, factors V and VIII and many other proteins. Cleavage of peptide bonds in fibrin and fibrinogen produces a variety of split (degradation) products (Fig. 24.12). Large amounts of the smallest fragments D and E can be detected in the plasma of patients with disseminated intravascular coagulation (see p. 355).

Inactivation of plasmin

Tissue plasminogen activator is inactivated by plasminogen activator inhibitor (PAI). Circulating plasmin is inactivated by potent inhibitors α_2-antiplasmin and α_2-macroglobulin.

Tests of haemostatic function

Defective haemostasis with abnormal bleeding may result from:

1 A vascular disorder;
2 Thrombocytopenia or a disorder of platelet function; or
3 Defective blood coagulation.

A number of simple tests are employed to assess the platelet, vessel wall and coagulation components of haemostasis.

Blood count and blood film examination

As thrombocytopenia is a common cause of abnormal bleeding, patients with suspected bleeding disorders should initially have a blood count including platelet count and blood film examination. In addition to establishing the presence of thrombocytopenia, the cause may be obvious (e.g. acute leukaemia).

Screening tests of blood coagulation

Screening tests provide an assessment of the 'extrinsic' and 'intrinsic' systems of blood coagulation and also the central conversion of fibrinogen to fibrin (Table 24.3).

The prothrombin time (PT) measures factors VII, X, V, prothrombin and fibrinogen. Tissue thromboplastin (a brain extract) or [synthetic] tissue factor with lipids and calcium is added to

Table 24.3 Screening tests used in the diagnosis of coagulation disorders.

Screening tests	Abnormalities indicated by prolongation	Most common cause of coagulation disorder
Thrombin time (TT)	Deficiency or abnormality of fibrinogen or inhibition of thrombin by heparin or FDPs	DIC Heparin therapy
Prothrombin time (PT)	Deficiency or inhibition of one or more of the following coagulation factors: VII, X, V, II, fibrinogen	Liver disease Warfarin therapy DIC
Activated partial thromboplastin time (APTT or PTTK)	Deficiency or inhibition of one or more of the following coagulation factors: XII, XI, IX (Christmas disease), VIII (haemophilia), X, V, II, fibrinogen	Haemophilia, Christmas disease (+ conditions above)
Fibrinogen quantitation	Fibrinogen deficiency	DIC, liver disease

DIC, disseminated intravascular coagulation; FDPs, fibrin degradation products.
NB. Platelet count and the tests of platelet function are also used in screening patients with a bleeding disorder (p. 328).

citrated plasma. The normal time for clotting is 10–14 s. It may be expressed as the international normalized ratio (INR) (see p. 375).

The activated partial thromboplastin time (APTT) measures factors VIII, IX, XI and XII in addition to factors X, V, prothrombin and fibrinogen. Three substances – phospholipid, a surface activator (e.g. kaolin) and calcium – are added to citrated plasma. The normal time for clotting is approximately 30–40 s.

Prolonged clotting times in the PT and APTT because of factor deficiency are corrected by the addition of normal plasma to the test plasma (50 : 50 mix). If there is no correction or incomplete correction with normal plasma, the presence of an inhibitor of coagulation is suspected.

The thrombin (clotting) time (TT) is sensitive to a deficiency of fibrinogen or inhibition of thrombin. Diluted bovine thrombin is added to citrated plasma at a concentration giving a clotting time of 14–16 s with normal subjects.

Specific assays of coagulation factors

Most factor assays are based on an APTT or PT in which all factors except the one to be measured are present in the substrate plasma. This usually requires a supply of plasma from patients with hereditary deficiency of the factor in question or artificially produced factor-deficient plasma. The corrective effect of the unknown plasma on the prolonged clotting time of the deficient substrate plasma is then compared with the corrective effect of normal plasma. Results are expressed as a percentage of normal activity.

A number of chemical, chromogenic and immunological methods are available for quantification of other proteins such as fibrinogen, VWF, factor Xa and factor VIII. Factor XIII activity can be assessed by testing for clot solubility in urea.

Bleeding time

The bleeding time was a useful test for abnormal platelet function including the diagnosis of VWF deficiency. The test involved the application of pressure to the upper arm with a blood pressure cuff, after which small incisions are made in the flexor surface forearm skin. Bleeding stops normally in 3–8 minutes. It has largely been replaced by specific platelet aggregation tests, platelet adhesion assays and the platelet function analysis-100 (PFA-100) test (see below). The bleeding time is prolonged in thrombocytopenia but is normal in vascular causes of abnormal bleeding.

Tests of platelet function

The most valuable investigation is platelet aggregometry which measures the fall in light absorbance in platelet-rich plasma as platelets aggregate. Initial (primary) aggregation is caused by an external agent, the secondary response by aggregating agents released from the platelets themselves. The five external aggregating agents most commonly used are ADP, collagen, ristocetin, arachidonic acid and adrenaline. The pattern of response to each agent helps to make the diagnosis (see Fig. 25.10). Flow cytometry is now increasingly used in routine practice to identify platelet glyoprotein defects.

In the PFA-100 test, citrated blood is aspirated through a capillary tube onto a membrane coated with collagen/ADP or collagen/adrenaline. Blood flow is maintained. Platelets begin to adhere and aggregate, primarily via VWF interactions with GPIb and GPIIb/IIIa, resulting in occlusion of the aperture.

The PFA-100 analysis may give false negative results with relatively common platelet defects. Full platelet function tests and VWF screening may be required to exclude abnormal platelet function, even if the PFA-100 test is normal.

Test of fibrinolysis

Increased levels of circulating plasminogen activator may be detected by demonstrating shortened euglobulin clot lysis times. A number of immunological methods are available to detect fibrinogen or fibrin degradation products (including D-dimers) in serum. In patients with enhanced fibrinolysis, low levels of circulating plasminogen may be detected.

SUMMARY

- Normal haemostasis requires vasoconstriction, platelet aggregation and blood coagulation. The intact endothelial cell normally separates collagen and other subendothelial connective tissues that would stimulate platelet aggregation from circulating blood. The endothelial cells also produce prostacyclin, nitric oxide and an ectonucleotidase which inhibit platelet aggregation.

- Platelets are produced from megakaryocytes in the bone marrow. They have surface glycoproteins which facilitate adherence via von Willebrand factor to collagen, to other platelets (aggregation) and to coagulation proteins. Platelets contain different types of storage granules which are released after platelet activation.

- Blood coagulation commences with tissue factor binding to clotting factor VII and this initiates a cascade which results in thrombin generation. Thrombin then activates factors VIII and V which greatly amplify the coagulation pathway resulting in a fibrin clot.

- Coagulation factor inhibitors include antithrombin, protein C and protein S.

- Dissolution of fibrin clots (fibrinolysis) occurs by activation of plasminogen to plasmin.

- Tests of haemostatic function include the thrombin time (TT), prothrombin time (PT), activated partial thromboplastin time (APTT) as well as individual coagulation factor assays and assay of von Willebrand factor. Tests of platelet function include the PFA-100 and platelet aggregation test.

Now visit www.wiley.com/go/essentialhaematology to test yourself on this chapter.

CHAPTER 25
Bleeding disorders caused by vascular and platelet abnormalities

Key topics

Essential Haematology, 6th Edition. © A. V. Hoffbrand and P. A. H. Moss. Published 2011 by Blackwell Publishing Ltd.

Abnormal bleeding

This may result from:

1 Vascular disorders
2 Thrombocytopenia
3 Defective platelet function or
4 Defective coagulation.

The pattern of bleeding is relatively predictable depending on the aetiology. Vascular and platelet disorders tend to be associated with bleeding from mucous membranes and into the skin whereas in coagulation disorders the bleeding is often into joints or soft tissue (Table 25.1).

The first three categories are discussed in this chapter and the disorders of blood coagulation follow in Chapter 26.

Table 25.1 Clinical differences between diseases of platelets/vessel wall or of coagulation factors.

	Platelets/vessel wall diseases	Coagulation diseases
Mucosal bleeding	Common	Rare
Petechiae	Common	Rare
Deep haematomas	Rare	Characteristic
Bleeding from skin cuts	Persistent	Minimal
Sex of patient	Equal	>80% male

Vascular bleeding disorders

The vascular disorders are a heterogeneous group of conditions characterized by easy bruising and spontaneous bleeding from the small vessels. The underlying abnormality is either in the vessels themselves or in the perivascular connective tissues. Most cases of bleeding caused by vascular defects alone are not severe. Frequently, the bleeding is mainly in the skin causing petechiae, ecchymoses or both (Fig. 25.1). In some disorders there is also bleeding from mucous membranes. In these conditions the standard screening tests are normal. The bleeding time is usually normal and the other tests of haemostasis are also normal. Vascular defects may be inherited or acquired.

Inherited vascular disorders

Hereditary haemorrhagic telangiectasia

This uncommon disease is transmitted as an autosomal dominant trait. Various genetic defects underlie the disease, e.g. of the endothelial protein, endoglin. There are dilated microvascular swellings which appear during childhood and become more numerous in adult life. These telangiectasia develop in the skin, mucous membranes (Fig. 25.1a) and internal organs. Pulmonary, hepatic, splenic and cerebral arteriovenous shunts are seen in a minority of cases. Recurrent epistaxes are frequent and recurrent gastrointestinal tract haemorrhage may cause chronic iron deficiency anaemia. Treatment is with embolization, laser treatment, oestrogens, tranexamic acid and iron supplementation.

Connective tissue disorders

In the Ehlers–Danlos syndromes there are hereditary collagen abnormalities with purpura resulting from defective platelet aggregation, hyperextensibility of joints and hyperelastic friable skin. Pseudoxanthoma elasticum is associated with arterial haemorrhage and thrombosis. Patients may present with superficial bruising and purpura following minor trauma or after the application of a tourniquet. Bleeding and poor wound healing after surgery may be a problem.

Giant cavernous haemangioma

These congenital malformations occasionally cause chronic activation of coagulation leading to laboratory features of disseminated intravascular coagulation (DIC) and in some cases thrombocytopenia.

Acquired vascular defects

1 Simple easy bruising is a common benign disorder which occurs in otherwise healthy women, especially those of child-bearing age.

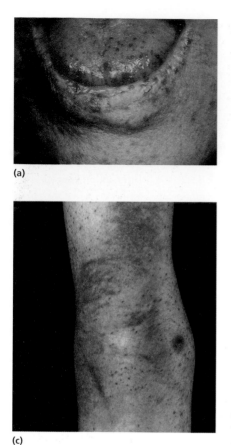

(a)

(c)

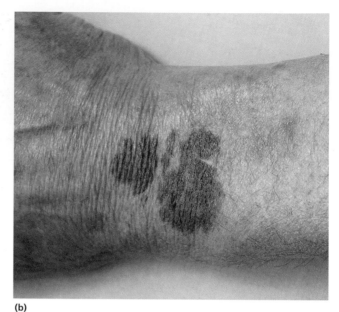

(b)

Figure 25.1 (a) Hereditary haemorrhagic telangiectasia: the characteristic small vascular lesions are obvious on the lips and tongue. **(b)** Senile purpura. **(c)** Characteristic perifollicular petechiae in vitamin C deficiency (scurvy).

2 Senile purpura caused by atrophy of the supporting tissues of cutaneous blood vessels is seen mainly on dorsal aspects of the forearms and hands (Fig. 25.1b).

3 Purpura associated with infections, mainly of bacterial, viral or rickettsial origins may cause purpura from vascular damage by the organism with DIC or as a result of immune complex formation (e.g. measles, dengue fever or meningococcal septicaemia).

4 The Henoch–Schönlein syndrome is usually seen in children and often follows an acute upper respiratory tract infection. It is an immunoglobulin A (IgA)-mediated vasculitis. The characteristic purpuric rash accompanied by localized oedema and itching is usually most prominent on the buttocks and extensor surfaces of the lower legs and elbows (Fig. 25.2). Painful joint swelling, haematuria and abdominal pain may also occur. It is usually a self-limiting condition but occasional patients develop renal failure.

5 Scurvy. In vitamin C deficiency, defective collagen may cause perifollicular petechiae, bruising and mucosal haemorrhage (Fig. 25.1c).

6 Steroid purpura. The purpura, which is associated with long-term steroid therapy or Cushing's syndrome, is caused by defective vascular supportive tissue.

Tranexamic acid and aminocaproic acid are useful antifibrinolytic drugs that may reduce bleeding resulting from vascular disorders or thrombocytopenia but are relatively contraindicated in the presence of haematuria because they might lead to clots obstructing the renal tract.

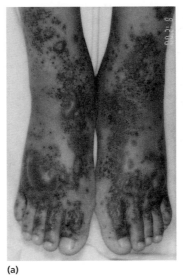

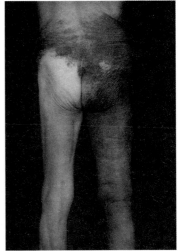

Figure 25.2 Henoch–Schönlein purpura: **(a)** unusually severe purpura on legs with bullous formation in a 6-year-old child; and **(b)** early urticarial lesions.

(a)

(b)

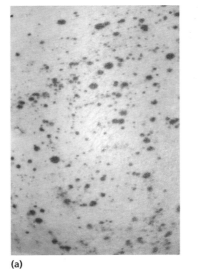

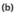

Figure 25.3 (a) Typical purpura; and **(b)** massive subcutaneous haemorrhage in a patient with drug-induced thrombocytopenia.

(a)

(b)

Thrombocytopenia

Abnormal bleeding associated with thrombocytopenia or abnormal platelet function is characterized by spontaneous skin purpura (Fig. 25.3) and mucosal haemorrhage and prolonged bleeding after trauma (Table 25.1). The main causes of thrombocytopenia are listed in Tables 25.2 and 25.3.

Failure of platelet production

This is the most common cause of thrombocytopenia and is usually part of a generalized bone marrow failure (Table 25.2). Selective megakaryocyte depression may result from drug toxicity or viral infection. Rarely, it is congenital as a result of mutation of the c-MPL thrombopoietin receptor, in

Table 25.2 Causes of thrombocytopenia.

Failure of platelet production
Selective megakaryocyte depression
  rare congenital defects (see text)
  drugs, chemicals, viral infections
Part of general bone marrow failure
  cytotoxic drugs
  radiotherapy
  aplastic anaemia
  leukaemia
  myelodysplastic syndromes
  myelofibrosis
  marrow infiltration (e.g. carcinoma, lymphoma,
    Gaucher's disease)
  multiple myeloma
  megaloblastic anaemia
  HIV infection

Increased consumption of platelets
Immune
  autoimmune
    idiopathic
    associated with systemic lupus erythematosus,
      chronic lymphocytic leukaemia or lymphoma;
      infections: *Helicobacter pylori*, HIV, other
      viruses, malaria
  drug-induced, e.g. heparin
  post-transfusional purpura
  feto–maternal alloimmune thrombocytopenia
Disseminated intravascular coagulation
Thrombotic thrombocytopenic purpura

Abnormal distribution of platelets
Splenomegaly (e.g. liver disease)

Dilutional loss
Massive transfusion of stored blood to bleeding
patients

HIV, human immunodeficiency virus.

Table 25.3 Thrombocytopenia as a result of
drugs or toxins.

Bone marrow suppression
Predictable (dose-related)
  ionizing radiation, cytotoxic drugs, ethanol
Occasional
  chloramphenicol, co-trimoxazole, idoxuridine,
    penicillamine, organic arsenicals, benzene, etc.

Immune mechanisms (proven or probable)
Analgesics, anti-inflammatory drugs
  gold salts
Antimicrobials
  penicillins, rifamycin, sulphonamides,
    trimethoprim, para-aminosalicylate
Sedatives, anticonvulsants
  diazepam, sodium valproate, carbamazepine
Diuretics
  acetazolamide, chlorathiazides, frusemide
Antidiabetics
  chlorpropamide, tolbutamide
Others
  digitoxin, heparin, methyldopa, oxyprenolol,
    quinine, quinidine

cal history, peripheral blood count, the blood film
and bone marrow examination.

Increased destruction of platelets

Autoimmune (idiopathic) thrombocytopenic purpura

Autoimmune (idiopathic) thrombocytopenic purpura (ITP) may be divided into chronic and acute forms.

Chronic idiopathic thrombocytopenic purpura

This is a relatively common disorder. The highest incidence has been considered to be in women aged 15–50 years although some reports suggest an increasing incidence with age. It is the most common cause of thrombocytopenia without anaemia or neutropenia. It is usually idiopathic but may be seen in association with other diseases such as systemic lupus erythematosus (SLE), human immunodefi-

association with absent radii, or in May–Hegglin anomaly with large inclusions in granulocytes, or in Wiskott–Aldrich syndrome (WAS) with eczema and immune deficiency. WAS is caused by mutation of the *WASP* gene, the protein being a regulator of signalling in haemopoietic cells. Diagnosis of these causes of thrombocytopenia is made from the clini-

ciency virus (HIV) infection or *Helicobacter pylori*, chronic lymphocytic leukaemia (CLL), Hodgkin lymphoma or autoimmune haemolytic anaemia (Table 25.2).

Pathogenesis

Platelet autoantibodies (usually IgG) result in the premature removal of platelets from the circulation by macrophages of the reticuloendothelial system, especially the spleen (Fig. 25.4). In many cases, the antibody is directed against antigen sites on the glycoprotein (GP) IIb–IIIa or Ib complex. The normal lifespan of a platelet is 7–10 days but in ITP this is reduced to a few hours. Total megakaryocyte mass and platelet turnover are increased in parallel to approximately five times normal.

Clinical features

The onset is often insidious with petechial haemorrhage, easy bruising and, in women, menorrhagia. Mucosal bleeding (e.g. epistaxes or gum bleeding) occurs in severe cases but fortunately intracranial haemorrhage is rare. The severity of bleeding in ITP is usually less than that seen in patients with comparable degrees of thrombocytopenia from bone marrow failure; this is attributed to the circulation of predominantly young, functionally superior platelets in ITP. Chronic ITP tends to relapse and remit spontaneously so the course may be difficult to predict. Many asymptomatic cases are discovered by a routine blood count.

The spleen is not palpable unless there is an associated disease causing splenomegaly.

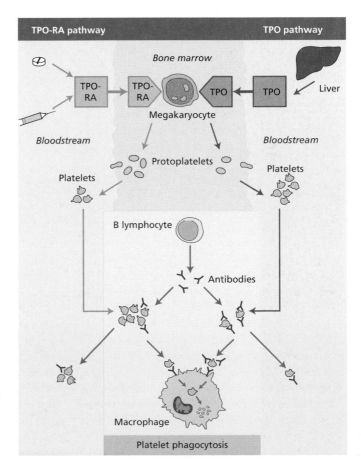

Figure 25.4 The pathogenesis of thrombocytopenia in autoimmune thrombocytopenic purpura. The actions of thrombopoietin (TPO) and thrombopoietin receptor agonists (TPO-RA) (thrombomimetics) are shown. These are orally active or given by injection. They increase platelet production. Platelets coated by antibodies are phagocytosed by macrophages.

Diagnosis

1 The platelet count is usually $10–100 \times 10^9/L$. The haemoglobin concentration and white cell count are typically normal unless there is iron deficiency anaemia because of blood loss.
2 The blood film shows reduced numbers of platelets, those present often being large. There are no morphological abnormalities in the other cell lines.
3 The bone marrow shows normal or increased numbers of megakaryocytes.
4 Sensitive tests are able to demonstrate specific antiglycoprotein GPIIb/IIIa or GPIb antibodies on the platelet surface or in the serum in most patients. Platelet-associated IgG assays are less specific. These tests are not usually used in clinical practice.

Treatment

As this is a chronic disease the aim of treatment should be to maintain a platelet count above the level at which spontaneous bruising or bleeding occurs with the minimum of intervention. In general, a platelet count above $50 \times 10^9/L$ does not require treatment.

1 *Corticosteroids* Eighty per cent of patients remit on high-dose corticosteroid therapy. Prednisolone 1 mg/kg/day is the usual initial therapy in adults and the dosage is gradually reduced after 10–14 days. In poor responders the dosage is reduced more slowly but alternative immunosuppression or splenectomy is considered.
2 *High dose intravenous immunoglobulin therapy* is able to produce a rapid rise in platelet count in the majority of patients. A regimen of 400 mg/kg/day for 5 days or 1 g/kg/day for 2 days is recommended. It is particularly useful in patients with life-threatening haemorrhage, in steroid-refractory ITP, during pregnancy or prior to surgery. The mechanism of action may be blockage of Fc receptors on macrophages or modification of autoantibody production.
3 *Immunosuppressive drugs* (e.g. vincristine, cyclophosphamide, azathioprine, mycophenolate mofetil or ciclosporin alone or in combination) are usually reserved for those patients who do not respond sufficiently to steroids, rituximab or splenectomy.
4 *Monoclonal antibody* Rituximab (anti-CD20) produces responses in approximately 50%, which are often durable and it is now usually tried before splenectomy.
5 *Thrombopoietin-receptor agonists* Romiplostim (subcutaneously) and eltrombopag (orally) are active non-peptide thrombopoietin-receptor agonists (thrombomimetics) (Fig. 25.4). They stimulate thrombopoiesis (Fig. 25.5). They are indicated for patients in whom steroids are contraindicated or who are refractory to steroids.
6 *Splenectomy* This operation was recommended in patients who have symptoms and still have platelets $<30 \times 10^9/L$ after 3 months of steroid therapy or who require unacceptably high doses of steroids to maintain a platelet count above $30 \times 10^9/L$. With the increase in number of alternative drugs, splenectomy is now performed less frequently for ITP than previously. Good results occur in most of the patients, but in patients with ITP refractory to steroids or immunoglobulin there may be little benefit. Splenunculi must be removed otherwise subsequent relapse of ITP can occur.
7 *Other treatments* that may elicit a remission include danazol (an androgen which may cause virilization in women) and intravenous anti-D immunoglobulin. It is often necessary to combine two drugs (e.g. danazol and an immunosuppressive agent). *Helicobacter pylori* infection should be treated as there are some reports that this may improve the platelet count.
8 *Platelet transfusions* Platelet concentrates are beneficial in patients with acute life-threatening bleeding. Their benefit will only last a few hours.
9 *Stem cell transplatation* has cured some severe cases.

Acute idiopathic thrombocytopenic purpura

This is most common in children. In approximately 75% of patients the episode follows vaccination or an infection such as chickenpox or infectious mononucleosis. Most cases are caused by non-specific immune complex attachments to platelets. Spontaneous remissions are usual but in 5–10% of cases the disease becomes chronic (lasting >6 months). Fortunately, morbidity and mortality in acute ITP is very low.

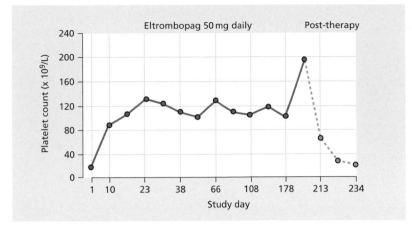

Figure 25.5 Response to eltrombopag in chronic immune thrombocytopenic purpura in a female aged 75 after failure of response to prednisolone. (Courtesy of Professor A. Newland.)

The diagnosis is one of exclusion and there is debate as to the need for bone marrow aspiration. If the platelet count is over 30×10^9/L no treatment is necessary unless the bleeding is severe. Those with counts below 20×10^9/L may be treated with steroids and/or intravenous immunoglobulin, especially if there is significant bleeding.

Infections

It seems likely that the thrombocytopenia associated with many viral and protozoal infections is immune-mediated. In HIV infection, reduced platelet production is also involved (see p. 390).

Post-transfusion purpura

Thrombocytopenia occurring approximately 10 days after a blood transfusion has been attributed to antibodies in the recipient developing against the human platelet antigen-1a (HPA-1a) (absent from the patient's own platelets) on transfused platelets. The reason why the patient's own platelets are then destroyed is unknown. Treatment is with intravenous immunoglobulin, plasma exchange or corticosteroids.

Drug-induced immune thrombocytopenia

An immunological mechanism has been demonstrated as the cause of many drug-induced throm-bocytopenias (Fig. 25.6). Quinine (including that in tonic water), quinidine and heparin are particularly common causes (Table 25.3).

The platelet count is often less than 10×10^9/L, and the bone marrow shows normal or increased numbers of megakaryocytes. Drug-dependent antibodies against platelets may be demonstrated in the sera of some patients. The immediate treatment is to stop all suspected drugs but platelet concentrates should be given to patients with dangerous bleeding.

Thrombotic thrombocytopenic purpura and haemolytic uraemic syndrome

Thrombotic thrombocytopenic purpura (TTP) occurs in familial or acquired forms. There is deficiency of the ADAMTS13 metalloprotease which breaks down ultra large von Willebrand factor multimers (ULVWF) (Fig. 25.7). In the familial forms more than 50 ADAMTS13 mutations have been reported whereas the acquired forms follow the development of an inhibitory IgG autoantibody, the presence of which may be stimulated by infection, autoimmune/connective tissue disease, certain drugs, stem cell transplantation or cardiac surgery. ULVWF multimeric strings secreted from Weibel–Palade bodies are anchored to the endothelial cells, and passing platelets adhere via their GPIb receptors. Increasing platelet aggregation onto the

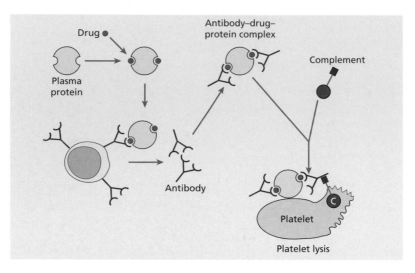

Figure 25.6 Usual type of platelet damage caused by drugs in which an antibody–drug–protein complex is deposited on the platelet surface. If complement is attached and the sequence goes to completion, the platelet may be lysed directly. Otherwise it is removed by reticuloendothelial cells because of opsonization with immunoglobulin and/or the C3 component of complement.

ULVWF multimeric strings has the potential to form large occlusive platelet thrombi. These strings are capable of embolizing to microvessels downstream contributing to organ ischemia (Fig. 25.8). In the closely related haemolytic uraemic syndrome (HUS) ADAMTS13 levels are normal.

TTP has traditionally been described as a pentad of thrombocytopenia, microangiopathic haemolytic anaemia, neurologic abnormalities, renal failure and fever. The microvascular thrombosis causes variable degrees of tissue ischaemia and infarction and is responsible for the microangiopathic haemolytic anaemia and thrombocytopenia (Fig. 25.8). In current clinical practice, thombocytopenia, schistocytosis and an impressively elevated serum lactate dehydrogenase (LDH) value are sufficient to suggest the diagnosis. The serum LDH is derived both from ischaemic or necrotic tissue cells and lysed red cells. Coagulation tests are normal in contrast to the findings in DIC (see Fig. 26.9). The serum LDH is raised. ADAMTS13 is absent or severely reduced in plasma.

Treatment is with plasma exchange, using fresh frozen plasma (FFP) or cryosupernatant. This removes the large molecular weight VWF multimers and the antibody and provides ADAMTS13.

The platelet count and serum LDH are useful for monitoring the response to treatment. Rituximab (anti-CD20) is also effective, used in conjunction with plasma infusions or with plasma exchange, and subsequently for reducing the risk of relapse. In refractory cases and chronic relapsing cases, high-dose corticosteroids, vincristine, intravenous immunoglobulin, rituximab and immunosuppressive therapy with azathioprine or cyclophosphamide have been used. In untreated cases mortality may approach 90%. Relapses are frequent.

HUS in children has many common features but organ damage is limited to the kidneys. There is also usually diarrhoea. Fits are frequent. Many cases are associated with *Escherichia coli* infection with the verotoxin 0157 strain or with other organisms, especially *Shigella*. Supportive renal dialysis and control of hypertension and fits are the mainstays of treatment. Platelet transfusions are contraindicated in HUS and TTP.

Disseminated intravascular coagulation

Thrombocytopenia may result from an increased rate of platelet destruction through consumption of platelets because of their participation in DIC (see p. 357).

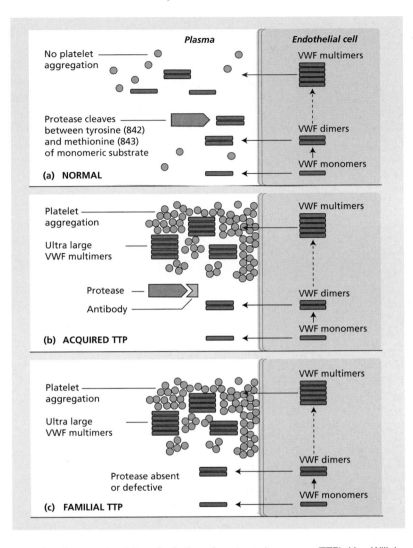

Figure 25.7 Proposed pathogenesis of thrombotic thrombocytopenic purpura (TTP). Von Willebrand factor (VWF) consists of a series of VWF multimers each of molecular weight (MW) 250 kDa which are covalently linked. **(a)** Under physiological circumstances a metalloprotease ADAMTS13 cleaves high molecular weight multimers at a Tyr-842–Met-843 bond and the resulting VWF has an MW of 500–20 000 kDa. **(b)** In non-familial TTP, an antibody develops to the metalloprotease and so blocks cleavage of VWF multimers. **(c)** In congenital forms of TTP, the protease appears to be absent. In both cases, the resultant ultra-large VWF multimers can bind platelets under high shear stress conditions and lead to platelet aggregation.

Increased splenic pooling

The major factor responsible for thrombocytopenia in splenomegaly is platelet 'pooling' by the spleen. In splenomegaly, up to 90% of platelets may be sequestered in the spleen whereas normally this accounts for approximately one-third of the total platelet mass (Fig. 25.9). Platelet lifespan is normal and in the absence of additional haemostatic defects, the thrombocytopenia of splenomegaly is not usually associated with bleeding.

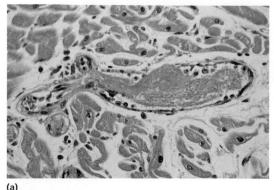

(a)

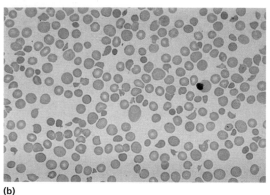

(b)

Figure 25.8 Thrombotic thrombocytopenic purpura.
(a) Platelet thrombus in a small cardiac vessel with
minor endothelial and inflammatory reaction.
(Courtesy of Dr J.E. McLaughlin.) **(b)** Peripheral blood
film showing red cell fragmentation.

Massive transfusion syndrome

Platelets are unstable in blood stored at 4°C and the
platelet count rapidly falls in blood stored for more
than 24 hours. Patients transfused with massive
amounts of stored blood (more than 10 units over
a 24-hour period) frequently show abnormal clotting and thrombocytopenia. These should be corrected by the use of platelet transfusions and FFP.

Disorders of platelet function

Disorders of platelet function are suspected in
patients who show skin and mucosal haemorrhage
despite a normal platelet count and normal levels
of VWF. These disorders may be hereditary or
acquired.

Hereditary disorders

Rare inherited disorders may produce defects at
each of the different phases of the platelet reactions
leading to the formation of the haemostatic platelet
plug.

Thrombasthenia (Glanzmann's disease)

This autosomal recessive disorder leads to failure of
primary platelet aggregation because of a deficiency

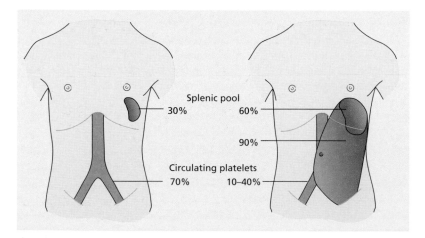

Splenic pool
30%   60%
             90%

Circulating platelets
70%   10–40%

Figure 25.9 The platelet distribution between the circulation and spleen in normal individuals (left), and in
patients with moderate or massive splenomegaly (right).

of the membrane glycoproteins IIb/IIIa which together form the VWF and fibrinogen receptor (see Fig. 24.5). It usually presents in the neonatal period and, characteristically, platelets fail to aggregate *in vitro* to any agonist except ristocetin.

Bernard–Soulier syndrome

In this disease the platelets are larger than normal and there is a deficiency of GPIb. There is defective binding to VWF, defective adherence to exposed subendothelial connective tissues and platelets do not aggregate with ristocetin. There is a variable degree of thrombocytopenia.

Storage pool diseases

In the rare grey platelet syndrome, the platelets are larger than normal and there is a virtual absence of α granules with deficiency of their proteins. In the more common δ-storage pool disease there is a deficiency of dense granules.

Platelet-dependent haemostasis is abnormal in von Willebrand disease because of an inherited defect in VWF (see p. 352).

Acquired disorders

Antiplatelet drugs

Aspirin therapy is the most common cause of defective platelet function. It produces abnormal closure times in the platelet function analysis-100 (PFA-100) test and, although purpura may not be obvious, the defect may contribute to the associated gastrointestinal haemorrhage. The cause of the aspirin defect is inhibition of cyclo-oxygenase with impaired thromboxane A_2 synthesis (see Fig. 27.8). There is consequent impairment of the release reaction and aggregation with arachidonic acid, collagen, adrenaline and adenosine diphosphate (ADP) (Fig. 25.10). After a single dose the defect lasts 7–10 days (i.e. the life of the platelet). Aspirin is contraindicated in patients with gastrointestinal or genitourinary bleeding, retinal bleeding, peptic ulcer, haemophilia or uncontrollable hypertension.

Dipyridamole inhibits platelet aggregation by blocking reuptake of adenosine and is usually used as an adjunct to aspirin. Clopidogrel inhibits binding of ADP to its platelet receptor (see Fig. 27.8), shown by impaired aggregation with ADP (Fig. 25.10) and is mainly used for prevention of thrombotic events (e.g. after coronary stenting or

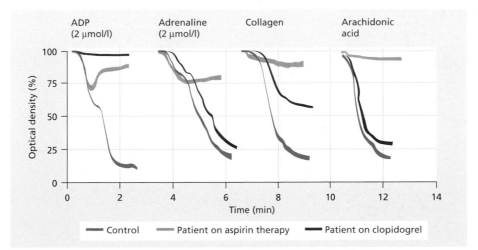

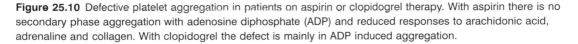

Figure 25.10 Defective platelet aggregation in patients on aspirin or clopidogrel therapy. With aspirin there is no secondary phase aggregation with adenosine diphosphate (ADP) and reduced responses to arachidonic acid, adrenaline and collagen. With clopidogrel the defect is mainly in ADP induced aggregation.

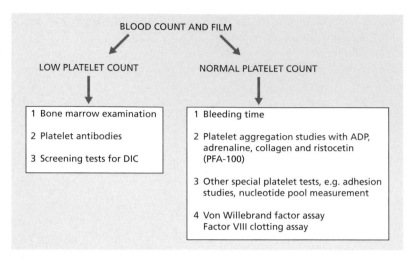

Figure 25.11 Laboratory tests for platelet disorders. NB. Some intrinsic platelet functional disorders are associated with thrombocytopenia (e.g. Bernard–Soulier syndrome). ADP, adenosine diphosphate; DIC, disseminated intravascular coagulation.

angioplasty) in patients with a history of symptomatic atherosclerotic disease. Intravenous agents abciximab, eptifibatide and tirofiban are inhibitors of GPIIb/IIIa receptor sites and may be used in patients undergoing percutaneous coronary intervention, with unstable angina and acute coronary syndromes. There is a risk of transient thrombocytopenia with these agents, especially with abciximab, and platelet transfusions may be needed.

Hyperglobulinaemia

Hyperglobulinaemia associated with multiple myeloma or Waldenström's disease may cause interference with platelet adherence, release and aggregation.

Myeloproliferative and myelodysplastic disorders

Intrinsic abnormalities of platelet function occur in many patients with essential thrombocythaemia, other myeloproliferative and myelodysplastic diseases and in paroxysmal nocturnal haemoglobinuria.

Uraemia

This is associated with various abnormalities of platelet function. Heparin, dextrans, alcohol and radiographic contrast agents may also cause defective function.

Diagnosis of platelet disorders

Patients with suspected platelet or blood vessel abnormalities should initially have a blood count and blood film examination (Fig. 25.11). Bone marrow examination is often needed in thrombocytopenic patients to determine whether or not there is a failure of platelet production. The marrow may also reveal one of the conditions associated with defective production (Table 25.2). In children and young adults with isolated thrombocytopenia, the marrow test is often not performed. In the elderly, the test is needed particularly to exclude myelodysplasia. In patients with thrombocytopenia, a negative drug history, normal or excessive numbers of marrow megakaryocytes and no other marrow abnormality or splenomegaly, ITP is the usual diagnosis. Testing for platelet antibodies in serum or on the surface of platelets has not proved reliable in distinguishing ITP from other causes of thrombocytopenia. Screening tests for DIC are also useful, as are tests for an underlying disease (e.g. SLE or HIV infection).

When the blood count, including platelet count and blood film examination, are normal, a PFA-100 or, much less frequently, a bleeding time is used to detect abnormal platelet function. In most patients with abnormal platelet function demonstrated by prolonged bleeding time, or the PFA-100 test, the defect is acquired and associated either with systemic disease (e.g. uraemia) or with aspirin therapy. The very rare hereditary defects of platelet function require more elaborate *in vitro* tests to define the specific abnormality. These include platelet aggregation studies (Fig. 25.10) and measurements of platelet nucleotide levels. If von Willebrand disease is suspected, assay of VWF and coagulation factor VIII are required.

Thrombomimetics

These are drugs that increase platelet production by activating the thrombopoietin receptor on megakaryocytes. Two such drugs are thromboplastin given subcutaneously once weekly and eltrombopag

active orally and given daily. They are used in ITP (Fig. 25.5) and are in trial in other conditions (e.g. post-chemotherapy, myelodysplasia, aplastic anaemia). They may cause disturbed liver function and increased bone marrow reticulin. Their long-term use may cause marrow fibrosis which is reversible by stopping the drug.

Platelet transfusions

Transfusion of platelet concentrates is indicated in the following circumstances:

1 Thrombocytopenia or abnormal platelet function when bleeding or before invasive procedures and where there is no alternative therapy available (e.g. steroids or high dose immunoglobulin). The platelet count should be above 50×10^9/L before, for example, liver biopsy or lumbar puncture.
2 Prophylactically in patients with platelet counts of less than $5{-}10 \times 10^9$/L. If there is infection, potential bleeding sites or coagulopathy, the count should be kept above 20×10^9/L).

The indications for transfusion of platelet concentrates are discussed further on p. 410. These indications may change with the wider use of thrombomimetic drugs.

SUMMARY

- Vascular bleeding disorders may be congenital including hereditary haemorrhagic telangiectasia and the Ehlers–Danlos syndrome.
- Acquired vascular disorders include fragile capillaries in healthy women, senile purpura, purpura associated with infections, Henoch–Schönlein syndrome, scurvy and steroid therapy.
- Thrombocytopenia, if severe, also causes skin and mucous membrane bleeding. It has a wide range of causes including: (i) failure of platelet production from a congenital cause, drugs or viral infection or a general bone marrow failure;

(ii) increased consumption of platelets. This may be acute or chronic autoimmune, drug-induced, caused by disseminated intravascular coagulation or thrombotic thrombocytopenic purpura.
- Chronic autoimmune thrombocytopenia is treated by immunosuppression with corticosteroids, rituximab, azathioprine, ciclosporin or by splenectomy.
- The platelet count may be raised by platelet transfusion or by the thrombomimetic drugs eltrombopag or romiplastin.
- Disorders of platelet function may be hereditary as in von Willebrand disease,

(Continued)

Glanzmann's thrombasthemia and Bernard–Soulier syndrome or acquired, most frequently caused by drugs (e.g. aspirin, clopidogrel and dipyridamole) but also non-steroidal anti-inflammatory drugs.

■ Platelet function analysis (PFA-100), platelet aggregation studies and VWF assays may be needed to diagnose platelet functional defects.

Now visit www.wiley.com/go/essentialhaematology to test yourself on this chapter.

CHAPTER 26
Coagulation disorders

Key topics

Hereditary coagulation disorders

Hereditary deficiencies of each of the coagulation factors have been described. Haemophilia A (factor VIII deficiency), haemophilia B (Christmas disease, factor IX deficiency) and von Willebrand disease (VWD) are the most frequent; the others are rarer.

Haemophilia A

Haemophilia A is the most common of the hereditary clotting factor deficiencies. The prevalence is of the order of 30–100 per million population. The inheritance is sex-linked (Fig. 26.1) but up to one-third of patients have no family history and result from recent mutation.

Molecular genetics

The factor VIII gene is situated near the tip of the long arm of the X chromosome (Xq2.8 region). It is extremely large and consists of 26 exons. The factor VIII protein includes a triplicated region $A_1A_2A_3$ with 30% homology with each other, a duplicated homology region C_1C_2 and a heavily glycosylated B domain which is removed when factor VIII is activated by thrombin. The protein is synthesized in the liver and endothelial cells.

The defect is an absence or low level of plasma factor VIII. Approximately half of the patients have missense or frameshift mutations or deletions in the factor VIII gene. In others a characteristic 'flip-tip' inversion is seen in which the factor VIII gene is broken by an inversion at the end of the X chromosome (Fig. 26.2). This mutation leads to a severe clinical form of haemophilia A.

Clinical features

Infants may develop profuse post-circumcision haemorrhage or joint and soft tissue bleeds and excessive bruising when they start to be active. Recurrent painful haemarthroses and muscle haematomas dominate the clinical course of severely affected patients and if inadequately treated lead to progressive joint deformity and disability (Figs 26.3–26.6). Local pressure can cause entrapment neuropathy or ischaemic necrosis. Prolonged bleeding occurs after dental extractions. Spontaneous haematuria and gastrointestinal haemorrhage, sometimes with obstruction resulting from intra-mucosal bleeding, can also occur. The clinical severity of the disease correlates inversely with the factor VIII level (Table 26.1). Operative and post-traumatic haemorrhage are life-threatening both in severely and mildly affected patients. Although not common, spontaneous intracerebral haemorrhage occurs more frequently than in the general population and is an important cause of death in patients with severe disease.

Haemophilic pseudotumours are large encapsulated haematomas with progressive cystic swelling from repeated haemorrhage. They are best visualized by magnetic resonance imaging (MRI) (Fig. 26.5b). They may occur in fascial and muscle planes, large muscle groups and in the long bones, pelvis and cranium. The latter result from repeated subperiosteal haemorrhages with bone destruction and new bone formation.

As a result of human immunodeficiency virus (HIV) present in concentrates made from human plasma during the early 1980s, over 50% of haemophiliacs treated in the USA or Western Europe

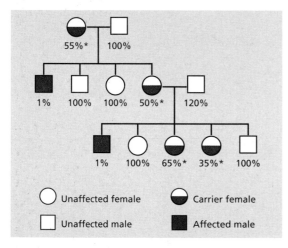

Figure 26.1 A typical family tree in a family with haemophilia. Note the variable levels of factor VIII activity in carriers (*) because of random inactivation of X chromosome (Lyonization). The percentages show the degree of factor VIII activity as a percentage of normal.

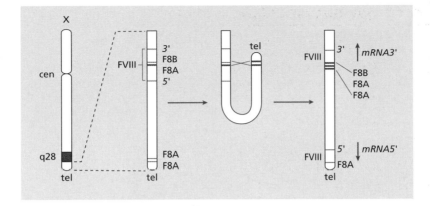

Figure 26.2 The mechanism of the flip-tip inversion leading to disruption of the factor VIII gene. **(Left)** The orientation of the factor VIII gene is shown with the three copies of gene A (F8A) in this region (one within an intron 22 and two near the telomere). **(Middle)** During spermatogenesis at meiosis, the single X pairs with the Y chromosome in the homologous regions. The X chromosome is longer than the Y and there is nothing to pair with most of the long arm of X. The chromosome undergoes homologous recombination between the A genes. **(Right)** The final result is that the factor VIII gene is disrupted. cen, centromeric end; tel, telomere; the arrows indicate the direction of transcription from the A gene.

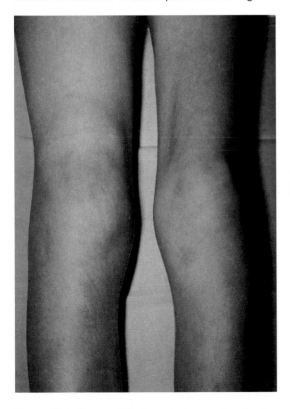

Figure 26.3 Haemophilia A: acute haemarthrosis of the right knee joint with swelling of the suprapatellar region. There is wasting of the quadriceps muscles, particularly on the left.

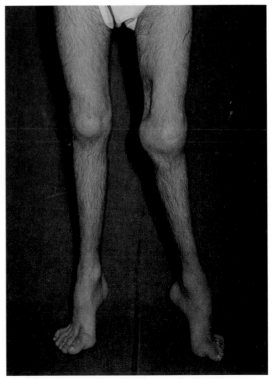

Figure 26.4 Haemophilia A showing severe disability. The left knee is swollen with posterior subluxation of the tibia on the femur. The ankles and feet show residual deformities of talipes equinus, with some cavus and associated toe clawing. There is generalized muscle wasting. The scar on the medial side of the left lower thigh is the site of a previously excised pseudotumour.

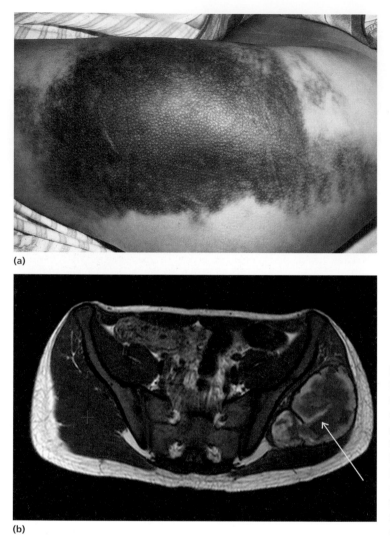

(a)

(b)

Figure 26.5 (a) Haemophilia A: massive haemorrhage in the area of the right buttock. **(b)** 15-year-old boy with sudden left hip pain and haemophilia A. Magnetic resonance imaging (MRI) axial image, T2 weighted, revealing large left spontaneous haematoma (yellow arrow) in left gluteus maximus muscle compared with normal right side (red cross). (Courtesy of Dr P. Wylie.)

became infected with HIV. Acquired immune deficiency syndrome (AIDS) has been a common cause of death in severe haemophilia. Thrombocytopenia from HIV infection may exacerbate bleeding episodes.

Many patients were infected with hepatitis C virus before testing of donors and blood products became possible. This has resulted in chronic hepatitis, cirrhosis and hepatoma. Hepatitis B transmission may also be a risk. Liver transplantation cures the haemophilia.

Laboratory findings (Table 26.2)

The following tests are abnormal:

1 Activated partial thromboplastin time (APTT).
2 Factor VIII clotting assay.

The platelet function analysis-100 (PFA-100) (and bleeding time) and prothrombin time (PT) are normal.

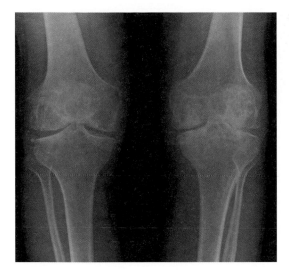

Figure 26.6 Haemophilia A: X-ray of the knee joints shows destruction and narrowing of the left joint space.

Table 26.1 Correlation of coagulation factor activity and disease severity in haemophilia A or B.

Coagulation factor activity (percentage of normal)	Clinical manifestations
<1	Severe disease Frequent spontaneous bleeding into joints, muscles, internal organs from early life Joint deformity and crippling if not adequately prevented or treated
1–5	Moderate disease Bleeding after minor trauma Occasional spontaneous episodes
>5	Mild disease Bleeding only after significant trauma, surgery

Carrier detection and antenatal diagnosis

Carriers are detected with DNA probes. A known specific mutation can be identified (Fig. 26.7) or restriction fragment length polymorphisms within or close to the factor VIII gene allow the mutant allele to be tracked. Chorionic biopsies at 8–10 weeks' gestation provide sufficient fetal DNA for analysis. Antenatal diagnosis is also possible following the demonstration of low levels of factor VIII in fetal blood obtained at 16–20 weeks' gestation from the umbilical vein by ultrasound-guided needle aspiration. This method is now only used if DNA analysis is uninformative (1% of carriers).

Treatment

Most patients in developed countries attend specialized haemophilia centres where there is a multidisciplinary team dedicated to their care. Bleeding episodes are treated with factor VIII replacement therapy and spontaneous bleeding is usually controlled if the patient's factor VIII level is raised to 30–50% of normal. Guidelines exist for the plasma level to be achieved for different types of haemorrhage. For major surgery, serious post-traumatic bleeding or when haemorrhage is occurring at a dangerous site, the factor VIII level should be elevated to 100% and then maintained above 50% when acute bleeding has stopped, until healing has occurred. On average, factor VIII infusion produces a plasma increment of 2 U/dL per unit infused per kilogram body weight. Roughly, the dose to be infused (units) = (weight (kg) × increment needed (U/dL))/2.

Recombinant factor VIII and plasma-derived purified factor VIII preparations, which are heat and solvent-detergent treated, are available for clinical use and have never transmitted viral infections.

1-Diamino-8-D-arginine vasopressin (DDAVP; desmopressin) provides an alternative means of increasing the plasma factor VIII level in milder haemophiliacs. Following the intravenous administration of this drug, there is a two- to fourfold rise maximum at 30–60 min in the patient's own factor

Table 26.2 Main clinical and laboratory findings in haemophilia A, factor IX deficiency (haemophilia B, Christmas disease) and von Willebrand disease.

	Haemophilia A	Factor IX deficiency	von Willebrand disease
Inheritance	Sex-linked	Sex-linked	Dominant (incomplete)
Main sites of haemorrhage	Muscle, joints, post-trauma or postoperative	Muscle, joints, post-trauma or postoperative	Mucous membranes, skin cuts, post-trauma or postoperative
Platelet count	Normal	Normal	Normal
PFA-100	Normal	Normal	Prolonged
Prothrombin time	Normal	Normal	Normal
Partial thromboplastin time	Prolonged	Prolonged	Prolonged or normal
Factor VIII	Low	Normal	May be moderately reduced
Factor IX	Normal	Low	Normal
VWF	Normal	Normal	Low or abnormal function (Table 26.3)
Ristocetin-induced platelet aggregation	Normal	Normal	Impaired

VWF, von Willebrand factor.

VIII by release from endothelial cells and this rise is proportional to the resting level. DDAVP may also be taken subcutaneously or nasally – this has been used as immediate treatment for mild haemophilia after accidental trauma or haemorrhage. DDAVP has an antidiuretic action and should be avoided in the elderly; fluid restriction is advised after its use.

Local supportive measures used in treating haemarthroses and haematomas include resting the affected part, application of ice and the prevention of further trauma.

Prophylactic treatment

The increased availability of factor VIII concentrates that may be stored in domestic refrigerators has dramatically altered haemophilia treatment. At the earliest suggestion of bleeding, the haemophilic child may be treated at home. This advance has reduced the occurrence of crippling haemarthroses and the need for inpatient care. Severely affected patients are now reaching adult life with little or no arthritis. After the first spontaneous joint bleed, most boys with severe haemophilia are started on prophylactic factor VIII three times a week, aiming to keep their factor VIII trough levels above 1%. This may require the placement of a vascular access device such as Port-a-Cath if venous access is difficult. A controlled trial has proven that regular prophylaxis is far superior to on-demand treatment as judged by progression of joint damage, which was virtually absent in children on prophylaxis but always seen in boys treated on-demand.

Haemophiliacs are advised to have regular conservative dental care. Haemophiliac children and their parents often require extensive help with social and psychological matters. With modern treatment the lifestyle of a haemophilic child can be almost normal but certain activities such as body extreme

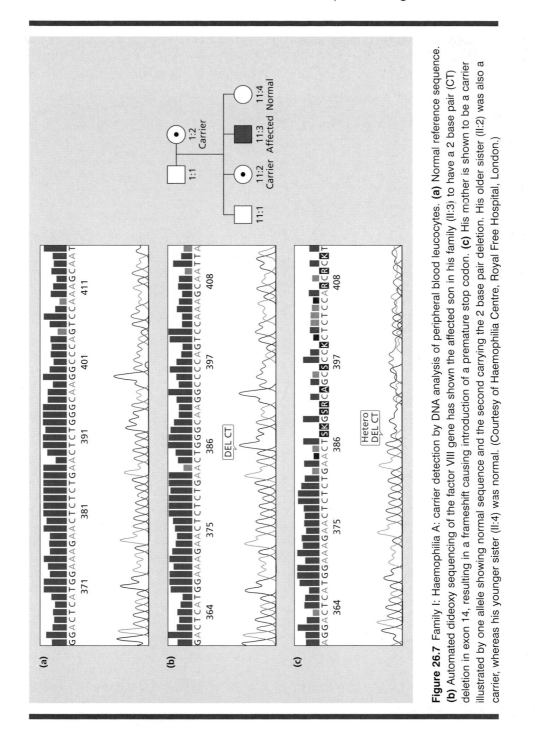

Figure 26.7 Family I: Haemophilia A: carrier detection by DNA analysis of peripheral blood leucocytes. **(a)** Normal reference sequence. **(b)** Automated dideoxy sequencing of the factor VIII gene has shown the affected son in his family (II:3) to have a 2 base pair (CT) deletion in exon 14, resulting in a frameshift causing introduction of a premature stop codon. **(c)** His mother is shown to be a carrier illustrated by one allele showing normal sequence and the second carrying the 2 base pair deletion. His older sister (II:2) was also a carrier, whereas his younger sister (II:4) was normal. (Courtesy of Haemophilia Centre, Royal Free Hospital, London.)

contact sports are to be avoided, or undertaken with extra prophylaxis.

Gene therapy

Because it is only necessary to maintain factor levels >1% to prevent most of the mortality and morbidity of factor VIII or IX deficiency, there is great interest in gene-based therapy. Various viral vectors (retroviral, adeno-associated) as well as non-viral vectors are being explored. Phase 1 trials are being carried out for both haemophilia A and B.

Inhibitors

One of the most serious complications of haemophilia is the development of antibodies (inhibitors) to infused factor VIII which occurs in 30–40% of severely effected patients, usually within the first 50 days of exposure. This renders the patient refractory to further replacement therapy. Immunosuppression and immune tolerance regimens have been used in an attempt to eradicate the antibody with success (at great cost) in about two-thirds of cases. Recombinant activated factor VII (VIIa) and activated prothrombin complex concentrates (FEIBA – factor VIII inhibitor bypassing activity) can be useful in the treatment of bleeding episodes.

Factor VIIa complexes with tissue factor exposed at the site of injury and produces local haemostasis. The process is independent of factor VIII or IX and is not affected by their inhibitors. Factor VIIa has a short half-life and therefore frequent doses may be needed. In the longer term, immunosuppression with cyclophosphamide, rituximab, intravenous immunoglobulin and high-dose factor VIII has also been successful.

Factor IX deficiency (Haemophilia B, Christmas disease)

The inheritance and clinical features of factor IX deficiency (Christmas disease, haemophilia B) are identical to those of haemophilia A. Indeed, the two disorders can only be distinguished by specific coagulation factor assays. The incidence is one-fifth that of haemophilia A. Factor IX is coded by a gene close to the gene for factor VIII near the tip of the long arm of the X chromosome at Xq2.6. Its synthesis,

like that of prothrombin, factor VII, factor X and protein C, is vitamin K-dependent. Carrier detection and antenatal diagnosis is performed as for haemophilia A. The principles of replacement therapy are similar to those of haemophilia A. Bleeding episodes are treated with high-purity factor IX concentrates. Because of its longer biological half-life, infusions do not have to be given as frequently as do factor VIII concentrates in haemophilia A. Recombinant factor IX is preferred, but higher doses are needed than with plasma-derived factor IX to attain the same response. Also the distribution and kinetics of clearance differ from the natural product, but it is certainly safe and effective.

Laboratory findings (Table 26.2)

The following tests are abnormal:

1 APTT;
2 Factor IX clotting assay.

As in haemophilia A, the PFA-100 (and bleeding time) and PT tests are normal.

Von Willebrand disease

In this disorder there is either a reduced level or abnormal function of von Willebrand factor (VWF) resulting from a missense mutation or null mutation. VWF is produced in endothelial cells and megakaryocytes. It has two roles (see Chapter 24). It promotes platelet adhesion to subendothelium at high shear rates and it is the carrier molecule for factor VIII, protecting it from premature destruction. The latter property explains the reduced factor VIII levels found in VWD.

Chronic elevation of VWF is part of the acute phase response to injury, inflammation, neoplasia or pregnancy. VWF is synthesized as a large 600-kDa dimeric protein which then forms multimers up to 20×10^6 Da in weight which are the largest molecules in blood. Three types of VWD have been described (Table 26.3). Type 2 is divided into four subtypes depending on the type of functional defect. Type 1 accounts for 75% of cases.

VWD is the most common inherited bleeding disorder. Usually, the inheritance is autosomal dominant. The severity of the bleeding is highly variable

Table 26.3 Classification of von Willebrand disease.

Type 1	Quantitative partial deficiency
Type 2	Functional abnormality
Type 3	Complete deficiency

Secondary classification of type 2 VWD

Subtype	Platelet-associated function	Factor VIII binding capacity	High MW VWF multimers
2A	Decreased	Normal	Absent
2B	Increased affinity for GPIb	Normal	Usually reduced/absent
2M	Decreased	Normal	Normal
2N	Normal	Reduced	Normal

GPIb, glycoprotein Ib; MW, molecular weight; VWD, von Willebrand disease; VWF, von Willebrand factor.

depending on mutation type and epistatic genetic effects such as ABO blood group. Women are worse affected than men at a given VWF level. Typically, there is mucous membrane bleeding (e.g. epistaxes, menorrhagia), excessive blood loss from superficial cuts and abrasions, and operative and post-traumatic haemorrhage. The severity is variable in the different types. Haemarthroses and muscle haematomas are rare, except in type 3 disease.

Laboratory findings (Table 26.2)

1 The PFA-100 test (see p. 328) is abnormal. This has largely replaced the bleeding time test.
2 Factor VIII levels are often low. If low, a factor VIII/VWF binding assay is performed.
3 The APTT may be prolonged.
4 VWF levels are usually low.
5 There is defective platelet aggregation by patient plasma in the presence of ristocetin (VWF: Rco). Aggregation to other agents (adenosine diphosphate (ADP), thrombin or adrenaline) is usually normal.
6 Collagen-binding function (VWF: CB) is usually reduced.
7 Multimer analysis is useful for diagnosing different subtypes (Table 26.3).
8 The platelet count is normal except for type 2B disease (where it is low).

Treatment

Options are as follows:

1 Local measures and antifibrinolytic agent (e.g. tranexamic acid for mild bleeding).
2 DDAVP infusion for those with type 1 VWD. This releases VWF from endothelial cells 30 min after intravenous infusion.
3 High-purity VWF concentrates for patients with very low VWF levels. Plasma-derived factor VIII/VWF concentrates are used. Recombinant VWF is now in phase II clinical trials.

Hereditary disorders of other coagulation factors

All these disorders (deficiency of fibrinogen, prothrombin, factors V, VII, combined V and VIII, factors X, XI, XIII) are rare. In all the inheritance is autosomal recessive except for factor XI deficiency where there is variable penetrance. Factor XI deficiency is seen mainly in Ashkenazi Jews and occurs in either sex. The bleeding risk shows incomplete correlation to severity of the deficiency, and bleeding only occurs after trauma such as surgery. Treatment is with fibrinolytic inhibitor, factor XI concentrate or fresh frozen plasma. Factor XIII deficiency produces a severe bleeding tendency, characteristically with umbilical stump bleeding. Plasma concentrates and recombinant preparation of factors VII and XIII are available.

Acquired coagulation disorders

The acquired coagulation disorders (Table 26.4) are more common than the inherited disorders. Unlike the inherited disorders, multiple clotting factor deficiencies are usual.

Vitamin K deficiency

Fat-soluble vitamin K is obtained from green vegetables and bacterial synthesis in the gut. Deficiency may present in the newborn (haemorrhagic disease of the newborn) or in later life.

Deficiency of vitamin K is caused by an inadequate diet, malabsorption or inhibition of vitamin K by drugs such as warfarin which act as vitamin K

Table 26.4 The acquired coagulation disorders.

Deficiency of vitamin K-dependent factors
Haemorrhagic disease of the newborn
Biliary obstruction
Malabsorption of vitamin K (e.g. tropical sprue, gluten-induced enteropathy)
Vitamin K-antagonist therapy (e.g. coumarins, indandiones)
Liver disease – complex dysregulation with synthetic failure of pro- and anticoagulant factors
Disseminated intravascular coagulation – consumption of all clotting factors and platelets

Inhibition of coagulation
Specific inhibitors (e.g. antibodies against factor VIII)
Non-specific inhibitors (e.g. antibodies found in systemic lupus erythematosus, rheumatoid arthritis which paradoxically cause thrombosis)

Miscellaneous
Diseases with M-protein production that interfere with haemostasis
L-Asparaginase
Therapy with heparin, defibrinating agents or thrombolytics
Massive transfusion syndrome

---

antagonists. Warfarin is associated with a decrease in the functional activity of factors II, VII, IX and X and proteins C and S, but immunological methods show normal levels of these factors. The non-functional proteins are called PIVKA (proteins formed in vitamin K absence). Conversion of PIVKA factors to their biologically active forms is a post-translational event involving carboxylation of glutamic acid residues in the N-terminal region where these factors show strong sequence homology (Fig. 26.8). Gamma-carboxylated glutamic acid binds calcium ions, inducing a reversible shape change in the N-termini of vitamin K dependent proteins. This exposes hydrophobic residues which bind to phospholipid. In the process of carboxylation, vitamin K is converted to vitamin K epoxide which is cycled back to the reduced form by a reductase (VKORC-1). Warfarin interferes with the action of vitamin K epoxide reductase leading to a functional vitamin K deficiency.

Haemorrhagic disease of the newborn

Vitamin K-dependent factors are low at birth and fall further in breast-fed infants in the first few days of life. Liver cell immaturity, lack of gut bacterial synthesis of the vitamin and low quantities in breast milk may all contribute to a deficiency which causes haemorrhage, usually on the second to fourth day of life, but occasionally during the first 2 months.

Diagnosis

The PT and APTT are both abnormal. The platelet count and fibrinogen are normal with absent fibrin degradation products.

Treatment

1 Prophylaxis. For many years vitamin K has been given to all newborn babies as a single intramuscular injection of 1 mg. This remains the most appropriate and safest treatment. Following epidemiological evidence suggesting a possible link between intramuscular vitamin K and an increased risk of childhood tumours (which has not been substantiated), some centres recommended an oral regimen but this has never been subjected to randomized controlled trial.

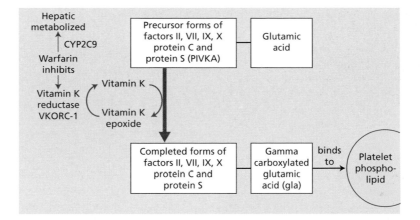

Figure 26.8 The action of vitamin K in γ-carboxylation of glutamic acid in coagulation factors which are then able to bind Ca²⁺ and attach to the platelet phospholipid. Warfarin inhibits vitamin K reductase. It is metabolized in the liver and genetic variations in the reductase enzyme VKORC-1 and in the cytochrome CYP2C9 largely account for wide variations in warfarin sensitivity of individuals.

2 In bleeding infants: vitamin K 1 mg intramuscularly is given every 6 hours with, initially, prothrombin complex concentrate if haemorrhage is severe.

Vitamin K deficiency in children or adults

Deficiency resulting from obstructive jaundice, pancreatic or small bowel disease occasionally causes a bleeding diathesis in children or adults.

Diagnosis
Both PT and APTT are prolonged. There are low plasma levels of factors II, VII, IX and X.

Treatment
1 Prophylaxis: vitamin K 5 mg/day orally.
2 Active bleeding or prior to liver biopsy: vitamin K 10 mg slowly intravenously. Some correction of PT is usual within 6 hours. The dose should be repeated on the next 2 days after which optimal correction is usual.
3 Rapid correction may be achieved by infusion of prothrombin complex concentrate.

Liver disease

Multiple haemostatic abnormalities contribute to a bleeding tendency and may exacerbate haemorrhage from oesophageal varices.

1 Biliary obstruction results in impaired absorption of vitamin K and therefore decreased synthesis of factors II, VII, IX and X by liver parenchymal cells.
2 With severe hepatocellular disease, in addition to a deficiency of these factors, there are often reduced levels of factor V and fibrinogen and increased amounts of plasminogen activator.
3 Functional abnormality of fibrinogen (dysfibrinogenaemia) is found in many patients.
4 Decreased thrombopoietin production from the liver contributes to thrombocytopenia.
5 Hypersplenism associated with portal hypertension frequently results in thrombocytopenia.
6 Disseminated intravascular coagulation (DIC; see below) may be related to release of thromboplastins from damaged liver cells and reduced concentrations of antithrombin, protein C and α₂-antiplasmin. In addition, there is impaired removal of activated clotting factors and increased fibrinolytic activity.
7 The net haemostatic inbalance in liver disease may be prothrombotic rather than haemorrhagic.

Disseminated intravascular coagulation

Widespread inappropriate intravascular deposition of fibrin with consumption of coagulation factors and platelets occurs as a consequence of many disorders that release procoagulant material into the circulation or cause widespread endothelial damage or platelet aggregation (Table 26.5). It may be associated with a fulminant haemorrhagic or thrombotic syndrome with organ dysfunction or run a less severe and more chronic course. The main clinical presentation is with bleeding but 5–10% of patients manifest thrombotic lesions (e.g. with gangrene of limbs).

Table 26.5 Causes of disseminated intravascular coagulation.

Infections
Gram-negative and meningococcal septicaemia
Clostridium welchii septicaemia
Severe falciparum malaria
Viral infection – varicella, HIV, hepatitis,
  cytomegalovirus

Malignancy
Widespread mucin-secreting adenocarcinoma
Acute promyelocytic leukaemia

Obstetric complications
Amniotic fluid embolism
Premature separation of placenta
Eclampsia; retained placenta
Septic abortion

Hypersensitivity reactions
Anaphylaxis
Incompatible blood transfusion

Widespread tissue damage
Following surgery or trauma
After severe burns

Vascular abnormalities
Kasabach–Merritt syndrome
Leaking prosthetic valves
Cardiac bypass surgery
Vascular aneurysms

Miscellaneous
Liver failure
Pancreatitis
Snake and invertebrate venoms
Hypothermia
Heat stroke
Acute hypoxia
Massive blood loss

Pathogenesis (Fig. 26.9)

The key event underlying DIC is increased activity of thrombin in the circulation that overwhelms its normal rate of removal by natural anticoagulants. This can come from tissue factor (TF) release into the circulation from damaged tissues present on tumour cells or from up-regulation of TF on circulating monocytes or endothelial cells in response to pro-inflammatory cytokines (e.g. interleukin-1, tumour necrosis factor, endotoxin).

1 DIC may be triggered by the entry of procoagulant material into the circulation in the following situations: severe trauma, amniotic fluid embolism, premature separation of the placenta, widespread mucin-secreting adenocarcinomas, acute promyelocytic leukaemia (t(15; 17)), liver disease, severe falciparum malaria, haemolytic transfusion reaction and some snake bites.
2 DIC may also be initiated by widespread endothelial damage and collagen exposure (e.g. endotoxaemia, Gram-negative and meningococcal septicaemia, septic abortion), certain virus infections and severe burns or hypothermia.

In addition to its role in the deposition of fibrin in the microcirculation, intravascular thrombin formation produces large amounts of circulating fibrin monomers which form complexes with fibrinogen and interfere with fibrin polymerization, thus contributing to the coagulation defect. Intense fibrinolysis is stimulated by thrombi on vascular walls and the release of split products interferes with fibrin polymerization, thus contributing to the coagulation defect. The combined action of thrombin and plasmin causes depletion of fibrinogen and all coagulation factors. Intravascular thrombin also causes widespread platelet aggregation in the vessels. The bleeding problems which may be a feature of DIC are compounded by thrombocytopenia caused by consumption of platelets.

Clinical features

These are usually dominated by bleeding, particularly from venepuncture sites or wounds (Fig. 26.10a). There may be generalized bleeding in the

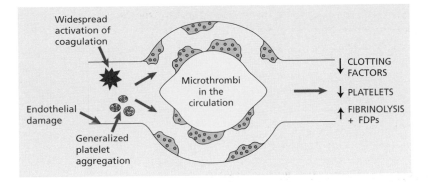

Figure 26.9 The pathogenesis of disseminated intravascular coagulation and the changes in clotting factors, platelets and fibrin degradation products (FDPs) that occur in this syndrome.

gastrointestinal tract, the oropharynx, into the lungs, urogenital tract and in obstetric cases, vaginal bleeding may be particularly severe. Less frequently, microthrombi may cause skin lesions, renal failure, gangrene of the fingers or toes (Fig. 26.10b) or cerebral ischaemia.

Some patients may develop subacute or chronic DIC, especially with mucin-secreting adenocarcinoma. Compensation by the liver may render some of the coagulation tests normal.

Laboratory findings (Table 26.6)

In many acute syndromes the blood may fail to clot because of gross fibrinogen deficiency.

Tests of haemostasis
1 The platelet count is low.
2 Fibrinogen concentration low.
3 The thrombin time is prolonged.
4 High levels of fibrin degradation products such as D-dimers are found in serum and urine.
5 The PT and APTT are prolonged in the acute syndromes.

Blood film examination
In many patients there is a haemolytic anaemia ('microangiopathic') and the red cells show prominent fragmentation because of damage caused when passing through fibrin strands in small vessels (see p. 85).

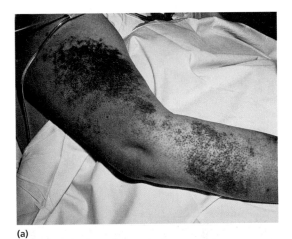

(a)

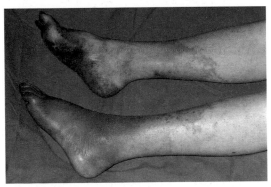

(b)

Figure 26.10 Clinical features of disseminated intravascular coagulation: **(a)** indurated and confluent purpura of the arm; **(b)** peripheral gangrene with swelling and discolouration of the skin of the feet in fulminant disease.

Table 26.6 Haemostasis tests: typical results in acquired bleeding disorders.

	Platelet count	Prothrombin time	Activated partial thromboplastin time	Thrombin time
Liver disease	Low	Prolonged	Prolonged	Normal (rarely prolonged)
DIC	Low	Prolonged	Prolonged	Grossly prolonged
Massive transfusion	Low	Prolonged	Prolonged	Normal
Coumarin anticoagulants	Normal	Grossly prolonged	Prolonged	Normal
Heparin	Normal (rarely low)	Mildly prolonged	Prolonged	Prolonged
Circulating anticoagulant	Normal	Normal or prolonged	Prolonged	Normal

DIC, Disseminated intravascular coagulation.

Treatment

Treatment of the underlying cause is most important. The management of patients who are bleeding differs from that of patients with thrombotic problems.

Bleeding

Supportive therapy with fresh frozen plasma (Table 26.7) and platelet concentrates is indicated in patients with dangerous or extensive bleeding. Cryoprecipitate provides a more concentrated source of fibrinogen and red cell transfusions may be required.

Thrombosis

The use of heparin or antiplatelet drugs to inhibit the coagulation process is considered in those with thrombotic problems such as skin ischaemia. Fibrinolytic inhibitors should not be considered because failure to lyse thrombi in organs such as the kidney may have adverse effects. Antithrombin concentrates or recombinant activated human protein C may be used to inhibit DIC in severe cases with sepsis (e.g. meningococcal septicaemia). There is reduced activated protein C (APC) in severe sepsis and recombinant human APC has been found to reduce mortality in this setting.

Table 26.7 Indications for the use of fresh frozen plasma (National Institutes of Health Consensus Guidelines).

Coagulation factor deficiency (PCC where specific or combined factor concentrate is not available)

Reversal of warfarin effect (PCC if available are highly effective compared to plasma which has almost no effect)

Multiple coagulation defects (e.g. in patients with liver disease, DIC) (PCC are much better, plasma is virtually useless)

Massive blood transfusion with coagulopathy and clinical bleeding

Thrombotic thrombocytopenic purpura

Deficiencies of antithrombin*, protein C* or protein S

Some patients with immunodeficiency syndromes

DIC, disseminated intravascular coagulation; PCC, prothrombin complex concentrates.
* Antithrombin and protein C concentrates now available.

Coagulation deficiency caused by antibodies

Circulating antibodies to coagulation factors are occasionally seen with an incidence of approximately 1 per million per year rising markedly with age. Alloantibodies to factor VIII occur in 5–10% of haemophiliacs. Factor VIII autoantibodies may also result in a bleeding syndrome. These immunoglobulin G (IgG) antibodies occur rarely postpartum, in certain immunological disorders (e.g. rheumatoid arthritis), in cancer and in old age. Treatment usually consists of a combination of immunosuppression and treatment with factor replacement, usually as human factor VIII, recombinant VIIa or activated prothrombin complex concentrate (FEIBA).

Another protein known as the **lupus anticoagulant** interferes with lipoprotein-dependent stages of coagulation and is usually detected by prolongation of the APTT test (Table 26.6). This inhibitor is detected in 10% of patients with systemic lupus erythematosus (SLE) and in patients with other autoimmune diseases who frequently have antibodies to other lipid-containing antigens (e.g. cardiolipin). The antibody is not associated with a bleeding tendency but there is an increased risk of arterial or venous thrombosis and, as with other causes of

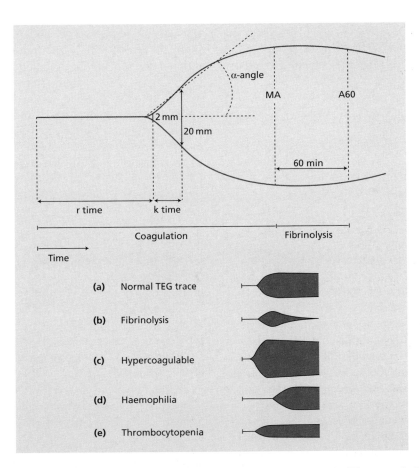

Figure 26.11 Thromboelastography (TEG): **(a–e)** normal trace and appearances in different pathological states. α-angle, speed of solid clot formation; A$_{60}$, measure of clot lysis or retraction at 60 min; k, clot formation time; MA, absolute strength of fibrin clot; r, rate of initial fibrin formation. (From Mallett S.V. and Cox D.J.A. (1992) *Br J Anaesth* **69**,307–13, with permission.)

thrombophilia, an association with recurrent miscarriage (see Chapter 27).

Massive transfusion syndrome

Many factors may contribute to a bleeding disorder following massive transfusion. Blood loss results in reduced levels of platelets, coagulation factors and inhibitors. Further dilution of these factors occurs during replacement with red cells.

Management

Platelet concentrates are given to maintain a platelet count >50×10^9/L or $80–100 \times 10^9$/L in cerebral injury or after trauma. The PT and APTT should be kept to less than 1.5 times normal with fresh frozen plasma given initially at 15 mL/kg. Cryoprecipitate is given to keep fibrinogen at least 1 g/L. Recombinant VIIa (RCT) is used in patients with massive blood loss after trauma or surgery to reduce haemorrhage but remains 'off label' as RCT in such situations has failed to unambiguously prove benefit and there is a significant rise of thrombosis in such patients.

The results of haemostasis screening tests in acquired bleeding disorders are shown in Table 26.6 and a summary of the indications for use of fresh frozen plasma in Table 26.7.

Thromboelastography: near-patient testing

Thromboelastography (TEG) is a technique for a global assessment of haemostatic function of a single blood sample in which the reaction of platelets with the protein coagulation cascade is observed from the time of the initial platelet fibrin interaction through platelet aggregation, clot strengthening and fibrin cross-linkage to eventual clot lysis. It is suited as a monitor of haemostasis in surgery (e.g. of the liver or heart) associated with haemostatic defects. Freshly drawn blood is placed in a cuvette which is oscillated, the motion being transferred to a pin which transmits deflection as torsion to a photoelectric detector with computerized data capture. As fibrin strands form, the fibrin clot affects movement of the pin. The normal trace shows the rate of initial fibrin formation, the time to formation of a clot (coagulation time), strength of the fibrin clot, clot lysis index or retraction. Typical patterns showing results in fibrinolysis, hypercoagulability, haemophilia and thrombocytopenia are shown in Fig. 26.11.

The PFA-100 may also be useful in testing platelet function before and during surgery (see p. 343) but it is not suitable to use as a stand alone screening test for primary haemostatic disorders.

SUMMARY

- Coagulation disorders may be inherited or acquired.
- Haemophilia A is the most common inherited deficiency of a clotting factor. It is severe if factor VIII activity in plasma is <1% of normal. It presents with excess bruising or prolonged bleeding after trauma and spontaneous bleeding, usually into muscles and joints, which can result in joint deformity.
- Many older patients are infected with hepatitis C or HIV as a result of receiving contaminated blood products.
- The APTT is prolonged and PT normal.
- Antenatal diagnosis is usually carried out by polymerase chain reaction (PCR)

techniques, the gene being carried on the X chromosome.
- Treatment is with recombinant or concentrates of factor VIII, or with drugs (e.g. DDAVP (desmopressin)).
- Factor IX deficiency has a similar pattern of inheritance and clinical manifestations.
- Von Willebrand disease (VWD) is the most frequent inherited bleeding disorder. Haemorrhage occurs from mucous membranes, skin cuts and post-trauma. It usually has a dominant inheritance. Platelet function is abnormal and VWF levels usually low.
- Acquired coagulation disorders include those caused by vitamin K deficiency (e.g.

in the newborn or with malabsorption) or caused by vitamin K antagonist therapy (e.g. warfarin).

- Other common coagulation abnormalities are those in liver disease caused by reduced synthesis of coagulation factors and in disseminated intravascular coagulation (DIC), which causes consumption of coagulation factors and platelets.

- Fresh frozen plasma is used in treatment of multiple coagulation defects, or specific defects if the appropriate concentrate is not available, and in therapy for thrombotic thrombocytopenic purpura.

Now visit www.wiley.com/go/essentialhaematology to test yourself on this chapter.

CHAPTER 27
Thrombosis and antithrombotic therapy

Key topics

Essential Haematology, 6th Edition. © A. V. Hoffbrand and P. A. H. Moss. Published 2011 by Blackwell Publishing Ltd.

Thrombi are solid masses or plugs formed in the circulation from blood constituents. Platelets and fibrin form the basic structure. Their clinical significance results from ischaemia from local vascular obstruction or distant embolization. Thrombi are involved in the pathogenesis of myocardial infarction, cerebrovascular disease, peripheral arterial disease, deep vein thrombosis (DVT) and pulmonary embolism (PE).

Thrombosis, both arterial and venous, is more common as age increases and is frequently associated with risk factors (e.g. surgery or pregnancy). The term thrombophilia is used to describe inherited or acquired disorders of the haemostatic mechanism that predispose to thrombosis.

Arterial thrombosis

Pathogenesis

Atherosclerosis of the arterial wall, plaque rupture and endothelial injury expose blood to subendothelial collagen and tissue factor. This initiates the formation of a platelet nidus on which platelets adhere and aggregate.

Platelet deposition and thrombus formation are important in the pathogenesis of atherosclerosis. Platelet-derived growth factor stimulates the migration and proliferation of smooth muscle cells and fibroblasts in the arterial intima. Regrowth of endothelium and repair at the site of arterial damage and incorporated thrombus result in thickening of the vessel wall.

As well as blocking arteries locally, emboli of platelets and fibrin may break away from the primary thrombus to occlude distal arteries. Examples are carotid artery thrombi leading to cerebral thrombosis and transient ischaemic attacks and heart valve and chamber thrombi leading to systemic emboli and infarcts (Fig. 27.1).

Clinical risk factors

The risk factors for arterial thrombosis are related to the development of atherosclerosis and are listed in Table 27.1. The identification of patients at risk is largely based on clinical assessment. A number of epidemiological studies have resulted in the con-

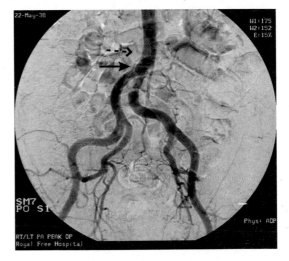

Figure 27.1 Arteriogram showing saddle embolus at the aortic bifurcation (dotted arrow) and embolus in the left common iliac artery (solid arrow).

Table 27.1 Risk factors for arterial thrombosis (atherosclerosis).
Positive family history
Male sex
Hyperlipidaemia
Hypertension
Diabetes mellitus
Gout
Polycythaemia
Hyperhomocysteinaemia
Cigarette smoking
ECG abnormalities
Elevated CRP, IL6, fibrinogen, lipoprotein-associated phospholipase A_2
Lupus anticoagulant
Collagen vascular diseases
Behçet's disease
CRP, C-reactive protein; ECG, electrocardiogram.

struction of coronary artery thrombosis risk profiles based on sex, age, elevated blood pressure, high levels of serum cholesterol, glucose intolerance, cigarette smoking and electrocardiogram abnormalities. These profiles have allowed presymptomatic assessment of young and apparently fit subjects and are valuable in counselling a change in lifestyle or for recommending medical therapy in individuals at risk. Epidemiological evidence implicates four inflammatory markers, fibrinogen, C-reactive protein, lipoprotein-associated phospholipase A_2 and interleukin-6 as predictive for coronary heart disease.

Venous thrombosis

Pathogenesis and risk factors

Virchow's triad suggests that there are three components that are important in thrombus formation:

1 Slowing down of blood flow;
2 Hypercoagulability of the blood; and
3 Vessel wall damage.

For venous thrombosis, increased systemic coagulability and stasis are most important, vessel wall damage being less important than in arterial thrombosis, although it may be important in patients with sepsis and indwelling catheters. Stasis allows the completion of blood coagulation at the site of initiation of the thrombus (e.g. behind the valve pockets of the leg veins in immobile patients).

Table 27.2 lists a number of recognized risk factors.

Hereditary disorders of haemostasis

The prevalence of inherited disorders associated with increased risk of thrombosis is higher than that of hereditary bleeding disorders. A hereditary 'thrombophilia' should be particularly suspected in young patients who develop spontaneous thrombosis, recurrent DVTs (Fig. 27.2) or an unusual site of thrombosis (e.g. axillary, splanchnic veins, sagittal sinus). Several abnormalities are now well characterized (Table 27.2).

Table 27.2 Hereditary and acquired risk factors for venous thrombosis.

Hereditary haemostatic disorders
Factor V Leiden
Prothrombin G20210A variant
Protein C deficiency
Antithrombin deficiency
Protein S deficiency
Dysfibrinogenaemia
ABO blood group

Hereditary or acquired haemostatic disorders
Raised plasma levels of factor VIII
Raised plasma levels of fibrinogen
Raised plasma levels of homocysteine

Acquired disorders
Lupus anticoagulant
Oestrogen therapy (oral contraceptive and HRT)
Heparin-induced thrombocytopenia
Pregnancy and puerperium
Surgery, especially abdominal, hip and knee surgery
Major trauma
Malignancy
Acutely ill hospitalized medical patients including cardiac or respiratory failure, infection, inflammatory bowel disorders
Myeloproliferative disease
Hyperviscosity, polycythaemia
Stroke
Pelvic obstruction
Nephrotic syndrome
Dehydration
Varicose veins
Age
Obesity
Paroxysmal nocturnal haemoglobinuria
Behçet's disease

HRT, hormone replacement therapy.

Factor V Leiden gene mutation (activated protein C resistance)

This is the most common inherited cause of an increased risk of venous thrombosis. It occurs in approximately 3–7% of Caucasian factor V alleles.

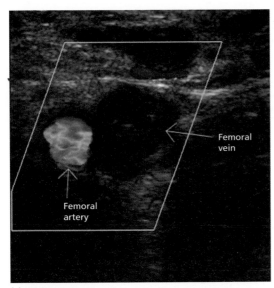

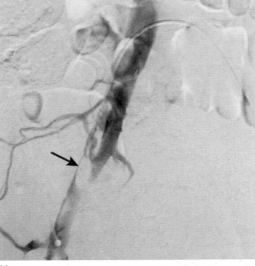

(a)

(b)

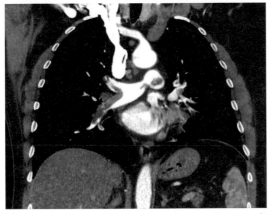

(c)

Figure 27.2 Diagnostic imaging of deep vein thrombosis (DVT) and pulmonary embolus (PE). **(a)** Colour power Doppler ultrasound of the right femoral vessels with compression shows normal flow in the femoral artery but absent flow in the vein because of thrombus. A normal vein would collapse with compression of the probe. (Courtesy of Dr Tony Young.) **(b)** Femoral venogram demonstrating extensive thrombus within the right external iliac vein. (Courtesy of Dr I.S. Francis and Dr A.Г. Watkinson.) **(c)** Computed tomography (CT) pulmonary angiography: a coronal image shows bilateral filling defects (green crosses) in the central central pulmonary arteries indicating pulmonary emboli. (Courtesy of Dr Tony Young.)

There is failure of activated protein C (APC) when added to plasma to prolong the activated partial thromboplastin time (APTT) test. Protein C, when activated, breaks down activated factor V so APC should slow the clotting reaction and prolong the APTT. APC resistance is caused by a genetic polymorphism in the factor V gene (replacement of arginine at position 506 with glutamine – Arg506Gln) which makes factor V less susceptible to cleavage by APC (Fig. 27.3). This is called the factor V Leiden mutation. The frequency of factor V Leiden in the general population in Western countries means that it cannot be regarded as a rare mutation but as a genetic polymorphism that is maintained in the population (Fig. 27.4). Presumably, individuals with this allele have been 'selected', probably because of a reduced bleeding tendency (e.g. post-partum). It does not increase the risk of arterial thrombosis.

Patients who are heterozygous for factor V Leiden are at an approximately five- to eight-fold increased risk of venous thrombosis compared to the general population but only 10% of carriers develop thrombosis during their lifetime.

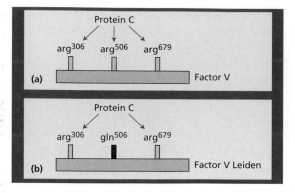

Figure 27.3 The genetic basis of factor V Leiden.
(a) Activated protein C (APC) inactivates factor Va by proteolytic cleavage at three sites in the Va heavy chain. **(b)** In the factor V Leiden mutation the Arg506Gln polymorphism leads to glutamine at position 506 with less efficient inactivation of factor V by APC and increased risk of thrombosis.

Individuals who are homozygous have a 30–140-fold risk. Following venous thrombosis they have a higher risk of re-thrombosis than individuals with DVT but normal factor V.

The incidence of factor V Leiden in patients with venous thrombosis is approximately 20–40%. Polymerase chain reaction (PCR) screening for the mutation is relatively simple and the test is widely performed. The absolute risk of thrombosis will depend on many other factors and it is difficult to advise individual patients of their risk. At present it is not recommended to start anticoagulation therapy in individuals with the Leiden mutation, even if homozygous, with no history of thrombosis. A small minority of patients with APC resistance do not have factor V Leiden but have other mutations of factor V.

Antithrombin deficiency

Inheritance is autosomal dominant. There are recurrent venous thromboses usually starting in early

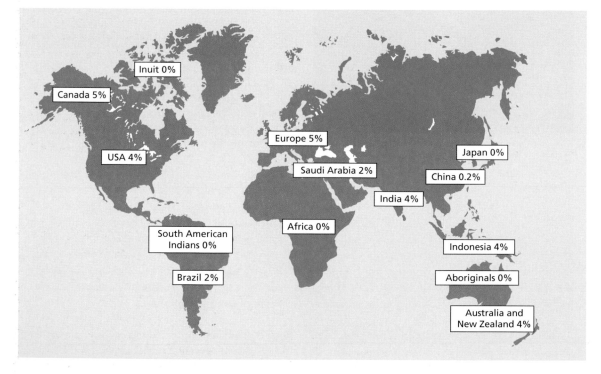

Figure 27.4 The incidence of carriers of factor V Leiden in different countries.

adult life. Arterial thrombi occur occasionally. Antithrombin concentrates are available and are used to prevent thrombosis during surgery or childbirth. Many molecular variants of antithrombin have been categorized and are associated with varying degrees of risk of thrombosis.

Protein C deficiency

Inheritance is autosomal dominant with variable penetrance. Protein C levels in heterozygotes are approximately 50% of normal. Characteristically, many patients develop skin necrosis as a result of dermal vessel occlusion when treated with warfarin, thought to be caused by reduction of protein C levels even further in the first day or two of warfarin therapy before reduction in the levels of the vitamin K-dependent clotting factors, especially factors II and X. Rarely, infants may be born with homozygous deficiency and characteristically present with severe disseminated intravascular coagulation (DIC) or purpura fulminans in infancy. APC concentrates are available and are used in selected acquired cases of severe sepsis with DIC as well as in genetic protein C deficiency. APC is also used in selected patients with multiorgan failure and sepsis for its anti-inflammitory, anticoagulant and pro-fibrinolytic effects.

Protein S deficiency

Protein S deficiency has been found in a number of families with a thrombotic tendency. It is a cofactor for protein C and the clinical features are similar to protein C deficiency, including a tendency to skin necrosis with warfarin therapy. The inheritance is autosomal dominant.

Prothrombin allele G20210A

Prothrombin allele G20210A is a variant (prevalence 2–3% in the population) that leads to increased plasma prothrombin levels and increases thrombotic risk by fivefold. It is probable that the cause of venous thrombosis with this mutation and with high levels of factors VIII, IX and XI is that sustained generation of thrombin results in pro-

longed down-regulation of fibrinolysis through activation of thrombin-activated fibrinolysis inhibitor (see p. 325).

Hyperhomocysteinaemia

Higher levels of plasma homocysteine may be genetic or acquired and are associated with increased risk for both venous and arterial thrombosis. However, recent large trials show little evidence that lowering the levels reduces these risks.

Homocysteine is derived from dietary methionine and is removed by either remethylation to methionine or conversion to cysteine via a *trans*-sulphuration pathway (Fig. 27.5). Classic homocystinuria is a rare autosomal recessive disorder caused by deficiency of cystathione β-synthase, the enzyme responsible for *trans*-sulphuration. Vascular disease and thrombosis are major features of the disease. Heterozygous cystathione β-synthase deficiency is present in approximately 0.5% of the population and leads to a moderate increase in homocysteine. Methylene tetrahydrofolate reductase is involved in the remethylation pathway and a common thermolabile variant of the enzyme may be responsible for mild homocysteinaemia (above $15\,\mu$mol/L) although this may only be seen in the presence of folate or vitamin B_{12} deficiency. Acquired risk factors for hyperhomocysteinaemia include deficiencies of folate, vitamin B_{12} or vitamin B_6, drugs (e.g. ciclosporin), renal damage and smoking. The levels also increase with age and are higher in men and post-menopausal females.

Defects of fibrinogen

Defects of fibrinogen are usually clinically silent or cause excess bleeding. Thrombosis is a rare association.

ABO blood group

Non-O blood group carriers have a higher risk of venous thrombosis or embolism than O carriers. This is related to their higher plasma levels of von Willebrand factor and factor VIII.

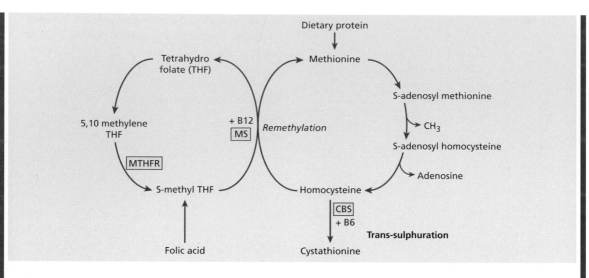

Figure 27.5 The metabolism of homocysteine. Homocysteine is derived from dietary methionine and is metabolized either by the *trans*-sulphuration or remethylation pathways. *Trans*-sulphuration proceeds using the cystathionine β-synthase (CBS) enzyme with vitamin B_6 as a cofactor. Remethylation involves the action of methionine synthase (MS) on 5-methyl-THF with vitamin B_{12} as a cofactor. In addition, methylene-tetrahydrofolate reductase (MTHFR) is involved in this cycle.

Hereditary or acquired disorders of haemostasis

High factor VIII or fibrinogen levels are also associated with venous thrombosis. The combination of multiple risk factors is associated with increased risk of thrombosis. If these are persistent they may represent a reason for extended anticoagulation.

Acquired risk factors

These may cause thrombosis in patients without another identifiable abnormality but are more likely to do so if an inherited predisposing abnormality (e.g. factor V Leiden) is also present.

Postoperative venous thrombosis

This is more likely to occur in the elderly, obese, those with a previous or family history of venous thrombosis, and in those in whom major abdominal or hip operations are performed. Elasticated stockings or mechanical methods (see p. 377) are used to reduce the risk of DVT.

Venous stasis and immobility

These factors are probably responsible for the high incidence of postoperative venous thrombosis and for venous thrombosis associated with congestive cardiac failure, myocardial infarction and varicose veins. In atrial fibrillation, thrombin generation from accumulation of activated clotting factors leads to a high risk clot formation in the atrial appendage and consequent systemic embolization. The use of muscle relaxants during anaesthesia may also contribute to venous stasis. Venous thrombosis also has a higher frequency after prolonged aeroplane journeys.

Malignancy

Patients with carcinoma of the ovary, brain and pancreas have a particularly increased risk of venous thrombosis but there is an increased risk with all cancers. The tumours produce tissue factor and a procoagulant that directly activates factor X. Mucin-secreting adenocarcinomas may be associated with DIC.

Inflammation

This up-regulates procoagulant factors, down-regulates anticoagulant pathways, particularly protein C. Thrombosis is particularly likely in inflammatory bowel disease, Behçet's disease, systemic tuberculosis, systemic lupus erythematosus (SLE) and diabetes.

Blood disorders

Increased viscosity, thrombocytosis, altered platelet membrane receptors and responses are possible factors for the high incidence of thrombosis in patients with polycythaemia vera and essential thrombocythaemia. Testing for the JAK2 V617F mutation may indicate an otherwise unsuspected myeloproliferative disease in patients with hepatic or portal vein thrombosis. There is a high incidence of venous thrombosis, including thrombi in large veins (e.g. the hepatic vein) in patients with paroxysmal nocturnal haemoglobinuria. An increased tendency to venous thrombosis has been observed in patients with sickle cell disease, with post-splenectomy thrombocytosis and those with a paraprotein.

Oestrogen therapy

Oestrogen therapy, particularly high dose therapy, is associated with increased plasma levels of factors II, VII, VIII, IX and X and depressed levels of antithrombin and tissue plasminogen activator in the vessel wall. There is a high incidence of postoperative venous thrombosis in women on high dose oestrogen therapy and full dose oestrogen-containing oral contraceptives. The risk is much less with low dose oestrogen contraceptive preparations. Hormone replacement therapy also increases the risk of thrombosis, largely obviated by the use of low oestrogen preparations.

The antiphospholipid syndrome

The antiphospholipid syndrome (APS) can be defined as the occurrence of venous and arterial thrombosis and/or recurrent miscarriage in association with laboratory evidence of persistent antiphospholipid antibody. The predominant antibodies in this disorder are directed against protein antigens that bind to anionic phospholipids, such as β_2-glycoprotein 1 (β_2-GPI-1) and prothrombin.

One antiphospholipid antibody is the 'lupus anticoagulant' (LA) which was initially detected in patients with SLE, and is identified by a prolonged plasma APTT which does not correct with a 50:50 mixture of normal plasma. Paradoxically, in view of its name, it is associated with venous and arterial thrombosis. A second test dependent on limiting quantities of phospholipid (e.g. the dilute Russell's viper venom test) is also used in diagnosis. Whereas lupus anticoagulants are reactive in the fluid phase, other antiphospholipid antibodies, such as anticardiolipin antibodies and antibodies to β_2-GPI-1, are identified by solid phase immunoassay. Both solid phase assays and coagulation tests for LA should be used in the diagnosis of APS.

As well as patients with SLE, antiphospholipid antibodies are also found in other autoimmune disorders particularly of connective tissues, lymphoproliferative diseases, post-viral infections, with certain drugs including phenothiazines and as an 'idiopathic' phenomenon in otherwise healthy subjects. Arterial thrombosis may cause peripheral limb ischaemia, stroke or myocardial infarct. Venous thrombosis includes DVT, PE and thrombosis in vessels supplying the abdominal organs. As with other causes of thrombophilia, recurrent abortion caused by placental infarction is also associated (Table 27.3). Thrombocytopenia may be present

Table 27.3 Clinical associations of lupus anticoagulant and anticardiolipin antibodies.

Venous thrombosis: deep venous thrombosis/pulmonary embolism, renal, hepatic, retinal veins
Arterial thrombosis
Recurrent fetal loss
Thrombocytopenia
Livedo reticularis
NB. Recurrent fetal loss may also occur in other types of thrombophilia.

and livedo reticularis is a frequent dermal manifestation.

Treatment is with anticoagulation where indicated. It is usual to maintain an international normalized ratio (INR) of between 2.0 and 3.0 with warfarin but higher levels may be needed if previous arterial or major DVT has occurred or recurrence of thrombosis occurs on warfarin therapy. Low dose heparin and aspirin are useful in the management of recurrent miscarriage.

Collagen vascular diseases and Behçet's syndrome are also associated with arterial and venous thrombosis, whether or not the lupus anticoagulant is present (see p. 369).

Investigation of thrombophilia

Many of the conditions associated with an increased thrombotic risk are obvious following clinical examination. A full assessment is indicated, particularly in patients who have recurrent or spontaneous DVT or PE, in patients who have thrombosis at a young age and in those patients with a familial tendency to thrombosis or thrombosis at an unusual site. It is also needed in women with recurrent fetal loss. With the increasing recognition of systemic causes of thrombophilia, the indications for thrombophilia screening are widening. The following laboratory tests are used in diagnosis.

Screening tests

1 Blood count and erythrocyte sedimentation rate – to detect elevation in haematocrit, white cell count, platelet count, fibrinogen and globulins.
2 Blood film examination – may provide evidence of myeloproliferative disorder; leucoerythroblastic features may indicate malignant disease.
3 Prothrombin time (PT) and APTT – a shortened APPT is often seen in thrombotic states and may indicate the presence of activated clotting factors. A prolonged APTT test, not corrected by the addition of normal plasma, suggests an LA or an acquired inhibitor to a coagulation factor.
4 Anticardiolipin and anti-β_2-GPI antibodies.

5 Thrombin time (and reptilase time) – prolongation suggests an abnormal fibrinogen.
6 Fibrinogen assay.
7 APC resistance test and DNA analysis for factor V Leiden.
8 Antithrombin – immunological and functional assays.
9 Protein C and protein S – immunological and functional assays.
10 Prothrombin gene analysis for the G20210A variant.
11 Plasma homocysteine estimation.
12 Test for CD59 and CD55 expression (paroxysmal nocturnal haemoglobinuria) in red cells if paroxysmal nocturnal haemoglobinuria is suspected.
13 Test for *JAK2 (V617F)* mutation if portal or hepatic vein thrombosis.
14 Protein electrophoresis for paraprotein.

Diagnosis of venous thrombosis

Deep vein thrombosis

Clinical suspicion DVT is suspected in those with previous DVT, cancer or confined to bed. In the leg, unilateral thigh or calf swelling or tenderness, pitting oedema and the presence of collateral superficial non-varicose veins are important signs. Homan's sign (pain in the calf on flexing the ankle) is usually positive.

Serial compression ultrasound This is a reliable and practical method for patients with first suspicion of DVT in the legs and other sites (Fig. 27.2a). It can be combined with spectral, colour (Fig. 27.2) or power Doppler (duplex) scanning which improves accuracy by focusing on individual veins. It does not distinguish between acute and chronic thrombi. Persisting venous obstruction detected by ultrasonography at the completion of warfarin therapy is associated with an increased risk of recurrent thrombosis.

Contrast venography This most sensitive procedure is reserved for patients with highly suggestive clinical findings but negative ultrasonography. Iodinated contrast medium is injected into a vein peripheral to the suspected DVT. This permits direct demonstration by X-ray of the site, size and extent of the thrombus (Fig. 27.2b). However, it is a painful invasive technique, with a risk of contrast reaction and procedure-induced DVT.

Plasma D-dimer concentration The concentration of these fibrin breakdown products is raised when there is a fresh thrombosis. It is a useful assay when venous thrombosis is suspected and with the help of clinical probability shown by the Wells score (Table 27.4). A negative result in emergency departments can be used to exclude DVT. D-dimer elevation in cancer, inflammation after surgery or trauma limits its usefulness.

Magnetic resonance imaging (MRI) This may also be used but is expensive. Impedance plethysmography is less sensitive and accurate and is falling out of use.

Pulmonary embolus

Clinical suspicion This is particularly suspected in patients with chest symptoms, especially if there are signs, or previous history of DVT, immobilization for more than 2 days or recent (<4 weeks) surgery, haemoptysis or cancer. Recurrent PE may lead to pulmonary hypertension.

Chest X-ray This is often normal but may show evidence of pulmonary infarction or pleural effusion.

Ventilation perfusion (VQ) scintigraphy This detects areas of the lung being ventilated but not perfused.

Computed tomography (CT) pulmonary angiography Fine slices of the lung are scanned by spiral CT so that filling defects in the pulmonary arteries are visualized (Fig. 27.2c).

Magnetic resonance pulmonary angiography Gadolinium-enhanced MRI is a relatively new, expensive but accurate technique.

Pulmonary angiography This is the traditional reference method but is invasive with complications, albeit uncommon, such as arrhythmia or contrast reaction.

Electrocardiogram This is performed to determine whether there is right heart 'strain' which occurs only in relatively severe cases.

Anticoagulant drugs

Anticoagulant drugs are used widely in the treatment of venous thromboembolic disease. Their value in the treatment of arterial thrombosis is less well established.

Heparin

This acidic unfractionated mucopolysaccharide of average molecular weight (MW) 15 000–18 000 is an inhibitor of blood coagulation because of its action in potentiating the activity of antithrombin (see below). As it is not absorbed from the gastrointestinal tract it must be given by injection. It is inactivated by the liver and excreted in the urine. The effective biological half-life is approximately 1 hour (Table 27.5).

Mode of action

Heparin dramatically potentiates the formation of complexes between antithrombin and activated serine protease coagulation factors, thrombin (IIa) and factors IXa, Xa and XIa (Fig. 27.6). This complex formation inactivates these factors

Table 27.4 Deep vein thrombosis: clinical assessment: the Wells score.

	Points
Active cancer (treatment ongoing or within previous 6 months or palliative)	1
Paralysis, plaster	1
Bed more than 3 days, surgery within 4 weeks	1
Tenderness along veins	1
Entire leg swollen	1
Pitting oedema	1
Collateral veins	1
Alternative diganosis likely	−2
Low probability 0–1	
High probability 2 or more	

Table 27.5 Comparison of unfractionated heparin with low molecular weight heparin.

	Unfractionated heparin	Low molecular weight heparin
Mean molecular weight in kilodaltons (range)	15 (4–30)	4.5 (2–10)
Anti-Xa : anti-IIa	1 : 1	2 : 1 to 4 : 1
Inhibits platelet function	Yes	No
Bioavailability	50%	100%

Half-life
  intravenous
  subcutaneous
	1 hour
	2 hours
		2 hours
		4 hours

Elimination	Renal and hepatic	Renal
Monitoring	APTT	Xa assay (usually not needed)
Frequency of heparin-induced thrombocytopenia	High	Low
Osteoporosis	Yes	Less frequent

APTT, activated partial thromboplastin time.

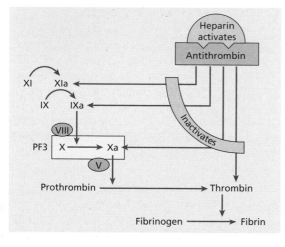

Figure 27.6 The action of heparin. This activates antithrombin which then forms complexes with activated serine protease coagulation factors (thrombin, Xa, IXa and XIa) and so inactivates them.

irreversibly. In addition, heparin impairs platelet function.

Low molecular weight heparin (LMWH) preparations (MW 2000–10 000) are produced by enzymatic or chemical depolymerization of unfractionated heparin. They have a greater ability to inhibit factor Xa than to inhibit thrombin and interact less with platelets than standard heparin, and so may have a lesser tendency to cause bleeding. They also have greater bioavailability and a more prolonged half-life in plasma, making once-daily administration in prophylaxis or treatment feasible (Table 27.4).

Indications

Heparin (usually LMWH) is routinely used in DVT, PE and unstable angina pectoris. It is also widely used in the prophylaxis of venous thrombosis and is the drug of choice for women requiring anticoagulation in pregnancy because it does not cross the placenta. It is also used during cardiopulmonary bypass surgery, for maintaining the patency of indwelling venous lines and in some case of DIC if the manifestations are predominantly vaso-occlusive. There is some evidence that LMWH (or warfarin) may improve the survival in cancer patients over and above the protection from venous thrombosis but the exact mechanisms, types of cancer improved and optimum treatment regimens remain to be elucidated.

Administration and laboratory control

Standard heparin

Continuous intravenous infusion This provides the smoothest control of heparin therapy and is the treatment of choice where rapid reversal of anticoagulation by protamine sulphate may be required (e.g. in surgical patients or late pregnancy). It is still used for treatment of acute PE but has largely been replaced for this indication and DVT by LMWH. In an adult, dosage of 30 000–40 000 units over 24 hours (1000–2000 units/hour with a loading dose of 5000 units) is usually satisfactory.

Therapy is monitored by maintaining the APTT usually at 1.5–2.5 times the upper limit of the normal value but laboratories need to establish local therapeutic ratios which can be from 1.6–2.7 to 3.7–6.2. It is usual to start warfarin therapy within 2 days of starting heparin therapy and to discontinue heparin when the INR has been above 2.0 on two successive days. For acute coronary syndromes, both unfractionated heparin and LMWH are of benefit when used with aspirin in the prevention of mural thrombosis, systemic embolization and venous thrombosis.

Low molecular weight heparin

LMWH (there are many commercial preparations) is given by subcutaneous injection and, as it has a longer half-life than standard heparin, it can be given once a day in prophylaxis, or once or twice a day in treatment (Table 27.5). Compared with unfractionated heparin, LMWH has a more predictable dose–response which avoids the need for routine monitoring. Many patients with uncomplicated DVTs may now be managed at home with regular LMWH injections once or twice daily according to the preparation. There is a 50% reduction in the risk of heparin-induced thrombocytopenia or osteoporosis.

It is now the treatment of choice for preventing or treating DVT and the preferred treatment for PE and unstable angina. Although routine monitoring is not required, measurement of anti-Xa peak levels 4 hours after injection allows dose adjustment in selected patients (e.g. in pregnancy, renal failure, gross obesity and in children). Typical treatment regimens are 200 anti-Xa units/kg once daily or 100 anti-Xa units/kg twice daily). LMWH is used for the prevention of DVT in both medical and surgical patients. It is also the preferred anticoagulant in pregnancy because it does not cross the placenta. Typical once-daily subcutaneous dosage in prophylaxis is 2000–2500 units (moderate risk patients), 4000–5000 units (high risk patients) and therapeutic doses (mechanical heart valves).

It is now mandatory for hospitals in England to have a policy for prevention of DVT and PE for all hospitalized patients. LMWHs are the gold standard pharmaceutical agents but oral anticoagulants (e.g. dabigatran and rivaroxaban) may supersede them.

Bleeding during heparin therapy

Bleeding may be because of excessive prolonged anticoagulation or due to an antiplatelet functional effect of heparin. Intravenous heparin has a half-life of less than 1 hour and it is usually only necessary to stop the infusion. Protamine is able to inactivate heparin immediately and for severe bleeding a dose of 1 mg/100 units heparin provides effective neutralization. However, protamine itself may act as an anticoagulant when in excess.

Heparin-induced thombocytopenia

A mild lowering of the platelet count may occur in the first 24 hours as a result of platelet clumping. This is of no clinical consequence (heparin-induced thombocytopenia (HIT) type 1). The important HIT, type 2, may occur in up to 5% of patients who are treated with unfractionated heparin and paradoxically presents with thrombosis. It results from the binding of heparin to platelet factor 4 (PF4) followed by the generation of an immunoglobulin G (IgG) antibody to the heparin–PF4 complex, which leads to platelet activation, throm-

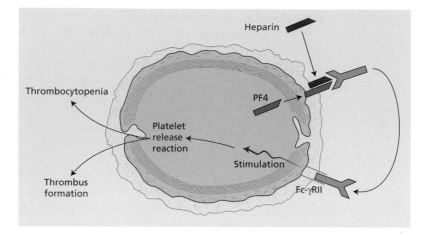

Figure 27.7 Mechanism of heparin-induced thrombocytopenia (HIT). Platelet factor 4 (PF4) is released from α granules and forms a complex on the platelet surface with heparin. Immunoglobulin G antibodies develop against this complex and can activate the platelet through the platelet immunoglobulin receptor Fc-γRII. This leads to platelet stimulation, further release of PF4 and the platelet release reaction with consequent thrombocytopenia and thrombus development.

bocytopenia and thrombosis (Fig. 27.7). Typically, it presents as a fall of >50% in the platelet count 5 or more days after starting heparin treatment or earlier if heparin has been given previously. Diagnosis is difficult but assays have recently been developed to allow the detection of antibodies to immobilized heparin–PF4 complex. Heparin therapy must be discontinued. Thrombin inhibitors such as hirudin or lepirudin may be used as alternatives and the heparinoid danaparoid may also be used. LMWH is less likely than unfractionated heparin to cause HIT but there is cross-reactivity of the antibody. Warfarin therapy in some cases causes skin necrosis and should be delayed until normalization of the platelet count has been achieved.

Osteoporosis

This occurs with long-term (>2 months) heparin therapy, especially in pregnancy. The drug complexes minerals from the bones but the exact pathogenesis is unknown.

Oral anticoagulants

Until recently there have been only derivatives of coumarin or phenindione. Warfarin, a coumarin, is most widely used. Coumarins are vitamin K antagonists (see p. 355) and so treatment results in decreased biological activity of the vitamin K-dependent factors II, VII, IX and X. They block the vitamin K induced post-ribosomal γ-carboxylation of glutamic acid residues of these proteins (Fig. 27.7). After warfarin is given, factor VII levels fall considerably within 24 hours but prothrombin has a longer plasma half-life and only falls to 50% of normal at 3 days; the patient is fully anticoagulated only after this period.

Principles of oral anticoagulation

A typical starting regimen for warfarin would be 10 mg on day 1, 5 mg on day 2 and then 5 mg on the third day. After this the dosage should be adjusted according to the PT. The initial dose can be 'tailor-made' using an algorithm based on clinical variables and genetic information on two genes involved in warfarin metabolism or action, cytochrome p450 (CYP2CP) and vitamin K epoxide reductase (see Fig. 26.8). The usual maintenance dosage of warfarin is 3–9 mg/day but individual responses vary greatly. Lower loading dosage is recommended for the elderly or those with liver disease.

International normalized ratio

The effect of oral anticoagulants is monitored by the PT. The INR is caculated from it and is based on the ratio of the patient's PT to a mean normal PT with correction for the 'sensitivity' of the thromboplastin used. This is calibrated against a primary World Health Organization (WHO) standard thromboplastin. The indications and recommended ranges for INR with warfarin treatment are summarized in Table 27.6.

Warfarin crosses the placenta and is teratogenic. Heparin is preferred for pregnant patients because it does not cross the placenta and its action is short-lived.

It is usual to continue warfarin for 3–6 months for established DVT, PE and following xenograft heart valves. Long-term therapy is given for recurrent venous thrombosis, for embolic complications of rheumatic heart disease or atrial fibrillation, and with prosthetic valves and arterial grafts and in selected patients with the APS.

Drug interactions

Approximately 97% of warfarin in the circulation is bound to albumin and only a small fraction of warfarin is free and can enter the liver parenchymal cells; it is this free fraction that is active. In the liver cells, warfarin is degraded in microsomes to an inactive water-soluble metabolite which is conjugated and excreted in the bile and partially reabsorbed to be also excreted in urine. Drugs that affect the albumin binding or excretion of warfarin (or of other oral anticoagulants) or those that decrease the absorption of vitamin K will interfere with the control of therapy (Table 27.7).

Management of warfarin overdose

If the INR is in excess of 4.5 without bleeding, warfarin should be stopped for 1 or 2 days and the dosage adjusted according to the INR. The long half-life of warfarin (40 hours) delays the full impact of dose changes for 4–5 days. If the INR is very high (e.g. >8) without bleeding, an oral dose of 0.5–2.5 mg vitamin K may be given. Mild bleeding usually only needs an INR assessment, drug withdrawal and subsequent dosage adjustment (Table 27.8). More serious bleeding may need cessation of therapy, vitamin K therapy or the infusion of fresh frozen plasma or prothrombin concentrates. Vitamin K is the specific antidote; an oral or intravenous dose of 2.5 mg is usually effective. Higher doses result in resistance to further warfarin therapy for 2–3 weeks.

Management of surgery

For minor surgery (e.g. dental extraction) anticoagulation can be maintained and mouth rinses with tranexamic acid given. For major surgery, warfarin is stopped to get an INR <1.5 and LMWH given when the INR falls to <2.0 (except on the day of surgery) and continued until the INR is >2.0 after restarting warfarin.

New anticoagulants

Traditional anticoagulant therapy has disadvantages. LMWH has to be given subcutaneously and warfarin requires frequent monitoring and dose adjustment and there is interaction with drugs and food.

Factor Xa inhibitors: fondaparinux, a synthetic analogue of the antithrombin-binding pentasaccharide of heparin, is an indirect irreversible

---

Table 27.6 Oral anticoagulant control tests. Target levels recommended by the British Society for Haematology.

Target INR	Clinical state
2.5 (2.0–3.0)	Treatment of DVT, pulmonary embolism, atrial fibrillation, recurrent DVT off warfarin; symptomatic inherited thrombophilia, cardiomyopathy, mural thrombus, cardioversion
3.0 (2.5–3.5)	Recurrent DVT while on warfarin, mechanical prosthetic heart valves, antiphospholipid syndrome (some cases)

DVT, deep venous thrombosis; INR, international normalized ratio.

Table 27.7 Drugs and other factors that interfere with the control of coumarin (e.g. warfarin) therapy.

Potentiation of coumarin anticoagulants	Inhibition of coumarin anticoagulants
Drugs that increase the effect of coumarins	**Drugs that depress the action of coumarins**
Reduced coumarin binding to serum albumin	*Acceleration of hepatic microsomal degradation of coumarin*
Sulphonamides	Barbiturates
	Rifampicin
Inhibition of hepatic microsomal degradation of coumarin	
Cimetidine	*Enhanced synthesis of clotting factors*
Allopurinol	Oral contraceptives
Tricyclic antidepressants	
Metronidazole	**Hereditary resistance to oral anticoagulants**
Sulphonamides	
	Pregnancy
Alteration of hepatic receptor site for drug	
Thyroxine	
Quinidine	
Decreased synthesis of vitamin K factors	
High doses of salicylates	
Some cephalosporins, other antibiotics	
Liver disease	
Decreased synthesis of vitamin K factors	
Decreased absorption of vitamin K	
e.g. Malabsorption, antibiotic therapy, laxatives	

NB. Patients are also more likely to bleed if taking antiplatelet agents (e.g. NSAIDs, dipyridamole or aspirin); alcohol in large amounts enhances warfarin action.

factor Xa inhibitor. It is given subcutaneously, has a plasma half-life of 17 hours and like the orally active factor Xa inhibitors does not require laboratory monitoring (by measuring factor Xa levels) except in especially obese patients, those with renal failure and children.

Rivaroxaban is an orally active irreversibile inhibitor of factor Xa. It has a rapid onset of action with a peak plasma level 2 hours after injection. It is given at a fixed dose and does not need monitoring.

Extensive trials have demonstrated that the Xa inhibitors are effective antithrombotic agent for prevention and treatment of both venous and arterial thromboembolic disorders. They may also reduce major bleeding and may improve long-term mortality and morbidity (e.g. in acute coronary syndromes).

Direct thrombin (factor II) inhibitors These include recombinant hirudins, bivalirudin, lepiruden, argatroban and dabigatran.

Bivalirudin and lepiruden have been used as an alternative to heparin in patients undergoing percutaneous coronary interventions and are associated with less bleeding and a reduced need for adjunctive treatment with glycoprotein IIb/IIIa antagonists in patients undergoing stenting.

Dabigatran is given twice daily by mouth at a fixed dose. It is as effective as conventional therapy in preventing venous thrombous in orthopoedic and general surgery without an increased risk of major haemorrhage. It has had similar success in the treatment of acute venous thrombosis and in the prevention of stroke and systemic arterial embolism in patients with atrial fibrillation. Like rivaroxaban, it has the potential to replace warfarin.

Table 27.8 Recommendations on the management of bleeding and excessive anticoagulation by the British Committee for Standards in Haematology (third edition 1998; 2005 update).

INR 3.0–6.0 (target INR 2.5)	Reduce warfarin dose or stop
INR 4.0–6.0 (target INR 3.5)	Restart warfarin when INR <5.0
INR 6.0–8.0	Stop warfarin*
No bleeding or minor bleeding	Restart when INR <5.0
INR >8.0	Stop warfarin*
No bleeding or minor bleeding	Restart warfarin when INR <5.0 If other risk factors for bleeding give 0.5–2.5 mg vitamin K orally
Major bleeding	Stop warfarin Give prothrombin complex concentrate 50 units/kg, in preference FFP 15 mL/kg (when available) Give 5 mg vitamin K (i.v. or oral)

FFP, fresh frozen plasma; INR, international normalized ratio; i.v., intravenous.
* 1 mg vitamin K may be given orally to rapidly reduce the INR to the therapeutic range within 24 hours in all patients with an INR above the therapeutic range and no bleeding.

Post-thrombotic syndrome

Thrombi that persist destroy venous valves and venous return is impaired. There is venous hypertension which is responsible for fluid accumulation in the extravascular space, with oedema and in the long-term skin atrophy, melanin pigmentation and, in severe cases, skin ulceration.

Mechanical methods of prophylaxis of DVT, PE

Graduated compression stockings

These are used postoperatively, past-partum and during long aeroplane flights to reduce the risk of DVT. After a DVT, if worn for 1–2 years they reduce the risk of the post-thrombotic syndrome. Knee high stockings are sufficient in the vast majority of cases. They should be compression class II and worn except when the patient is recumbent.

Intermittent compression devices

Intermittent pneumatic compression and mechanical foot pumps are used in some hospitals in high risk patients in whom bleeding as a result of LMWH is likely.

Inferior vena cava filter

This can provide protection against pulmonary embolism when a DVT in the legs is diagnosed but anticoagulation is contraindicated (e.g. ongoing or very recent intracranial or gastrointestinal bleeding or where there is recurrent PE despite adequate anticoagulation).

Fibrinolytic agents

Two fibrinolytic agents, streptokinase and tissue plasminogen activator, are most frequently used to lyse fresh thrombi, although other agents are available. These drugs may be used systemically for patients with acute myocardial infarction, major PE or iliofemoral thrombosis, and locally in patients with acute peripheral arterial occlusion.

Administration of thrombolytic agents has been simplified with standardized dosage regimens. The therapy is most effective in the first 6 hours after symptoms begin but is still of benefit up to 24 hours. Aspirin therapy is also given and the value of additional heparin therapy is under study.

The use of laboratory tests for monitoring and control of short-term thrombolytic therapy is now considered unnecessary. However, certain clinical complications exclude the use of thrombolytic agents (Table 27.9).

Table 27.9 Contraindications to thrombolytic therapy.

Absolute contraindications	Relative contraindications
Active gastrointestinal bleeding	Traumatic cardiopulmonary resuscitation
Aortic dissection	Major surgery in the past 10 days
Head injury or cerebrovascular accident in the past 2 months	Past history of gastrointestinal bleeding
Neurosurgery in the past 2 months	Recent obstetric delivery
Intracranial aneurysm or neoplasm	Prior arterial puncture
Proliferative diabetic retinopathy	Prior organ biopsy
	Serious trauma
	Severe arterial hypertension (systolic pressure >200 mmHg, diastolic pressure >110 mmHg)
	Bleeding diathesis

Table 27.10 Antiplatelet therapy in patients with an acute coronary syndrome and in those undergoing percutaneous coronary intervention (PCI). (After Lange R.A. and Hillis L.D. (2004) *N Engl J Med* **350**, 277–80.)

Drug	Target/patient group	Duration
Acute coronary syndrome		
Aspirin	All	Life-long
Clopidogrel	All	9–12 months
Glycoprotein IIb/IIIa inhibitors		
Abciximab	None	–
Eptifibatide	High risk	48–72 hours
Tirofiban	High risk	48–72 hours
Patients undergoing PCI		
Aspirin	All	Life-long
Clopidogrel	All	9–12 months
Abciximab	High risk	12 hours after PCI
Eptifibatide	High risk	18–24 hours after PCI
Tirofiban	None	–

Recombinant tissue plasminogen activator has a particularly high affinity for fibrin and this allows lysis of thrombi with less systemic activation of fibrinolysis.

Antiplatelet drugs

Antiplatelet agents are gaining an increasing role in clinical medicine. It is now clear that aspirin is valuable in the secondary prevention of vascular disease. Several other agents are being used for different indications (Table 27.10). The sites of action of the antiplatelet drugs are illustrated in Fig. 27.8.

Aspirin Aspirin inhibits platelet cyclo-oxygenase irreversibly, thus reducing the production of platelet thromboxane A_2. Low-dose therapy (e.g. 75 mg/day) has lesser risk of gastrointestinal bleeding and is most commonly used in patients who have a history of coronary artery or cerebrovascular disease. It may also be useful in preventing thrombosis in patients with thrombocytosis.

Clopidogrel This adenosine diphospate (ADP) receptor antagonist (Fig. 27.8) is an antiplatelet agent used for reduction of ischaemic events in patients with ischaemic stroke, myocardial infarction or peripheral vascular disease. It is used after coronary artery stenting or angioplasty and in patients requiring long-term antiplatelet therapy who are intolerant or allergic to aspirin.

Dipyridamole (Persantin®) This drug is a phosphodiesterase inhibitor thought to elevate cyclic adenosine monophosphate levels in circulating platelets which decreases their sensitivity to activating stimuli. Dipyridamole has been shown to reduce thromboembolic complications in patients with prosthetic heart valves and to improve the results in coronary bypass operations.

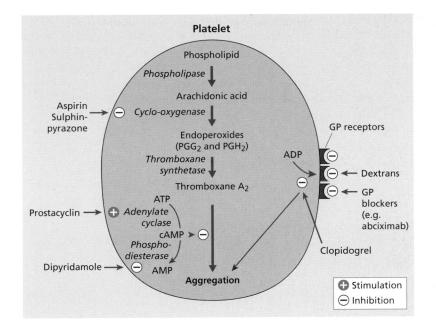

Figure 27.8 Sites of action of antiplatelet drugs. Aspirin acetylates the enzyme cyclo-oxygenase irreversibly. Sulphinpyrazone inhibits cyclo-oxygenase reversibly. Dipyridamole inhibits phosphodiesterase, increases cyclic adenosine monophosphate (cAMP) levels and inhibits aggregation. Clopidogrel, GP blockers inhibition of adenosine uptake by red cells allows adenosine accumulation in plasma which stimulates platelet adenylate cyclase. Prostacyclin (epoprostenol) stimulates adenylate cyclase. The lipid-soluble β-blockers inhibit phospholipase. Calcium-channel antagonists block the influx of free calcium ions across the platelet membrane. Dextrans coat the surface interfering with adhesion and aggregation. GP, glycoprotein.

Glycoprotein IIb/IIIa inhibitors: abciximab, eptifibatide, tirofiban These drugs are monoclonal antibodies that inhibit the platelet GPIIb/IIIa receptor. They are used in conjunction with heparin, aspirin and clopidogral for the prevention of ischaemic complications in high-risk patients undergoing percutaneous transluminal coronary angioplasty. They can be used once only.

- Thrombosis is the formation of solid masses of platelets and fibrin in the circulation. It may be arterial or venous.
- Arterial thrombosis is mainly related to atherosclerosis of the vessel wall with risk factors such as hypertension, hyperlipidemia, smoking and diabetes.
- Venous thrombosis is related to genetic coagulation factor abnormalities (e.g. factor V Leiden), stasis of the circulation or to an acquired increase in coagulation factors (e.g. oestrogen therapy, postoperative, pregnancy) or to unknown factors (e.g. age or obesity).
- Diagnosis of deep vein thrombosis is with serial compression ultrasound combined with Doppler (duplex) scanning, contrast venography or MRI imaging. Plasma D-dimer concentration assay may help.
- Pulmonary embolus is diagnosed by chest X-ray, electrocardiogram, ventilation perfusion scintigraphy or CT angiography.
- Anticoagulant drugs are used to prevent or treat venous thrombosis. Heparin can be given in the unfractionated form. Much more frequently low molecular weight heparin is given subcutaneously.

SUMMARY

(Continued)

- Warfarin is the most frequently used oral anticoagulant, the dose usually aimed to raise the international normalized ratio (INR) between 2.0 and 3.0. There are frequent drug interactions that affect the dose.
- New anticoagulants include the factor X_a inhibitor, rivaroxaban and factor II (prothrombin) inhibitor, dabigatran.

- Thrombi, if fresh, may be dissolved by fibrinolytic agents (e.g. streptokinase) or recombinant tissue plasminogen activator. Antiplatelet drugs – aspirin, clopidogrel and dipyrimadole – are used to treat arterial disorders.

Now visit www.wiley.com/go/essentialhaematology to test yourself on this chapter.

CHAPTER 28
Haematological changes in systemic disease

Key topics

Anaemia of chronic disorders

Many of the anaemias seen in clinical practice occur in patients with systemic disorders and are the result of a number of contributing factors. The anaemia of chronic disorders (also discussed on p. 46) is of central importance and occurs in patients with a variety of chronic inflammatory and malignant diseases (Table 28.1). Usually, both the erythrocyte sedimentation rate (ESR) and C-reactive protein (CRP) are raised. It may be complicated by additional haematological changes caused by the disease. The serum iron and total iron binding capacity (transferrin) are both low; serum ferritin can be normal or raised. The characteristic features are described in Chapter 3.

The pathogenesis of this anaemia appears to be related to the decreased release of iron from macrophages to plasma and so to erythroblasts, caused by hepcidin, reduced red cell lifespan and an inadequate erythropoietin response to anaemia. The plasma levels of various cytokines, especially interleukin-1 (IL-1), IL-6 and tumour necrosis factor (TNF) are raised and reduce erythropoietin secretion. The anaemia is corrected by the successful treatment of the underlying disease. It does not respond to iron therapy despite the low serum iron. Responses to recombinant erythropoietin therapy may be obtained (e.g. in rheumatoid arthritis or cancer). In many conditions the anaemia is complicated by anaemia from other causes (e.g. iron or folate deficiency, renal failure, bone marrow infiltration, hypersplenism or endocrine abnormality).

Table 28.1 Causes of anaemia of chronic disorders.

Chronic inflammatory diseases
Infectious (e.g. pulmonary abscess, tuberculosis, osteomyelitis, pneumonia, bacterial endocarditis)
Non-infectious (e.g. rheumatoid arthritis, systemic lupus erythematosus and other connective tissue diseases, sarcoid, Crohn's disease, cirrhosis)

Malignant disease
(e.g. carcinoma, lymphoma, sarcoma, myeloma)

Malignant diseases (other than primary bone marrow diseases)

Anaemia

Contributing factors include anaemia of chronic disorders, blood loss and iron deficiency, marrow infiltration (Fig. 28.1) often associated with a leuco-erythroblastic blood film (see p. 118), folate deficiency, haemolysis and marrow suppression from radiotherapy or chemotherapy (Table 28.2).

Microangiopathic haemolytic anaemia (see p. 85) occurs with mucin-secreting adenocarcinoma (Fig. 28.2), particularly of the stomach, lung and breast. Less common forms of anaemia with malignant disease include autoimmune haemolytic anaemia with malignant lymphoma and rarely with other tumours; primary red cell aplasia with thymoma or lymphoma; and myelodysplastic syndromes secondary to chemotherapy. There is also an association of pernicious anaemia with carcinoma of the stomach.

The anaemia of malignant disease may respond partly to erythropoietin but this may accelerate tumour growth. Folic acid should only be given if there is definite megaloblastic anaemia caused by the deficiency; it might 'feed' the tumour.

Polycythaemia

Secondary polycythaemia is occasionally associated with renal, hepatic, cerebellar and uterine tumours (see p. 208).

White cell changes

Leukaemoid reactions (see p. 117) may occur with tumours showing widespread necrosis and inflammation. Hodgkin lymphoma is associated with a variety of white cell abnormalities including eosinophilia, monocytosis and leucopenia. In non-Hodgkin lymphoma, malignant cells may circulate in the blood (see p. 260).

Platelet and blood coagulation abnormalities

Patients with malignant disease may show either thrombocytosis or thrombocytopenia. Disseminated

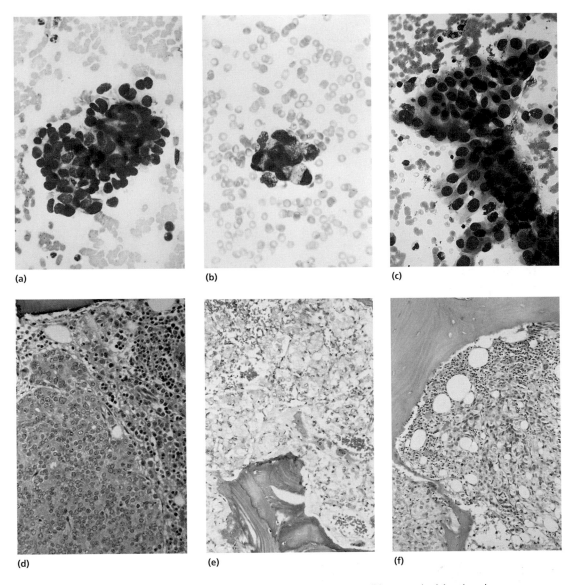

Figure 28.1 Metastatic carcinoma in bone marrow aspirates: **(a)** breast; **(b)** stomach; **(c)** colon; bone marrow trephine biopsies: **(d)** prostate; **(e)** stomach; **(f)** kidney.

tumours, particularly mucin-secreting adenocarcinomas, are associated with disseminated intravascular coagulation (DIC; see p. 355) and generalized haemostatic failure. Activation of fibrinolysis occurs in some patients with carcinoma of the prostate. Occasional patients with malignant disease have spontaneous bruising or bleeding caused by an acquired inhibitor of one or other coagulation factor, most frequently factor VIII, or to a paraprotein interfering with platelet function.

Cancer patients have a high incidence (estimated at 15%) of venous thromboembolism. This is increased by surgery and some drugs (e.g. thalidomide). It is most common in ovarian, brain, pancreatic and colon cancers. It may be difficult to manage with oral anticoagulation because of

Table 28.2 Haematological abnormalities in malignant disease.

Haematological abnormality	Tumour or treatment associated
Pancytopenia	
Marrow hypoplasia	Chemotherapy, radiotherapy
Myelodysplasia	Chemotherapy, radiotherapy
Leucoerythroblastic	Metastases in marrow
Megaloblastic	Folate deficiency
	B_{12} deficiency (carcinoma of stomach)
Red cells	
Anaemia of chronic disorders	Most forms
Iron deficiency anaemia	Especially gastrointestinal, uterine
Pure red cell aplasia	Thymoma
Immune haemolytic anaemia	Lymphoma, ovary, other tumours
Microangiopathic haemolytic anaemia	Mucin-secreting carcinoma
Polycythaemia	Kidney, liver, cerebellum, uterus
White cells	
Neutrophil leucocytosis	Most forms
Leukaemoid reaction	Disseminated tumours, those with necrosis
Eosinophilia	Hodgkin lymphoma, others
Monocytosis	Various tumours
Platelets and coagulation	
Thrombocytosis	Gastrointestinal tumours with bleeding, others
Disseminated intravascular coagulation	Mucin-secreting carcinoma, prostate
Activation of fibrinolysis	Prostate
Acquired inhibitors of coagulation	Most forms
Paraprotein interfering with platelet function	Lymphomas, myeloma
Tumour cell procoagulants – tissue factor and cancer procoagulant (activates factor X)	Especially ovarian, pancreas, brain, colon

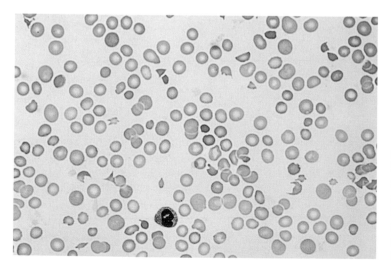

Figure 28.2 Peripheral blood film in metastatic mucin-secreting adenocarcinoma of the stomach showing red cell polychromasia and fragmentation and thrombocytopenia. The patient had disseminated intravascular coagulation.

bleeding, interruptions with chemotherapy and thrombocytopenia, anorexia or vomiting. Liver disease and drug interactions can cause further complications so daily low molecular weight heparin injections may be preferable to oral anticoagulants.

Rheumatoid arthritis (and other connective tissue disorders)

In patients with rheumatoid arthritis, the anaemia of chronic disorders is proportional to the severity of the disease. It is complicated in some patients by iron deficiency caused by gastrointestinal bleeding related to therapy with salicylates, other non-steroidal anti-inflammatory agents or corticosteroids. Bleeding into inflamed joints may also be a factor. Marrow hypoplasia may follow therapy with gold. In Felty's syndrome, splenomegaly is associated with neutropenia (Fig. 28.3). Anaemia and thrombocytopenia may also be present.

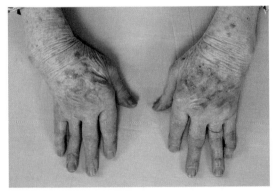

(a)

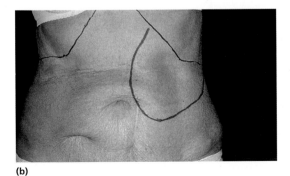

(b)

Figure 28.3 Felty's syndrome: **(a)** the typical deformities of rheumatoid arthritis of the hand; and **(b)** splenomegaly.

In systemic lupus erythematosus (SLE) there may be anaemia of chronic disorders and 50% of patients are leucopenic with reduced neutrophil and lymphocyte counts often associated with circulating immune complexes. Renal impairment and drug-induced gastrointestinal blood loss also contribute to the anaemia. Autoimmune haemolytic anaemia (typically with immunoglobulin G (IgG) and the C3 component of complement on the surface of the red cells) occurs in 5% of patients and may be the presenting feature of the syndrome. There may be autoimmune thrombocytopenia in 5% of patients. The lupus anticoagulant is described on p. 369. This circulating anticardiolipin interferes with blood coagulation by altering the binding of coagulation factors to platelet phospholipid and predisposes to both arterial and venous thrombosis and recurrent abortions. The antibody may be responsible for a false positive Wassermann reaction. Tests for anti-nuclear factor and anti-DNA antibodies are usually positive.

Patients with temporal arteritis and polymyalgia rheumatica have a markedly elevated ESR, pronounced red cell rouleaux in the blood film and a polyclonal immunoglobulin response. These and other collagen vascular disorders are associated with anaemia of chronic disorders.

Renal failure

Anaemia

A normochromic anaemia is present in most patients with chronic renal failure. Generally, there is a 2 g/dL fall in haemoglobin level for every 10 mmol/L rise in blood urea. There is impaired red cell production as a result of defective erythropoietin secretion (see Fig. 2.5). Uraemic serum has also been shown to contain factors that inhibit proliferation of erythroid progenitors but, in view of the excellent response to erythropoietin in most patients, the clinical relevance of these is doubtful. Variable shortening of red cell lifespan occurs and in severe uraemia the red cells show abnormalities including spicules (spurs) and 'burr' cells (Fig. 28.4). Increased red cell 2,3-diphosphoglycerate (2,3-DPG) levels in response to the anaemia and hyperphosphataemia result in decreased oxygen

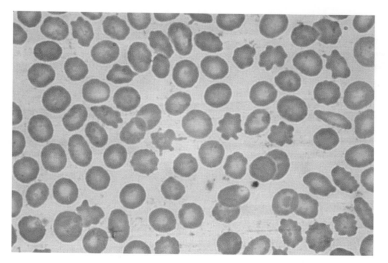

Figure 28.4 Peripheral blood film in chronic renal failure showing red cell acanthocytosis and numerous 'burr' cells.

affinity and a shift of the haemoglobin oxygen dissociation curve to the right (see p. 21), which is augmented by uraemic acidosis. The patient's symptoms are therefore relatively mild for the degree of anaemia.

Other factors may complicate the anaemia of chronic renal failure (Table 28.3): the anaemia of chronic disorders, iron deficiency from blood loss during dialysis or caused by bleeding because of defective platelet function, and folate deficiency in some chronic dialysis patients. Aluminium excess in patients on chronic dialysis also inhibits erythropoiesis. Patients with polycystic kidneys usually have retained erythropoietin production and may have less severe anaemia for the degree of renal failure.

Treatment

Erythropoietin therapy has been found to correct the anaemia in patients on dialysis or in chronic renal failure, providing that iron and folate deficiency, aluminium excess and infections have been corrected. The dosage of erythropoietin usually required is 50–150 units/kg three times a week by subcutaneous infusion. Maintenance by 75 units/kg/week subcutaneously is typical. New preparations of erythropoietin are now used fortnightly

Table 28.3 Haematological abnormalities in renal failure.

Anaemia
Reduced erythropoietin production
Aluminium excess in dialysis patients
Anaemia of chronic disorders
Iron deficiency
  blood loss (e.g. dialysis, venesection, defective platelet function)
Folate deficiency
  chronic haemodialysis without replacement therapy

Abnormal platelet function

Thrombocytopenia
Immune complex-mediated (e.g. systemic lupus erythematosus, polyarteritis nodosa)
Some cases of acute nephritis and following allograft
Haemolytic uraemic syndrome and thrombotic thrombocytopenic purpura

Thrombosis
Some cases of the nephrotic syndrome

Polycythaemia
In renal allograft recipients
Rarely in renal cell carcinoma, cysts, arterial disease

(a heavily glycosylated derivative) or monthly (a pegolated derivative). Complications of therapy have been initial transient flu-like symptoms, hypertension, clotting of the dialysis lines and, rarely, fits. A poor response to erythropoietin suggests iron or folate deficiency, infection, aluminium toxicity or hyperparathyroidism. Intravenous iron is often needed to correct iron deficiency shown by serum ferritin, percentage saturation of total iron-binding capacity or percentage hypochromic red cells in the blood.

Platelet and coagulation abnormalities

A bleeding tendency with purpura, gastrointestinal or uterine bleeding occurs in 30–50% of patients with chronic renal failure and is marked in patients with acute renal failure. The bleeding is out of proportion to the degree of thrombocytopenia and has been associated with abnormal platelet or vascular function, which can be reversed by dialysis. Correction of the anaemia with erythropoietin also improves the bleeding tendency. Immune complex-mediated thrombocytopenia occurs in some patients with acute nephritis, SLE and polyarteritis nodosa and also following renal allografts. Renal allografts may also lead to polycythaemia in 10–15% of patients.

The haemolytic uraemic syndrome and thrombotic thrombocytopenic purpura are discussed on p. 337. Patients with the nephrotic syndrome have an increased risk of venous thrombosis.

Congestive heart failure

Anaemia is common in congestive heart failure due to a variety of causes. These include haemodilution, chronic kidney disease, release of cytokines increasing hepcidin synthesis and so reducing iron absorption and recycling of iron from macrophages, and reducing erythropoetin secretion and erythropoietin responsiveness of erythroblasts. Iron deficiency may develop. Treatment with oral or intravenous iron may reduce anaemia, fatigue and increase cardiac function, exercise capacity and quality of life.

Liver disease

The haematological abnormalities in liver disease are listed in Table 28.4. Chronic liver disease is associated with anaemia that is mildly macrocytic and often accompanied by target cells, mainly as a result of increased cholesterol in the membrane (Fig. 28.5a). Contributing factors to the anaemia may include blood loss (e.g. bleeding varices) with iron deficiency, dietary folate deficiency and direct suppression of haemopoiesis by alcohol.

Haemolytic anaemia may occur in patients with alcohol intoxication (Zieve's syndrome) (Fig. 28.5b) and in Wilson's disease (caused by copper oxidation of red cell membranes); autoimmune haemolytic anaemia is found in some patients with chronic immune hepatitis. Haemolysis may also occur in end-stage liver disease because of abnormal red cell membranes resulting from lipid changes. Viral hep-

Table 28.4 Haematological abnormalities in liver disease.

Liver failure ± obstructive jaundice ± portal hypertension
Refractory anaemia– usually mildly macrocytic, often with target cells; may be associated with:
Blood loss and iron deficiency
Alcohol (± ring sideroblastic change)
Folate deficiency
Haemolysis (e.g. Zieve's syndrome, Wilson's disease, immune hypersplenism from portal hypertension)

Bleeding tendency
Deficiency of vitamin K-dependent factors; also of factor V and fibrinogen
Thrombocytopenia hypersplenism, immune platelet function defects
Functional abnormalities of fibrinogen
Increased fibrinolysis
Portal hypertension – haemorrhage from varices

Viral hepatitis
Aplastic anaemia

Tumours
Polycythaemia
Neutrophil leucocytosis and leukaemoid reactions

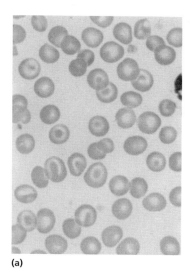

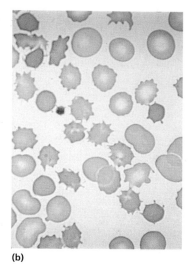

(a) (b)

Figure 28.5 Liver disease: peripheral blood film showing: **(a)** macrocytosis and target cells; and **(b)** marked acanthocytosis and echinocytosis in Zieve's syndrome.

atitis (usually non-A, non-B, non-C) is associated with aplastic anaemia.

The acquired coagulation abnormalities associated with liver disease are described on p. 355. There are deficiencies of vitamin K-dependent factors (II, VII, IX and X) and, in severe disease, of factor V and fibrinogen. Thrombocytopenia may occur from hypersplenism or from immune complex-mediated platelet destruction. Abnormalities of platelet function may also be present. Dysfibrinogenaemia with abnormal fibrin polymerization may occur as a result of excess sialic acid in the fibrinogen molecules. A consumptive coagulopathy may be superimposed. These haemostatic defects may contribute to major blood loss from bleeding varices caused by portal hypertension.

Hypothyroidism

A moderate anaemia is usual and may be caused by lack of thyroxine. T_3 and T_4 potentiate the action of erythropoietin. There is also a reduced oxygen need and thus reduced erythropoietin secretion. The anaemia is often macrocytic and the mean corpuscular volume falls with thyroxine therapy. Autoimmune thyroid disease, especially myxoedema or Hashimoto's disease, is associated with pernicious anaemia. Iron deficiency may also be present, particularly in women with menorrhagia.

Infections

Haematological abnormality is usually present in patients with infections of all types (Table 28.5). The effect of inflammation as a prothrombotic stimulus is also discussed on p. 369.

Bacterial infections

Acute bacterial infections are the most common cause of neutrophil leucocytosis. Toxic granulation, Döhle bodies and metamyelocytes may be present in the blood. Leukaemoid reactions with a white cell count $>50 \times 10^9$/L and granulocyte precursors in the blood may occur in severe infections, particularly in infants and young children. Mild anaemia is common if the infection is prolonged. Severe haemolytic anaemia occurs in bacterial septicaemias, particularly those caused by Gram-negative organisms, where there is usually associated DIC (see p. 355). DIC dominates the clinical picture

Table 28.5 Blood abnormalities associated with infections.

Haematological abnormality	Infection associated
Anaemia	
Anaemia of chronic disorders	Chronic infections especially tuberculosis
Aplastic anaemia	Viral hepatitis
Transient red cell aplasia	Human parvovirus
Marrow fibrosis	Tuberculosis
Immune haemolytic anaemia	Infectious mononucleosis, *Mycoplasma pneumoniae*
Direct red cell damage or microangiopathic	Bacterial septicaemia (associated DIC), *Clostridium perfringens*, malaria, bartonellosis
	Viruses – haemolytic uraemic syndrome and TTP
Hypersplenism	Chronic malaria, tropical splenomegaly syndrome, leishmaniasis, schistosomiasis
White cell changes	
Neutrophil leucocytosis	Acute bacterial infections
Leukaemoid reactions	Severe bacterial infections particularly in infants
	Tuberculosis
Eosinophilia	Parasitic diseases (e.g. hookworm, filariasis, schistosomiasis, trichinosis)
	Recovery from acute infections
Monocytosis	Chronic bacterial infections: tuberculosis, brucellosis, bacterial endocarditis, typhoid
Neutropenia	Viral infections – HIV, hepatitis, influenza
	Fulminant bacterial infections (e.g. typhoid, miliary tuberculosis)
Lymphocytosis	Infectious mononucleosis, toxoplasmosis, cytomegalovirus, rubella, viral hepatitis, pertussis, tuberculosis, brucellosis
Lymphopenia	HIV infection
	Legionella pneumophila
Thrombocytopenia	
Megakaryocytic depression, immune complex-mediated and direct interaction with platelets	Acute viral infections particularly in children (e.g. measles, varicella, rubella, malaria, severe bacterial infection)
Prothrombotic state	All with prolonged inflammation

DIC, disseminated intravascular coagulation; HIV, human immunodeficiency virus; TTP, thrombotic thrombocytopenic purpura.

with certain infections (e.g. bacterial meningitis). The acute phase response to infections is accompanied by a rise in coagulation factors and a fall in natural anticoagulants.

Clostridium perfringens organisms produce an α toxin, a lecithinase acting directly on the circulating red cells (Fig. 28.6). Haemolysis in bartonellosis (Oroya fever) is caused by direct red cell infection. With severe acute bacterial infections there may be thrombocytopenia. *Mycoplasma pneumoniae* infections are associated with autoimmune haemolytic anaemia of the 'cold' type (see p. 84).

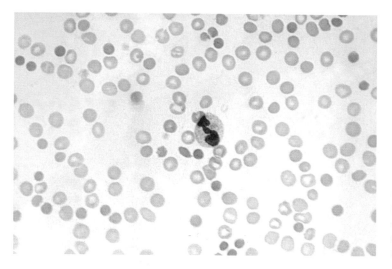

Figure 28.6 Peripheral blood film in a patient with haemolytic anaemia in clostridial septicaemia showing red cell contraction and spherocytosis.

Chronic bacterial infections are associated with the anaemia of chronic disorders. In tuberculosis, additional factors in the pathogenesis of anaemia include marrow replacement and fibrosis associated with miliary disease and reactions to antituberculous therapy (e.g. isoniazid is a pyridoxine antagonist and may cause sideroblastic anaemia). Disseminated tuberculosis is associated with leukaemoid reactions and patients with involvement of bone marrow may show leucoerythroblastic changes in the peripheral blood film (see Fig. 8.9).

Viral infections

Acute viral diseases are often associated with a mild anaemia. An immune haemolytic anaemia with an anti-i autoantibody is associated with infectious mononucleosis (see p. 138). Viral infections, as well as syphilis, have been associated with paroxysmal cold haemoglobinuria (see p. 84). Viruses have also been linked to the pathogenesis of the haemolytic uraemic syndrome, thrombotic thrombocytopenic purpura (see p. 337) and the haemophagocytic syndrome (see p. 121). Aplastic anaemia may occur with viral A or more usually non-A, non-B, non-C hepatitis. Transient red cell aplasia is associated with human parvovirus infection and this may result in severe anaemia in patients with a haemolytic anaemia because of the shortened red cell survival (e.g. in hereditary spherocytosis or sickle cell disease; see p. 78, Fig. 22.5).

Acute thrombocytopenia is not uncommon in rubella, morbilli and varicella infections. Rubella and cytomegalovirus (CMV) infections may cause a reactive lymphocytosis similar to that found in infectious mononucleosis. CMV may be responsible for a post-transfusion mononucleosis-like syndrome, CMV being transmitted by leucocytes. CMV infections in infants are associated with massive hepatosplenomegaly. In bone marrow transplant recipients or other immunosuppressed patients, CMV infections may cause pancytopenia as well as other severe disorders (e.g. pneumonitis or hepatitis; see p. 309).

HIV infection

This is associated with a wide range of haematological changes. These are caused by marrow defects and immune cytopenias directly resulting from HIV infection, the effects of opportunistic infections or lymphoma and the side-effects of drugs used to treat HIV itself or drugs for the complicating infection or lymphoma.

Thrombocytopenia and neutropenia may be immune or secondary to marrow dysfunction. The marrow may be hypercellular with prominent plasma cells and lymphocytes, normocellular, hypocellular or fibrotic. Dysplastic features are common, with ineffective thrombopoiesis or granulocyte formation accounting at least in part for the cytopenia. The myelodysplasia does not show the chromosome abnormalities found in classic myelodysplasia and does not appear to be pre-leukaemic. Thrombocytopenia is treated if necessary by corticosteroids, high-dose gammaglobulin infusions or by other therapies for immune thrombocytopenia (see p. 336), or by antiretroviral therapy.

Anaemia is also common, like the other cytopenias, and more severe as the disease progresses. It is usually multifactorial in origin – the anaemia of chronic disorders, marrow dysplasia and drug therapy, especially zidovudine. Serum vitamin B_{12} is often low, most likely because of intestinal malabsorption, but the anaemia does not respond to vitamin B_{12} therapy. Blood transfusions or recombinant erythropoietin injections are needed.

Increased plasma cells in the marrow and polyclonal increase in immunoglobulins are frequent. A paraprotein is present in 5–10% but appears benign. Non-Hodgkin lymphoma, in over 90% high grade, both systemically and in the central nervous system, occurs in HIV infected individuals with over 100 times the frequency expected in the general population. Diffuse large B-cell lymphomas are most common, with 20% confined to the central nervous system; a substantial minority are Burkitt lymphoma. Hodgkin lymphoma, usually of poor prognosis type, is also increased in frequency. EBV infection appears to usually underlie this as well as Burkitt lymphoma.

Treatment of lymphomas in the setting of HIV is with standard regimens. Continuation of antiretroviral therapy exaggerates the tendency to cytopenia induced by chemotherapy so prophylaxis against opportunistic infections is important. The bone marrow may indeed reveal the presence of opportunistic infection (Fig. 28.7a,b).

Malaria

Some degree of haemolysis is seen in all types of malarial infection. The most severe abnormalities are found in *Plasmodium falciparum* infections (Fig. 28.8). In the worst cases, DIC occurs and intravascular haemolysis is marked with haemoglobinuria. This may be associated with quinine therapy ('blackwater fever'). Thrombocytopenia is commonly found in acute malaria. Patients with chronic malaria have an anaemia of chronic disorders; hypersplenism may contribute to the anaemia and result in moderate thrombocytopenia and neutropenia. Tropical splenomegaly (see p. 144) is probably a chronic immune reaction to malaria. Dyserythropoiesis in the marrow, folate deficiency and protein-caloric malnutrition may contribute to anaemia.

Toxoplasmosis

Toxoplasmosis in children and adults is associated with lymphadenopathy and large numbers of atypical lymphocytes in the blood. Congenital disease may be confused with hydrops fetalis in a severely anaemic hydropic infant with gross hepatosplenomegaly, thrombocytopenia or a leucoerythroblastic blood film.

Kala-azar (visceral leishmaniasis)

The visceral form of leishmaniasis is associated with pancytopenia, hepatosplenomegaly and lymphadenopathy. Bone marrow or splenic aspirates may show large numbers of parasitized macrophages (Fig. 28.9).

Other parasitic diseases

In the acute phase of both African and South American trypanosomiasis, organisms are found in the peripheral blood (Fig. 28.10). Microfilariae of bancroftian filariasis and loiasis are also detected during blood film examination (Fig. 28.11). In chronic schistosomiasis, hypersplenism follows the splenic enlargement associated with portal hypertension. In many parasitic diseases there is eosinophilia (Table 28.5).

Osteopetrosis

Osteopetrosis is a rare genetic disorder in which there is an increase in bone mass with skeletal abnormality and bone marrow failure. It is caused by defects in a

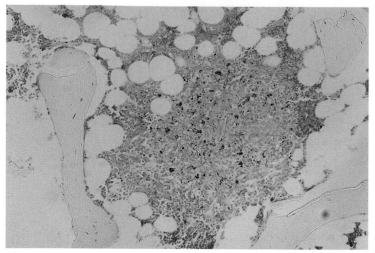

(a)

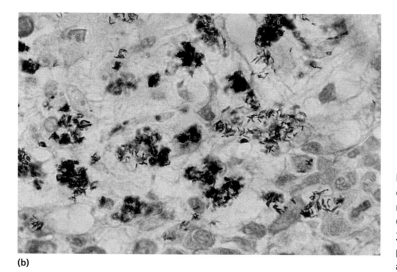

(b)

Figure 28.7 Human immunodeficiency virus (HIV) infection: bone marrow trephine biopsy. **(a)** Granuloma showing positivity with Ziehl–Nielsen stain. **(b)** Higher power shows large numbers of acid-fast bacilli.

variety of genes affecting osteoclast function. The bones are brittle, there is extramedullary haemopoiesis with enlargement of the liver and spleen. The only cure is by stem cell transplantation.

Non-specific monitoring of systemic disease

The inflammatory response to tissue injury includes changes in plasma concentrations of proteins known as acute phase proteins. These include fibrinogen and other clotting factors, complement compo-

nents and CRP (see p. 395), haptoglobin, serum amyloid A (SAA) protein, ferritin and others. The rise in these liver-derived proteins is part of a wider response which includes fever, leucocytosis and increased immune reactivity. The acute phase response is mediated by cytokines (e.g. IL-1; see Fig. 8.4) and TNF, released from macrophages and possibly other cells. Patients with chronic disease may show periodic or continuous evidence of the acute phase response depending upon the extent of inflammation. Quantitative measurements of acute phase proteins are valuable indicators of the

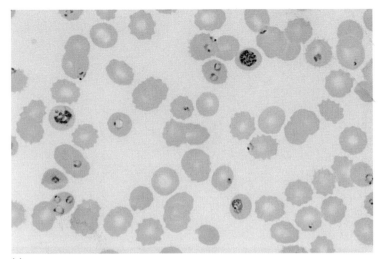

(a)

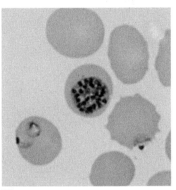

(b)

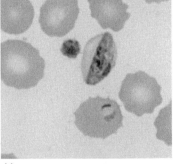

(c)

Figure 28.8 Malaria: peripheral blood in severe *Plasmodium falciparum* infection showing: **(a)** many ring forms and a meront; and at higher magnification: **(b)** a meront; and **(c)** a gametocyte.

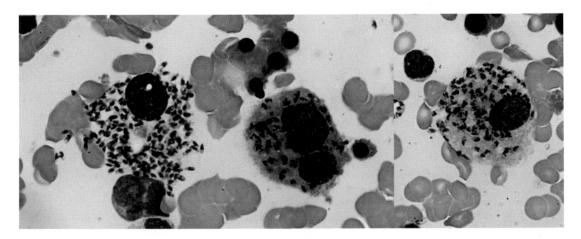

Figure 28.9 Kala-azar: bone marrow aspirates showing macrophages containing Leishman–Donovan bodies.

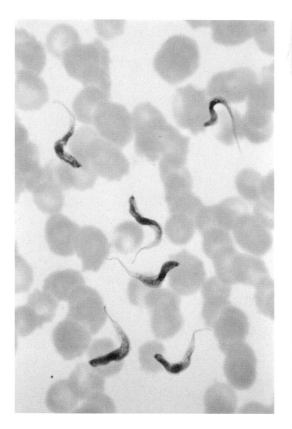

Figure 28.10 African trypanosomiasis: blood film showing *Trypanosoma brucei*.

Table 28.6 Advantages and disadvantages of the tests used to monitor the acute phase response.	
Advantages	**Disadvantages**
CRP*	
Specific test of acute phase protein	More than one protein required to measure acute (CRP) and chronic inflammation
Fast response (6 hours) to change in disease activity	Costly when assayed in small numbers
High sensitivity – owing to large incremental change	Sophisticated equipment and antisera required
Can be measured on stored serum	
Small sample volumes	
Automated analysis	
ESR and plasma viscosity	
Useful in chronic disease	Not sensitive to acute changes (<24 hours)
ESR inexpensive, easy, no electrical power required	Not specific for acute phase response
Plasma viscosity – result obtained quickly (15 min)	Slow to change with alteration in disease activity and insensitive to small changes in activity
Plasma viscosity not affected by anaemia	Fresh samples (<2 hours) required for ESR

ESR, erythrocyte sedimentation rate.
* C-reactive protein (CRP) is normally present in low concentrations (<5 mg/L). Levels are not influenced by anaemia, pregnancy or heart failure. During severe acute infection the plasma concentration may rise 100-fold.

presence and extent of inflammation and of its response to treatment. When short-term (less than 24 hours) changes in the inflammatory response are expected CRP is the test of choice (Table 28.6). Long-term changes in the acute phase proteins are monitored by either the ESR or plasma viscosity. These tests are influenced by plasma proteins which are either slowly responding acute phase reactants (e.g. fibrinogen) or are not acute phase proteins (e.g. immunoglobulins).

Erythrocyte sedimentation rate

This commonly used but non-specific test measures the speed of sedimentation of red cells in plasma over a period of 1 hour. The speed is mainly dependent on the plasma concentration of large proteins (e.g. fibrinogen and immunoglobulins). The normal range in men is 1–5 mm/hour and in women 5–15 mm/hour but there is a progressive increase in old age. The ESR is raised in a wide variety of systemic inflammatory and neoplastic diseases and in pregnancy. It is useful for diagnosing and monitor-

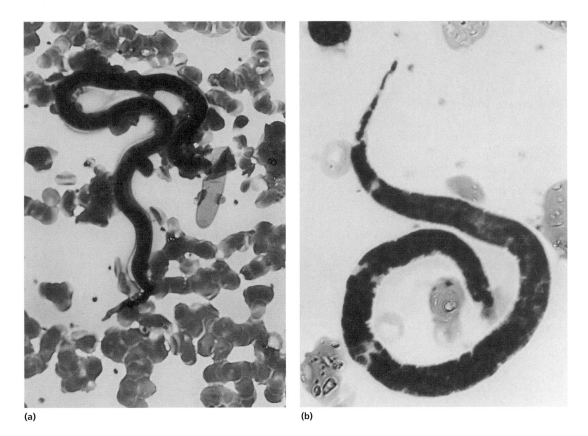

(a) (b)

Figure 28.11 Peripheral blood films showing microfilariae of: **(a)** *Wuchereria bancrofti*; and **(b)** *Loa loa*.

ing temporal arteritis and polymyalgia rheumatica and for monitoring patients with Hodgkin disease. High values (>100 mm/hour) have a 90% predictive value for serious disease including infections, collagen vascular disease or malignancy (particularly myeloma). A raised ESR is associated with marked rouleaux formation of red cells in the peripheral blood film (see Fig. 21.5). Changes in the ESR can be used to monitor the response to therapy.

Lower than expected readings occur in polycythaemia vera because of the high red cell concentration. Higher than expected values may occur in severe anaemia because of the low red cell concentration.

Plasma viscosity

In many laboratories measurement of ESR has been replaced by plasma viscosity measurement. Plasma viscosity is affected by the concentration of plasma proteins of large molecular size, especially those with pronounced axial asymmetry – fibrinogen and some immunoglobulins. Normal values at room temperature are usually in the range of 1.50–1.70 mPa/second. Lower levels are found in neonates because of lower levels of proteins, particularly fibrinogen. Viscosity increases only slightly in the elderly as fibrinogen increases. There is no difference in values between men and women. Other advantages over the ESR test include independence from the effects of anaemia and results that are available within 15 minutes.

C-reactive protein

Phylogenetically CRP is a crude 'early' immunoglobulin that initiates the inflammatory reaction.

CRP–antigen complexes can substitute for antibody in the fixation of Clq and trigger the complement cascade initiating the inflammatory response to antigens or tissue damage, Subsequent binding of C3b on the surface of micro-organisms opsonizes them for phagocytosis.

After tissue injury, an increase in CRP, SAA protein and other acute phase reactants may be detected within 6–10 hours. Increase in fibrinogen may not occur until 24–48 hours following injury. Immunoassays of CRP are now widely used for early detection of acute inflammation or tissue injury and for the monitoring of remission (e.g. response of infection to an antibiotic).

Table 28.6 lists the advantages and disadvantages of the tests used to assess the acute phase response.

SUMMARY

- Chronic inflammation or malignant disorders cause anaemia with low serum iron and iron binding capacity, normal or raised serum ferritin, an inadequate response to erythropoietin and reduced red cell lifespan. The degree of anaemia relates to the severity of the underlying disease. It does not respond to iron therapy.
- This anaemia may be complicated by other causes of anaemia (e.g. iron or folate deficiencies, renal failure, bone marrow infiltration, haemolysis, hypersplenism).
- Polycythaemia is a much less frequent complication of systemic diseases (e.g. renal).
- White cell changes are also frequent in systemic diseases. These include neutrophil leucocytosis especially in bacterial infections, leucoerythroblastic or leukaemoid reactions, and in viral and connective tissue diseases, neutropenia.
- Eosinophilia occurs with certain infections, particularly parasitic and allergic disease. Monocytosis is associated with chronic bacterial infections (e.g. tuberculosis, brucellosis).
- Lymphocytosis is a feature of viral infections and some bacterial infections e.g. Bordetella pertussis.
- Platelets may be increased or low in malignant, infectious and other systemic diseases. Disseminated intravascular coagulation is a major cause of thrombocytopenia and fall in coagulation factors.
- C-reactive protein can be used for non-specific monitoring of systemic disease for short term (hours or days) and erythrocyte sedimentation rate (or plasma viscosity) over weeks or months.

Now visit www.wiley.com/go/essentialhaematology to test yourself on this chapter.

CHAPTER 29
Blood transfusion

Key topics

Essential Haematology, 6th Edition. © A. V. Hoffbrand and P. A. H. Moss. Published 2011 by Blackwell Publishing Ltd.

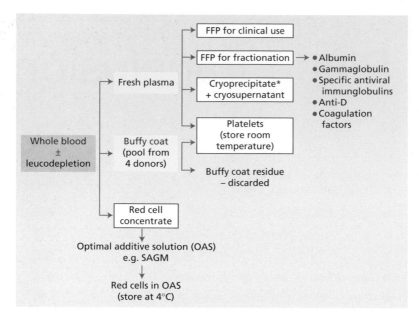

Figure 29.1 The preparation of blood components from whole blood. FFP, fresh frozen plasma; SAGM, saline-adenine-glucose-mannitol. *Cryoprecipitate is mainly a source of fibrinogen. Cryosupernatant is used for plasma exchange in thrombotic thrombocytopenic purpura.

Blood transfusion aims at the safe transfer of blood components (Fig. 29.1) from a donor to a recipient. In the UK, all Blood Banks are inspected by the Medicines and Healthcare Regulatory Agency (MHRA). All adverse events involving blood products must be reported to the Serious Adverse Blood Reactions and Events (SABRE) scheme. Errors in the transfusion process including SABRE reportable events are reported to the Serious Hazards of Transfusion (SHOT) scheme.

Blood donation

This should be voluntary. The measures to protect donors and for donor selection are listed in Table 29.1.

Red cell antigens and blood group antibodies

Approximately 400 red blood cell group antigens have been described. The clinical significance of blood groups in blood transfusion is that individuals who lack a particular blood group antigen may produce antibodies reacting with that antigen which may lead to a transfusion reaction. The different blood group antigens vary greatly in their clinical significance with the ABO and Rh (formerly Rhesus) groups being the most important. Some other systems are listed in Table 29.2.

Blood group antibodies

Naturally occurring antibodies occur in the plasma of subjects who lack the corresponding antigen and who have not been transfused or been pregnant (Table 29.3). The most important are anti-A and anti-B. They are usually immunoglobulin M (IgM), and react optimally at cold temperatures (4°C) so, although reactive at 37°C, are called cold antibodies.

Immune antibodies develop in response to the introduction – by transfusion or by transplacental passage during pregnancy – of red cells possessing antigens that the subject lacks. These antibodies are commonly IgG, although some IgM antibodies may also develop – usually in the early phase of an immune response. Immune antibodies react optimally at 37°C (warm antibodies). Only IgG

Table 29.1 Measures to protect the donor and for donor selection.

Donor selection

Age 17–70 years (maximum 60 at first donation)

Weight above 50 kg (7 st 12 lb)

Haemoglobin >13 g/dL for men, >12 g/dL for women

Minimum donation interval of 12 weeks (16 weeks advised) and three donations per year maximum

Pregnant and lactating women excluded because of high iron requirements; donation deferred for 9 months post pregnancy

Exclusion of those with:
  known cardiovascular disease, including
    hypertension
  significant respiratory disorders
  epilepsy and other CNS disorders
  gastrointestinal disorders with impaired
    absorption
  previous blood transfusions in the UK

Insulin-dependent diabetes

Chronic renal disease

Ongoing medical investigation or clinical trials

Exclusion of any donor returning to occupations such as driving bus, plane or train, heavy machine or crane operator, mining, scaffolding, etc. because delayed faint would be dangerous

Defer for 6 months after body piercing or tattoo, after acupuncture

Defer for 2 months after vaccinations, e.g. measles, mumps

CNS, central nervous system.

Table 29.2 Donor testing in England and Wales.

1 Blood group, Rh status
2 Microbiological tests
3 Human immunodeficiency virus (HIV) 1 and 2
4 Hepatitis B virus (HBV)
5 Hepatitis C virus (HCV)
6 Human T-cell leukaemia viruses (HTLV)
7 Cytomegalovirus (CMV) – for immunosuppressed recipients
8 Malaria – antibody screening of potentially exposed donors
9 Chagas' disease – antibody screening of potentially exposed donors
10 Bacteria – all donations tested for antibody to syphilis

antibodies are capable of transplacental passage from mother to fetus. The most important immune antibody is the Rh antibody, anti-D.

ABO system

This consists of three allelic genes: A, B and O. The A and B genes control the synthesis of specific enzymes responsible for the addition of single carbohydrate residues (*N*-acetyl galactosamine for group A and D-galactose for group B) to a basic antigenic glycoprotein or glycolipid with a terminal sugar L-fucose on the red cell, known as the H substance (Fig. 29.2). The O gene is an amorph and does not transform the H substance. Although there are six possible genotypes, the absence of a specific anti-O prevents the serological recognition of more than four phenotypes (Table 29.4). The two major subgroups of A (A_1 and A_2) complicate the issue but are of minor clinical significance. A_2 cells react more weakly than A_1 cells with anti-A and patients who are A_2B can be wrongly grouped as B.

The A, B and H antigens are present on most body cells including white cells and platelets. In the 80% of the population who possess secretor genes, these antigens are also found in soluble form in secretions and body fluids (e.g. plasma, saliva, semen and sweat).

Naturally occurring antibodies (usually IgM, occasionally IgG) to A and/or B antigens are found in the plasma of subjects whose red cells lack the corresponding antigen (Table 29.4; Fig. 29.3).

Rh system

The Rh blood group locus (previously known of as the rhesus system) is composed of two related structural genes, *RhD* and *RhCE*, which encode the

Table 29.3 Clinically important blood group systems.

Systems (abbr)	Frequency of antibodies	Cause of haemolytic transfusion reaction	Cause of haemolytic disease of newborn
ABO (ABO)	Almost universal	Yes (common)	Yes (usually mild)
Rh (RH)	Common	Yes (common)	Yes
Kell (KEL)	Occasional	Yes (occasional)	Anaemia not haemolysis
Duffy (Fy)	Occasional	Yes (occasional)	Yes (occasional)
Kidd (JK)	Occasional	Yes (occasional)	Yes (occasional)
Lutheran (LU)	Rare	Yes (rare)	No
Lewis (LE)	Occasional	Yes (rare)	No
P (PI)	Occasional	Yes (rare)	Yes (rare)
MNS (MNS)	Rare	Yes (rare)	Yes (rare)

Table 29.4 The ABO blood group system.

Phenotype	Genotype	Antigens	Naturally occurring antibodies	Frequency (UK) (%)
O	OO	O	Anti-A, anti-B	46
A	AA or AO	A	Anti-B	42
B	BB or BO	B	Anti-A	9
AB	AB	AB	None	3

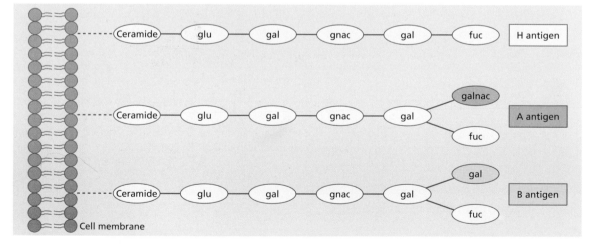

Figure 29.2 Structure of ABO blood group antigens. Each consists of a chain of sugars attached to lipids or proteins which are an integral part of the cell membrane. The H antigen of the O blood group has a terminal fucose (fuc). The A antigen has an additional *N*-acetyl galactosamine (galnac), and the B antigen has an additional galactose (gal). glu, glucose.

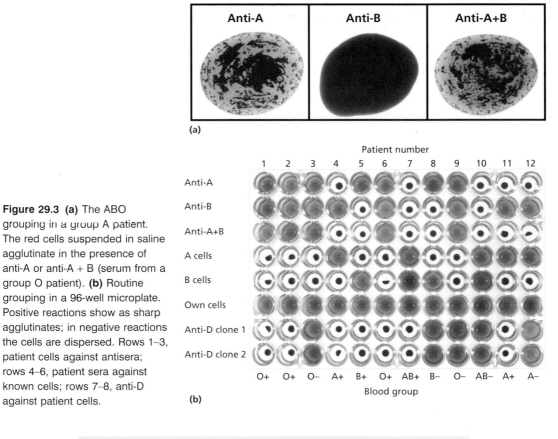

(a)

(b)

Figure 29.3 (a) The ABO grouping in a group A patient. The red cells suspended in saline agglutinate in the presence of anti-A or anti-A + B (serum from a group O patient). **(b)** Routine grouping in a 96-well microplate. Positive reactions show as sharp agglutinates; in negative reactions the cells are dispersed. Rows 1–3, patient cells against antisera; rows 4–6, patient sera against known cells; rows 7–8, anti-D against patient cells.

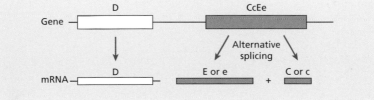

Figure 29.4 Molecular genetics of the Rhesus blood group. The locus consists of two closely linked genes, *RhD* and *RhCcEe*. The *RhD* gene codes for a single protein which contains the RhD antigen whereas *RhCcEe* mRNA undergoes alternative splicing to three transcripts. One of these encodes the E or e antigen whereas the other two (only one is shown) contain the C or c epitope. A polymorphism at position 226 of the *RhCcEe* gene determines the Ee antigen status whereas the C or c antigens are determined by a four amino acid allelic difference. Some individuals do not have an *RhD* gene and are therefore Rh D–.

membrane proteins that carry the D, Cc and Ee antigens. The *RhD* gene may be either present or absent, giving the Rh D+ or Rh D– phenotype, respectively. Alternative RNA splicing from the *RhCE* gene generates two proteins, which encode the C or c and the E or e antigens (Fig. 29.4). A shortened nomenclature for Rh phenotype is commonly used (Table 29.5).

Rh antibodies rarely occur naturally; most are immune (i.e. they result from previous transfusion or pregnancy). Anti-D is responsible for most of the clinical problems associated with the system and a

Table 29.5 The most common Rh genotypes in the UK population.

CDE nomenclature	Short symbol	Caucasian frequency (%)	Rh D status
cde/cde	Rr	15	Negative
CDe/cde	R_1r	31	Positive
CDe/CDe	R_1R_1	16	Positive
cDE/cde	R_2r	13	Positive
CDe/cDE	R_1R_2	13	Positive
cDE/cDE	R_2R_2	3	Positive
Other genotypes		9	Positive (almost all)

simple subdivision of subjects into Rh D+ and Rh D− using anti-D is sufficient for routine clinical purposes. Anti-C, anti-c, anti-E and anti-e are occasionally seen and may cause both transfusion reactions and haemolytic disease of the newborn. Anti-d does not exist. Rh haemolytic disease of the newborn is described in Chapter 30.

Other blood group systems

Other blood group systems are less frequently of clinical importance. Although naturally occurring antibodies of the P, Lewis and MN system are not uncommon, they usually only react at low temperatures and hence are of no clinical consequence. Immune antibodies against antigens of these systems are detected infrequently. Many of the antigens are of low antigenicity and others (e.g. Kell), although comparatively immunogenic, are of relatively low frequency and therefore provide few opportunities for isoimmunization except in multiply transfused patients.

Hazards of allogeneic blood transfusion

A large number of measures are taken to protect the recipient (Table 29.6).

Infection

Donor selection and testing of all donations are designed to prevent transmission of diseases (Tables

Table 29.6 Measures to protect the recipient.

Donor selection (Table 29.1)

Donor deferral/exclusion (Table 29.1)

Stringent arm cleaning

Microbiological testing of donations (Table 29.2)

Immunohaematological testing of donations

Diversion of first 20–30 mL blood collected

Leucodepletion of cellular products

Post-collection viral inactivation

Monitoring and testing for bacterial contamination

Pathogen inactivation

Safest possible sources of donor for plasma products

29.1 and 29.2). The main risk is from viruses that have long incubation periods and especially those that are carried for many years by asymptomatic individuals. Some viruses that are transfusion transmissible show cell-associated latency and, if in white cells, can cause infection in the recipient after allogeneic transfusion. Live viruses causing acute infection can be transmitted in the pre-symptomatic viraemic phase if blood is collected during that short period.

Individual infections

Hepatitis

Donors with a history of hepatitis are deferred for 12 months. If there is a history of jaundice, they can be accepted if markers for hepatitis B virus (HBV) and hepatitis C virus (HCV) are negative (Table 29.7).

Human immunodeficiency virus

This can be transmitted by cells or plasma. Male homosexuals, bisexuals, intravenous drug users and prostitutes are excluded, as are their sexual partners and partners of haemophiliacs. Inhabitants of large areas of sub-Saharan Africa and South-East Asia where HIV infection is particularly common are

---

Table 29.7 Infectious agents reported to have been transmitted by blood transfusion.

Viruses

Hepatitis viruses	Hepatitis A virus (HAV)
	Hepatitis B virus (HBV)
	Hepatitis C virus (HCV)
	Hepatitis D virus (HDV) (requires coinfection with HBV)
Retroviruses	Human immunodeficiency virus (HIV) 1, 2 (other subtypes)
	Human T-cell leukaemia virus (HTLV) I, II
Herpes viruses	Human cytomegalovirus (CMV)
	Epstein–Barr virus (EBV)
	Human herpesvirus 8 (HHV-8)
Parvoviruses	Parvovirus B19
Miscellaneous viruses	GBV-C – previously referred to as hepatitis G virus (HGV)
	Transfusion transmitted virus (TTV)
	West Nile virus

Bacteria

Endogenous	*Treponema pallidum* (syphilis)
	Borrelia burgdorferi (Lyme disease)
	Brucella melitensis (brucellosis)
	Yersinia enterocolitical/Salmonella spp.
Exogenous	Environmental species – *Staphyloccocal* spp./*Pseudomonas*/*Serratia* spp.
Rickettsiae	*Rickettsia rickettsii* (Rocky Mountain spotted fever)
	Coxiella burnettii (Q fever)

Protozoa

	Plasmodium spp. (malaria)
	Trypanosoma cruzi (Chagas' disease)
	Toxoplasma gondii (toxoplasmosis)
	Babesia microti/divergens (babesiosis)
	Leishmania spp. (leishmaniasis)

Prions

	New variant Creutzfeldt–Jakob disease (nvCJD)

NB. The microbiological testing of donations in the UK is detailed in Table 29.2.

also excluded. Rare transmission occurs when the donor is incubating the infection but has not yet developed the antibody that is detected in the laboratory test used (window period transmission).

Human T-cell leukaemias viruses

Human T-cell leukaemias virus type I (HTLVI) is associated with adult T-cell leukaemia or tropical spastic paraparesis. Human T-cell leukaemia virus type II (HLTVII) has no known association with any clinical condition. Screening for both is mandatory in the UK despite the low prevalence, approximately 1 in 50 000 untested donors.

Cytomegalovirus

Post-infusion cytomegalovirus (CMV) infection is usually subclinical but may give an infectious mononucleosis syndrome. Immunosuppressed individuals are at risk of pneumonitis and a potentially fatal disease. These are premature babies (<1500 g), stem cell and other organ transplant recipients, patients who have received alemtuzumab (anti-CD52, Campath) and pregnant women (the fetus is at risk). For such recipients, CMV negative blood or blood components must be given if they are CMV negative.

Other infections

Syphilis is more likely to be transmitted by platelets (stored at room temperature) than blood (stored at 4°C). However, all donations are tested. Malarial parasites are viable in blood stored at 4°C, so in endemic areas all recipients are given antimalarial drugs. In non-endemic areas donors are carefully vetted for travel to tropical areas and in some centres tests for malarial antibodies are performed. Chagas' disease is a significant problem with blood transfusion in Latin America. **Bacterial infections** resulting from skin commensals are most frequently transmitted by platelets stored for more than 3 days.

Prions The risk of new variant Creutzfeldt–Jakob disease (nvCJD) is considered a threat to blood safety only in the UK. Plasma for fractionation and fresh frozen plasma (FFP) for infants or children is obtained from the USA. It is unknown how many people could be infected with nvCJD. There are rare reports of transmission by blood transfusion, so recipients of blood or blood components are now excluded as blood donors in the UK. No screening tests for prions are yet available.

Techniques in blood group serology

The most important technique is based on the agglutination of red blood cells. Saline agglutination is important in detecting IgM antibodies, usually at room temperature and 4°C (e.g. anti-A, anti-B; Fig. 29.3). Addition of colloid to the incubation or proteolytic enzyme treatment of red cells increases the sensitivity of the indirect antiglobulin test (see below), as does low ionic strength saline. These latter methods can detect a range of IgG antibodies.

The antiglobulin test is a fundamental and widely used test in both blood group serology and general immunology. Antihuman globulin (AHG) is produced in animals following the injection of human globulin, purified complement or specific immunoglobulin (e.g. IgG, IgA or IgM). Monoclonal preparations are also now available. When AHG is added to human red cells coated with immunoglobulin or complement components, agglutination of the red cells indicates a positive test (Fig. 29.5).

The antiglobulin test may be either direct or indirect. The direct antiglobulin test is used for

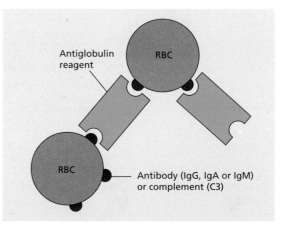

Figure 29.5 The antiglobulin test for antibody or complement on the surface of red blood cells (RBC). The antihuman globulin (Coombs') reagent may be broad spectrum or specific for immunoglobulin G (IgG), IgM, IgA or complement (C3).

detecting antibody or complement on the red cell surface where sensitization has occurred *in vivo*. The AHG reagent is added to washed red cells and agglutination indicates a positive test. A positive test occurs in haemolytic disease of the newborn, autoimmune haemolytic anaemia and haemolytic transfusion reactions.

The indirect antiglobulin test is used to detect antibodies that have coated the red cells *in vitro*. It is a two-stage procedure: the first step involves the incubation of test red cells with serum; in the second step, the red cells are washed and the AHG reagent is added. Agglutination implies that the original serum contained antibody which has coated the red cells *in vitro*. This test is used as part of the routine antibody screening of the recipient's serum prior to transfusion and for detecting blood group antibodies in a pregnant woman.

Most of the above methods were originally developed for tube techniques. These were replaced by 96-well microplates but most laboratories now use gel-based technology (Fig. 29.6).

Cross-matching and pre-transfusion tests

A number of steps are taken to ensure that patients receive compatible blood at the time of transfusion.

From the patient

1 The ABO and Rh blood group is determined.
2 Serum is screened for important antibodies by an indirect antiglobulin test on a large panel of antigenically typed group O red cells.

If a red cell alloantibody is discovered in the recipient, donor blood is selected lacking the relevant antigen. The most likely are Rh D, C, c, E, e and K.

From the donor

An appropriate ABO and Rh unit is selected. Donor (blood) testing is described on p. 399.

The cross-match

The techniques that may be used are described in Table 29.8.

Electronic cross-match

In this, a patient has group and antibody screen performed as two separate occasions. If both are negative and no blood has been transfused between the test, ABO and Rh compatible blood is issued directly without wet testing.

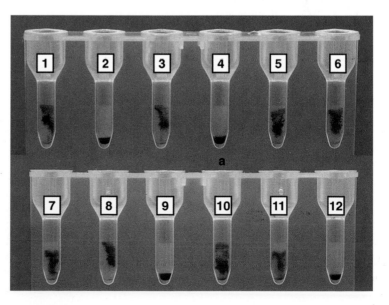

Figure 29.6 Patient antibody screening using the microcolumn (gel) system: 10 tests with two controls (tube 11 is the positive control and tube 12 the negative control) are shown. The patient's serum is tested against screening cells with known red cell phenotype. Tubes 1, 3, 5–8 and 10 show positive results. The patient's serum contained anti-Fy^a. (Courtesy of Mr G. Hazlehurst.)

Table 29.8 Techniques used in compatibility testing. Donor cells tested against recipient serum and agglutination detected visually or microscopically after mixing and incubation at the appropriate temperature.

For detecting clinically significant IgM antibodies
Saline 37°C

For detecting immune antibodies (mainly IgG)
Indirect antiglobulin test at 37°C
Low ionic strength saline at 37°C
Enzyme-treated red cells at 37°C

Ig, immunoglobulin.

Complications of blood transfusion (Table 29.9)

Haemolytic transfusion reactions

Haemolytic transfusion reactions may be immediate or delayed. Immediate life-threatening reactions associated with massive intravascular haemolysis are the result of complement-activating antibodies of IgM or IgG classes, usually with ABO specificity. Reactions associated with extravascular haemolysis (e.g. immune antibodies of the Rh system that are unable to activate complement) are generally less severe but may still be life-threatening. The cells become coated with IgG and are removed in the reticuloendothelial system. In mild cases, the only signs of a transfusion reaction may be a progressive unexplained anaemia with or without jaundice. In some cases where the pre-transfusion level of an antibody was too low to be detected in a cross-match, a patient may be reimmunized by transfusion of incompatible red cells and this will lead to a delayed transfusion reaction (most often caused by anti-c or anti-JK) with accelerated clearance of the red cells. There may be rapid appearance of anaemia with mild jaundice.

Clinical features of a major haemolytic transfusion reaction

Haemolytic shock phase This may occur after only a few millilitres of blood have been transfused

Table 29.9 Complications of blood transfusion.

Early	Late
Haemolytic reactions: immediate or delayed	Transmission of infection (Table 29.7)
Reactions caused by infected blood	Transfusional iron overload (see Chapter 4)
Allergic reactions to white cells, platelets or proteins	Immune sensitization, e.g. to red cells, platelets or Rh D antigen
Pyrogenic reactions (to plasma proteins or caused by HLA antibodies)	Transfusion-associated graft-versus-host disease
Circulatory overload	
Bacterial contamination	
Air embolism	
Thrombophlebitis	
Citrate toxicity	
Hyperkalaemia	
Clotting abnormalities (after massive transfusion)	
TRALI	
Post-transfusion purpura	

HLA, human leucocyte antigen; TRALI, transfusion-related acute lung injury.

or up to 1–2 hours after the end of the transfusion. Clinical features include urticaria, pain in the lumbar region, flushing, headache, precordial pain, shortness of breath, vomiting, rigours, pyrexia and a fall in blood pressure. If the patient is anaesthetized this shock phase is masked. There is increasing evidence of red cell destruction and haemoglobin-uria, jaundice and disseminated intravascular coag-ulation (DIC) may occur. Moderate leucocytosis (e.g. $15–20 \times 10^9/L$ is usual.

The oliguric phase   In some patients with a haemolytic reaction there is renal tubular necrosis with acute renal failure.

Diuretic phase   Fluid and electrolyte imbal-ance may occur during the recovery from acute renal failure.

Investigation of an immediate transfusion reaction

If a patient develops features suggesting a severe transfusion reaction the transfusion should be stopped and investigations for blood group incom-patibility and bacterial contamination of the blood must be initiated.

1 Most severe reactions occur because of clerical errors in the handling of donor or recipient blood specimens. Therefore it must be established that the identity of the recipient (from the patient's wristband) is the same as that on the compatibil-ity label and that this corresponds with the actual unit being transfused.

2 The unit of donor blood and post-transfusion samples of the patient's blood should be sent to the laboratory who will:

  (a) repeat the group on pre- and post-transfusion samples and on the donor blood, and repeat the cross-match;

  (b) perform a direct antiglobulin test on the post-transfusion sample;

  (c) check the plasma for haemoglobinaemia;

  (d) perform tests for DIC; and

  (e) examine the donor sample directly for evi-dence of gross bacterial contamination and set up blood cultures from it at 20 and 37°C. If the clinical picture is suggestive of bacterial infection blood cultures must be taken from the patient and broad-spectrum intravenous antibodies started.

3 A post-transfusion sample of urine must be examined for haemoglobinuria.

4 Further samples of blood are taken 6 hours and/or 24 hours after transfusion for a blood count and bilirubin, free haemoglobin and methaemal-bumin (see p. 76) estimations.

5 In the absence of positive findings, the patient's serum is examined 5–10 days later for red cell or white cell antibodies.

Management of patients with major haemolysis

The principal object of initial therapy is to maintain the blood pressure and renal perfusion. Intravenous dextran, plasma or saline and frusemide are some-times needed. Hydrocortisone 100 mg intrave-nously and an antihistamine may help to alleviate shock. In the event of severe shock, support with intravenous adrenaline 1 : 10 000 in small incremental doses may be required. Further com-patible transfusions may be required in severely affected patients. If acute renal failure occurs this is managed in the usual way, if necessary with dialysis until recovery occurs.

Other transfusion reactions

Febrile reactions because of white cell anti-bodies   Human leucocyte antigen (HLA) antibod-ies (see below and Chapter 23) are usually the result of sensitization by pregnancy or a previous transfu-sion. They produce rigors, pyrexia and, in severe cases, pulmonary infiltrates. They are minimized by giving leucocyte-depleted (i.e. filtered) packed cells (see below).

Febrile or non-febrile non-haemolytic allergic reactions   These are usually caused by hypersensi-tivity to donor plasma proteins and if severe can result in anaphylactic shock. The clinical features are urticaria, pyrexia and, in severe cases, dyspnoea, facial oedema and rigors. Immediate treatment is with antihistamines and hydrocortisone. Adrenaline is also useful. Washed red cells or frozen red cells may be needed for further transfusions if the majority of plasma-removed blood (e.g. saline, adenine, glucose, mannitol (SAGM) blood) causes reactions.

Post-transfusion circulatory overload   The management is that of cardiac failure. These reac-tions are prevented by a slow transfusion of packed red cells or of the blood component required, accompanied by diuretic therapy.

Transfusion of bacterially contaminated blood This is very rare but may be serious. It can present with circulatory collapse.

Graft-versus-host disease (GVHD) This may occur when live lymphocytes are transfused to an immunocompromised patient. It is prevented by irradiation of the blood product. It is almost uniformly fatal.

Hyperhaemolysis syndrome Some patients particularly with sickle cell anaemia, haemolyse donor blood even though no alloantibodies to red cells can be detected. The haemolysis appears to be caused by overactivity of the recipient's macrophages. It is prevented by infusion of gammaglobulin and corticosteriod therapy.

Transfusion-related acute lung injury (TRALI) This presents within 6 hours of an infusion as pulmonary infiltrates with chest symptoms depending on severity. It is caused by positive transfer of HLA antibodies in donor plasma causing endothelial and epithelial injury. Most of the donors are multiparous women. Management is supportive.

Post-transfusion purpura This is a rare problem of severe thrombocytopenia 7–10 days after transfusion of a platelet-containing product, usually red cells. It is caused by an antibody in the recipient (previously transfused or pregnant) anti HPA-1a against a platelet-specific antigen HPA-Ia (PI^{AI}). Both transfused and recipient platelets are destroyed by the immune complexes. It is usually self-limiting but immunoglobulin or plasma exchange may be needed.

Viral transmission Post-transfusion hepatitis may be caused by one of the hepatitis viruses, although CMV and Epstein–Barr virus have also been implicated. Post-transfusion hepatitis and HIV infection is seen rarely now because of routine screening of all blood donations.

Other infections Toxoplasmosis, malaria and syphilis may be transmitted by blood transfusion. Transfusion-transmitted nvCJD has probably occurred in three cases in the UK.

Post-transfusional iron overload Repeated red cell transfusions over many years, in the absence of blood loss, cause deposition of iron initially in reticuloendothelial tissue at the rate of 200–250 mg/unit of red cells. After 50 units in adults, and lesser amounts in children, the liver, myocardium and endocrine glands are damaged with clinical consequences. This is a major problem in thalassaemia major and other severe chronic refractory anaemias (see Chapter 4).

Reduction of blood product use

In the light of transfusion risks, and limited resources, appropriate use of blood components is of increasing importance.

Preoperative correction of anaemia (particularly iron deficiency) and cessation of antiplatelet therapies (e.g. aspirin) where possible, together with lower trigger levels for red cell transfusions (7–8 g/dL in most surgical patients) can all help to reduce blood use.

In surgery the use of alternative fluid replacement, intraoperative or postoperative cell salvage, biological alternatives (e.g. erythropoetin, recombinant clotting factors, recombinant activated clotting factor VII (VIIa) or fibrin glue) all may help.

Blood components

A blood donation is taken by an aseptic technique into plastic bags containing an appropriate amount of anticoagulant – usually citrate, phosphate, dextrose (CPD). The citrate anticoagulates the blood by combining with the blood calcium. Three components are made by initial centrifugation of whole blood: red cells, buffy coat and plasma (Fig. 29.1).

Red cells are stored at 4–6°C for up to to 35 days, depending on the preservative. After the first 48 hours there is a slow progressive K$^+$ loss from the red cells into the plasma. In cases where infusion of K$^+$ could be dangerous, fresh blood should be used (e.g. for exchange transfusion in haemolytic disease of the newborn). During red cell storage there is a fall in 2,3-diphosphoglycerate (2,3-DPG) but after transfusion 2,3-DPG levels return to normal within 24 hours. Optimum additive solutions have been developed to increase the shelf life of plasma-depleted red cells by maintaining both adenosine triphosphate (ATP) and 2,3-DPG levels.

Platelets and plasma may also be collected by apharesis (and centrifuging).

Leucodepletion

In many countries, including Britain, blood products are now routinely filtered to remove the majority of white cells, a process known as leucodepletion. This is usually performed soon after collection and prior to processing and is more effective than filtration of blood at the bedside. A blood component is defined as leucocyte depleted if there are less than 5×10^6/L white cells present.

Leucodepletion reduces the incidence of febrile transfusion reactions and HLA alloimmunization. It is effective at preventing transmission of CMV infection and in addition should reduce the theoretical possibility of transmission of nvCJD in countries where this has been reported.

Red cells

Packed (plasma-depleted) red cells are the treatment of choice for most transfusions (Fig. 29.7a). In older subjects, a diuretic is often given simultaneously and the infusion should be sufficiently slow to avoid

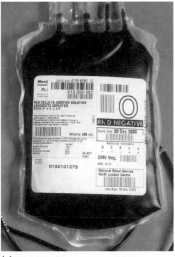

(a)

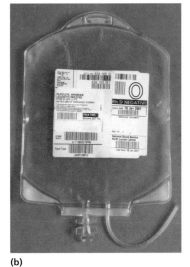

(b)

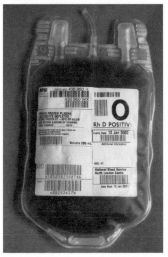

(c)

Figure 29.7 Blood components: **(a)** plasma-depleted red cells; **(b)** platelets; and **(c)** fresh frozen plasma.

circulatory overload. Iron chelation therapy, to avoid iron overload, should be considered with patients on a regular transfusion programme (see Chapter 4).

Erythropoietin is widely used to reduce transfusion requirements (e.g. in patients with renal failure, on dialysis, cancer patients and myelodysplasia). Factor VIIa can reduce transfusion need in patients with major haemorrhage (e.g. at surgery or after trauma).

Red cell substitutes are under development but have not yet proven clinically valuable. These synthetic oxygen-carrying substitutes are often fluorinated hydrocarbons and stromal-free pyridoxylated and polymerized haemoglobin solutions.

Autologous donation and transfusion

Anxiety over HIV and other infections has increased the demand for autotransfusion. There are three ways of administering an autologous transfusion:

1 *Predeposit* Blood is taken from the potential recipient in the weeks immediately prior to elective surgery.
2 *Haemodilution* Blood is removed immediately prior to surgery once the patient has been anaesthetized and then reinfused at the end of the operation.
3 *Salvage* Blood lost during the operation is collected during heavy blood loss and then reinfused.

Autotransfusion is the safest form of transfusion with regard to transmission of viral disease though it has a higher risk of bacterial contamination and of clerical errors. For predeposit, the individual must be fit enough to donate blood and the predicted operative replacement transfusion should be 2–4 units. Larger replacement transfusions would require blood to be collected over a longer period and red cells stored in the frozen state, which is even more labour intensive and expensive. The high cost and initial restriction of its use to patients undergoing elective surgery means that it can benefit only a minor proportion of the total number of blood recipients. Preoperative autotransfusion is largely reserved for those patients with

multiple antibodies for whom it is difficult to identify matching donor blood.

Granulocyte concentrates

These are prepared as buffy coats or on blood cell separators from normal healthy donors or from patients with chronic myeloid leukaemia. They have been used in patients with severe neutropenia ($<0.5 \times 10^9$/L) who are not responding to antibiotic therapy but it is not usually possible to give sufficient amounts. They may transmit CMV infection and must be irradiated to eliminate the risk of causing GVHD.

Platelet concentrates

These are harvested by cell separators or from individual donor units of blood (Fig. 29.7b). They are stored at room temperature. Platelet transfusion is used in patients who are thrombocytopenic or have disordered platelet function and who are actively bleeding (therapeutic use) or are at serious risk of bleeding (prophylactic use).

For prophylaxis, the platelet count should be kept above $5–10 \times 10^9$/L unless there are additional risk factors such as sepsis, drug use or coagulation disorders for which the threshold should be higher. For invasive procedures (e.g. liver biopsy or lumbar puncture) the platelet count should be raised to above 50×10^9/L. For brain or eye surgery the count should be $>100 \times 10^9$/L.

Therapeutic use is indicated in bleeding associated with platelet disorders. In massive haemorrhage the count should be kept above 50×10^9/L.

Platelet transfusions should be avoided in autoimmune thrombocytopenic purpura unless there is serious haemorrhage. They are contraindicated in heparin-induced thrombocytopenia, thrombotic thrombocytopenic purpura and haemolytic uraemic syndrome (see p. 337).

Refractoriness to platelet transfusions is defined by a poor platelet increment post-transfusion ($<7.5 \times 10^9$/L at 1 hour or $<4.5 \times 10^9$/L at 24 hours). The causes are either immunological (mostly HLA alloimmunization) or non-immunological (sepsis, hypersplenism, DIC, drugs). Platelets express HLA class I (but not class II) antigens and

HLA-matched or cross-match-compatible platelets are needed for patients with HLA antibodies.

Platelet transfusions are likely to be reduced with the introduction of direct stimulators of platelet production (e.g. romiplostim or amino acid/group).

Preparations from human plasma

Fresh frozen plasma

Rapidly frozen plasma separated from fresh blood is stored at less than −30°C. Frozen plasma is usually prepared from single donor units although pooled products are also available. Its main use is for the replacement of coagulation factors (e.g. when specific concentrates are unavailable) or after massive transfusions, in liver disease and DIC, after cardiopulmonary by-pass surgery, to reverse a warfarin effect and in thrombotic thrombocytopenic purpura (see p. 337). Virally inactivated forms of FFP are now available. Male donors are preferred to reduce the risk of TRALI (see p. 408).

Human albumin solution (4.5%)

This is a useful plasma volume expander when a sustained osmotic effect is required prior to the administration of blood, but it should not be given in excess. It is also used for fluid replacement in patients undergoing plasmapheresis and sometimes for fluid replacement in selected patients with hypoalbuminaemia.

Human albumin solution (20%) (salt-poor albumin)

This may be used in severe hypoalbuminaemia when it is necessary to use a product with minimal electrolyte content. Principal indications for its use are patients with nephrotic syndrome or liver failure.

Cryoprecipitate

This is obtained by thawing FFP at 4°C and contains concentrated factor VIII and fibrinogen. It is stored at less than −30°C or, if lyophylized, at 4–6°C, and was used widely as replacement therapy in those with haemophilia A and von Willebrand disease before more purified preparations of factor VIII became available. Its main use is in fibrinogen replacement in DIC or massive transfusion or hepatic failure.

Freeze-dried factor VIII concentrates

These are also used for treating haemophilia A or von Willebrand disease. The small volume makes them ideal for children, surgical cases, patients at risk from circulatory overload and for those on home treatment. Their use has declined since recombinant forms of factor VIII became widely available.

Freeze-dried factor IX–prothrombin complex concentrates

A number of preparations are available that contain variable amounts of factors II, VII, IX and X. They are mainly used for treating factor IX deficiency (Christmas disease) but are also used in patients with liver disease or with haemorrhage following overdose with oral anticoagulants or in patients with factor VIII inhibitors. There is a risk of thrombosis.

Protein C concentrate

This is used in severe sepsis with DIC (e.g. meningococcal septicaemia) to reduce thrombosis resulting from depletion of protein C.

Immunoglobulin

Pooled immunoglobulin is a valuable source of antibodies against common viruses. It is used in hypogammaglobulinaemia from whatever cause for protection against viral and bacterial disease. It may also be used in immune thrombocytopenia and other acquired immune disorders (e.g. post-transfusion purpura or alloimmune neonatal thrombocytopenia).

Specific immunoglobulin

This may be obtained from donors with high titres of antibody (e.g. anti-RhD, anti-hepatitis B, anti-herpes zoster or anti-rubella).

Acute blood loss

After a single episode of blood loss, there is initial vasoconstriction with a reduction in total blood volume. The plasma volume rapidly expands and the haemoglobin and packed cell volume fall and there is a rise in neutrophils and platelets. The reticulocyte response begins on the second or third day and lasts 8–10 days. The haemoglobin begins to rise by about the seventh day but, if iron stores have become depleted, the haemoglobin may not rise subsequently to normal. Clinical assessment is needed to gauge whether blood transfusion is needed. This is usually unnecessary in adults at losses less than 500 mL unless haemorrhage is continuing and may not be needed with losses of up to 1.5 L. Blood transfusion is not without risks and should not be undertaken lightly. The problems of massive blood loss and massive transfusion are considered on p. 360.

SUMMARY

- Blood transfusion involves the safe transfer of blood components from a donor to a recipient. Most commonly this is red cells and the red cells must be matched between recipient and donor.
- Careful donor selection and microbiological testing help to protect both donor and recipient.
- Red cells contain over 400 antigens. It is the ABO and Rh systems that are most important in transfusion. Subjects lacking an antigen (e.g. group A or B) may develop a naturally occurring antibody to it, usually IgM. These antibodies in a recipient may haemolyse or opsonize donor red cells if these contain the antigen.
- Antibodies may also develop from exposure to the antigen by a transfusion or pregnancy. Cross-matching of donor red cells with recipient plasma is therefore carried out to ensure they are compatible.
- Complications of blood transfusion include haemolytic reactions, febrile reactions to white cells or proteins, circulatory overload, transmission of infections, especially viral, and, in the longer term, iron overload.
- Blood components other than red cells can also be transfused. These include platelets and protein products including fresh frozen plasma, albumin solutions, coagulation factor concentrates and immunoglobulin.

Now visit www.wiley.com/go/essentialhaematology to test yourself on this chapter.

CHAPTER 30

Pregnancy and neonatal haematology

Key topics

Haematology of pregnancy

Pregnancy places extreme stresses on the haematological system and an understanding of the physiological changes that result is obligatory in order to interpret any need for therapeutic intervention.

Physiological anaemia

Physiological anaemia is the term often used to describe the fall in haemoglobin (Hb) concentration that occurs during normal pregnancy (Fig. 30.1). Blood plasma volume increases by approximately 1250 mL, or 45%, above normal by the end of gestation and although the red cell mass itself increases by some 25% this still leads to a fall in Hb concentration. Values below 10 g/dL are probably abnormal and require investigation.

Iron deficiency anaemia

Up to 600 mg iron is required for the increase in red cell mass and a further 300 mg for the fetus. Despite an increase in iron absorption, few women avoid depletion of iron reserves by the end of pregnancy.

In uncomplicated pregnancy, the mean corpuscular volume (MCV) typically rises by approximately 4 fL. A fall in red cell MCV is the earliest sign of iron deficiency. Later, the mean corpuscular haemoglobin (MCH) falls and finally anaemia results. Early iron deficiency is likely if the serum ferritin is below 15 μg/L together with serum iron <10 μmol/L and should be treated with oral iron supplements. The use of routine iron supplementation in pregnancy is debated but iron is probably better avoided until the Hb falls below 10 g/dL or MCV below 82 fL in the third trimester.

Folate deficiency

Folate requirements are increased approximately twofold in pregnancy and serum folate levels fall to approximately half the normal range with a less dramatic fall in red cell folate. In some parts of the world, megaloblastic anaemia during pregnancy is common because of a combination of poor diet and exaggerated folate requirements. Given the protective effect of folate against neural tube defects (NTDs) as well as against anaemia, 400 μg/day folic acid (5 mg if there has been a previous NTD pregnancy) should be taken periconceptually and throughout pregnancy. Food fortification with folate is now being practised in many countries (not the UK) and has been associated with a fall in incidence of NTDs. Vitamin B_{12} deficiency is rare during pregnancy although serum vitamin B_{12} levels

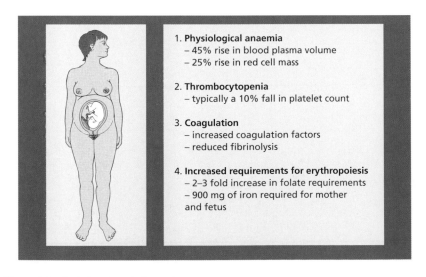

1. **Physiological anaemia**
   – 45% rise in blood plasma volume
   – 25% rise in red cell mass

2. **Thrombocytopenia**
   – typically a 10% fall in platelet count

3. **Coagulation**
   – increased coagulation factors
   – reduced fibrinolysis

4. **Increased requirements for erythropoiesis**
   – 2–3 fold increase in folate requirements
   – 900 mg of iron required for mother and fetus

Figure 30.1 Haematological changes during pregnancy.

fall to below normal in 20–30% of pregnancies and low values are sometimes the cause of diagnostic confusion.

Thrombocytopenia

The platelet count typically falls by approximately 10% in an uncomplicated pregnancy. In approximately 7% of women this fall is more severe and can result in thrombocytopenia (platelet count $<140 \times 10^9$/L). In over 75% of cases this is mild and of unknown cause, a condition referred to as *incidental thrombocytopenia of pregnancy*. Approximately 21% of cases are secondary to a hypertensive disorder and 4% are associated with immune thrombocytopenic purpura (ITP; Fig. 30.2).

Incidental thrombocytopenia of pregnancy This is a diagnosis of exclusion and is usually detected at the time of delivery. The platelet count is always $>70 \times 10^9$/L and recovers within 6 weeks. No treatment is required and the infant is not affected.

Thrombocytopenia of hypertensive disorders This is variable in severity but the platelet count rarely falls to $<40 \times 10^9$/L. It is more severe when associated with pre-eclampsia and if severe the primary treatment is as rapid delivery as possible.

The platelet count falls for a day or two after delivery and then recovers rapidly. The HELLP syndrome (haemolysis, elevated liver enzymes and low platelets) is a subtype of this category. It is associated with prolongation of the prothrombin time (PT) and activated partial thromboplastin time (APTT).

Idiopathic (autoimmune) thrombocytopenic purpura (see p. 334) In pregnancy, ITP represents a particular problem, both to the mother and to the fetus, as the antibody crosses the placenta and the fetus may become severely thrombocytopenic.

Like all adults, pregnant women with ITP and platelet counts $>50 \times 10^9$/L do not usually need treatment. Treatment is required for women with platelet counts $<10 \times 10^9$/L and for those with platelet counts of $10–30 \times 10^9$/L who are in their second or third trimester or who are bleeding. Treatment is with steroids, intravenous immunoglobulin G (IgG), rituximab and splenectomy as appropriate.

At delivery, umbilical vein blood sampling or fetal scalp vein sampling to measure the fetal platelet count may be offered although their exact role is unclear. In general, caesarean section is not indicated when the maternal platelet count is $>50 \times 10^9$/L unless the fetal platelet count is known to be $<20 \times 10^9$/L. Platelet transfusion may be

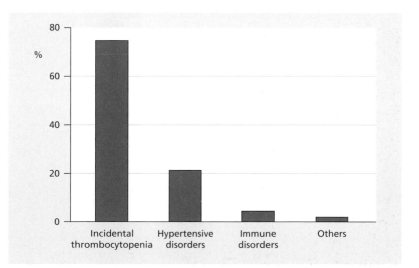

Figure 30.2 Causes of thrombocytopenia during pregnancy.

given to mothers in labour with very low platelet counts or who are actively bleeding. Caesarean section may be indicated to protect the fetus.

Newborns of mothers with ITP should have a blood count measured for the first 4 days of life as the platelet count may progressively drop. A count $>50 \times 10^9$/L is reassuring. Cerebral ultrasounds may be performed to look for intracranial haemorrhage (ICH). In newborns without evidence of ICH, treatment with intravenous IgG is appropriate if the infant's platelet count is $<20 \times 10^9$/L. Neonates with thrombocytopenia and ICH should be treated with steroids and intravenous IgG therapy.

Haemostasis and thrombosis

Pregnancy leads to a hypercoaguable state with consequent increased risks of thromboembolism and disseminated intravascular coagulation (DIC; see p. 355). There is an increase in plasma factors VII, VIII, X and fibrinogen with shortening of PT and APTT, and fibrinolysis is suppressed. These changes last for up to 2 months into the puerperal period and the incidence of thrombosis during this period is increased. There is an association between thrombophilic conditions in the mother and with recurrent fetal loss. This is presumed to result from placental thrombosis and infarction.

Treatment of thrombosis

Warfarin has no role in management. It crosses the placenta and in addition is associated with embryopathy, especially between 6 and 12 weeks' gestation. Heparin does not cross the placenta but a significant side-effect of prolonged use is maternal osteoporosis. Low molecular weight heparin is now the treatment of choice because it can be given once daily and is less likely to cause osteoporosis.

Neonatal haematology

Normal blood count

The cord blood Hb varies between approximately 16.5 and 17 g/dL and is influenced by the timing of cord clamping (Fig. 30.3). The reticulocyte count

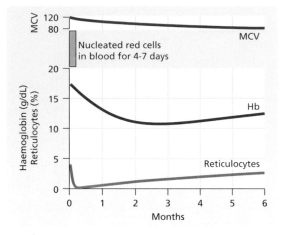

Figure 30.3 Typical profile of the blood count in the neonatal period. MCV, mean corpuscular volume.

is initially high (2–6%) but falls to below 0.5% at 1 week as erythropoiesis is suppressed in response to the marked increase in the oxygenation of tissues after birth. This is associated with a progressive fall in Hb to approximately 10–11 g/dL at 8 weeks from which point it recovers to 12.5 g/dL at around 6 months. The lower limit of normal during childhood is 11.0 g/dL. In the blood film, nucleated red cells will be seen for the first 4 days and for up to 1 week in preterm infants. Numbers are increased in cases of hypoxia, haemorrhage or haemolytic disease of the newborn (HDN). MCV averages 119 fL but falls to adult levels by around 9 weeks. By 1 year, the MCV has fallen to around 70 fL and rises throughout childhood again to reach adult levels at puberty. Preterm infants have a more dramatic fall in Hb to 7–9 g/dL at 8 weeks and are more prone to iron and folate deficiency in the first few months of life. Neutrophils are initially high at birth and fall to plateau at 4 days – from this point on the lymphocyte count is higher than neutrophils throughout childhood.

Anaemia in the neonate

This should be considered for Hb <14 g/dL at birth. The clinical significance of anaemia is compounded by the high (70–80%) levels of HbF at birth, as this is less effective than HbA at releasing oxygen to the tissues. Causes include the following (Fig. 30.4):

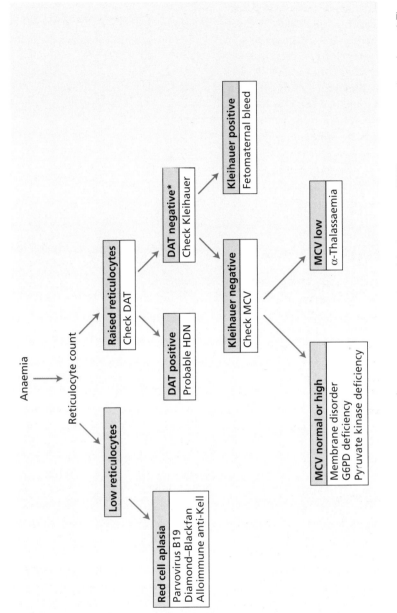

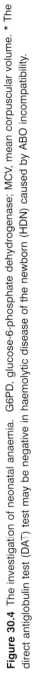

Figure 30.4 The investigation of neonatal anaemia. G6PD, glucose-6-phosphate dehydrogenase; MCV, mean corpuscular volume. * The direct antiglobulin test (DAT) test may be negative in haemolytic disease of the newborn (HDN) caused by ABO incompatibility.

1 *Haemorrhage* Fetomaternal, twin–twin, cord, internal, placenta.
2 *Increased destruction* Haemolysis (immune or non-immune) or infection.
3 *Decreased production* Congenital red cell aplasia, infection (e.g. parvovirus). Anti-Kell causes alloimmune anaemia of the fetus and newborn with decreased erythropoiesis.

Generally, anaemia at birth is usually secondary to immune haemolysis or haemorrhage; non-immune causes of haemolysis appear within 24 hours. Impaired red cell production is usually not apparent for at least 3 weeks. Haemolysis is often associated with severe jaundice and the causes include HDN, autoimmune haemolytic anaemia in the mother and congenital disorders of the red cell membrane or metabolism.

Red cell transfusion may be needed for symptomatic anaemia with Hb <10.5 g/dL or a higher threshold if there is severe cardiac or respiratory disease.

Anaemia of prematurity

Premature infants have a more marked fall in Hb after birth and this is termed *physiological anaemia of prematurity*. Features include a slowly falling Hb, normal blood film and reticulocytopenia. It can be minimized by ensuring adequate iron and folate replacement and limiting phlebotomy. Erythropoietin is used in some centres.

Neonatal polycythaemia

This is defined as a venous haematocrit over 0.65 and can occur with twin–twin transfusion, intrauterine growth restriction and maternal hypertension or diabetes. If symptoms are present it should be treated with partial exchange transfusion using a crystalloid solution.

Fetomaternal alloimmune thrombocytopenia

Fetomaternal alloimmune thrombocytopenia results from an immunological process similar to that of

HDN. Fetal platelets that possess a paternally inherited antigen (HPA-1a in 80%; HPA-5b in 15%) that is not present on maternal platelets can sensitize the mother to make antibodies that cross the placenta, coat the platelets which are then destroyed by the reticuloendothelial system and lead to serious bleeding, including ICH. Alloimmune thrombocytopenia differs from HDN in that 50% of cases occur in the first pregnancy. Its incidence is approximately 1 in 1000–5000 births.

Thrombocytopenia can lead to serious, sometimes fatal, bleeding *in utero* or after birth. Treatment is unsatisfactory. Severe postnatal cases may be treated with a platelet transfusion that is negative for the relevant antigen. Antenatal treatment may be either maternal intravenous immunoglobulin or fetal transfusion with HPA-compatible platelets.

Coagulation

Standard tests need to be interpreted with caution in the neonate. The APTT and PT are prolonged because of reduced levels of the vitamin K-dependent factors II, VII, IX and X, and become normal at around 6 months. The thrombin time (TT) is comparable with adult values. Neonates have an increased risk of thrombosis. This is a result of physiologically low levels of inhibitors of coagulation and the use of indwelling vascular catheters. Antithrombin and protein C levels are approximately 60% of normal for the first 3 months. Homozygous protein C deficiency is associated with fulminant purpura fulminans in early life. Therapeutic protein C concentrates are now available. Homozygous antithrombin deficiency usually presents later in childhood but arterial and venous thrombosis may also occur in the neonate.

Haemolytic disease of the newborn

HDN is the result of *red cell alloimmunization* in which IgG antibodies passage from the maternal circulation across the placenta into the circulation of the fetus where they react with fetal red cells and lead to their destruction. Anti-D antibody is responsible for most cases of severe HDN although anti-c, anti-E, anti-K and a wide range of other antibodies are found in occasional cases (see Table 29.2). Although antibodies against the ABO blood group system are most frequent cause of HDN this is usually mild.

Rh haemolytic disease of the newborn

When an Rh D-negative woman has a pregnancy with an Rh D-positive fetus, Rh D-positive fetal red cells cross into the maternal circulation (especially at parturition and during the third trimester) and sensitize the mother to form anti-D. The mother could also be sensitized by a previous miscarriage, amniocentesis or other trauma to the placenta or by blood transfusion. Anti-D crosses the placenta to the fetus during the next pregnancy with an Rh D-positive fetus, coats the fetal red cells and results in reticuloendothelial destruction of these cells, causing anaemia and jaundice. If the father is heterozygous for D antigen, there is a 50% probability that the fetus will be D-positive. The fetal Rh D genotype can be established by polymerase chain reaction (PCR) analysis for the presence of Rh D in a maternal blood sample.

The main aim of management is to *prevent* anti-D antibody formation in Rh D-negative mothers. This can be achieved by the administration of small amounts of anti-D antibody which 'mop up' and destroy Rh D-positive fetal red cells before they can sensitize the immune system of the mother to produce anti-D.

Prevention of Rh immunization

At the time of booking, all pregnant women should have their ABO and Rh group determined and serum screened for antibodies at least twice during the pregnancy. All non-sensitized Rh D-negative women should be given at least 500 units (100 μg) of anti-D at 28 and 34 weeks' gestation to reduce the risk of sensitization from fetomaternal haemorrhage. Fetal Rh D typing from DNA in maternal blood can be used before 28 weeks. If the fetus is Rh D-negative, no further anti-D prophylaxis is needed. In addition, at birth the babies of Rh D-negative women who do not have antibodies must have their cord blood grouped for ABO and Rh. If the baby's blood is Rh D-negative, the mother will require no further treatment. If the baby is Rh D-positive, prophylactic anti-D should be administered at a minimum dose of 500 units intramuscularly within 72 hours of delivery. A **Kleihauer test** is performed. This uses differential staining to estimate the number of fetal cells in the maternal circulation (Fig. 30.5a). If the Kleihauer is positive many centres will perform flow cytometry for a more accurate estimate of the volume of fetomaternal haemorrhage (FMH) (Fig 30.5b). The chance of developing antibodies is related to the number of fetal cells found. The dose of anti-D is increased if there is >4 mL transplacental haemorrhage. Anti-D IgG (125 units) is given for each 1 mL of FMH greater than 4 mL.

Sensitizing episodes during pregnancy
Anti-D IgG should be given to Rh D-negative women who have potentially sensitizing episodes during pregnancy: 250 units is given if the event occurs up to week 20 of gestation and 500 units thereafter, followed by a Kleihauer test. Potentially sensitizing events include therapeutic termination of pregnancy, spontaneous miscarriage after 12 weeks' gestation, ectopic pregnancy and invasive antenatal diagnostic procedures.

Treatment of established anti-D sensitization
If anti-D antibodies are detected during pregnancy they should be quantified at regular intervals. The clinical severity is related to the strength of anti-D present in maternal serum but is also affected by such factors as the IgG subclass, rate of rise of antibody and past history. The development of haemolytic disease in the fetus can be assessed by velocimetry of the fetal middle cerebral artery by Doppler ultrasonography as increased velocities correlate with fetal anaemia (Fig. 30.6). If anaemia is detected, fetal blood sampling and intrauterine transfusion of irradiated Rh D-negative packed red cells may be indicated.

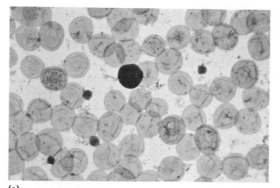

(a)

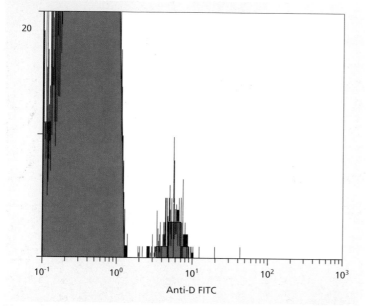

(b)

Figure 30.5 (a) Kleihauer test for fetal red cells; a deeply eosin-staining cell containing fetal haemoglobin is seen at the centre. Haemoglobin has been eluted from the other red cells by an incubation at acid pH and these appear as colourless ghosts. **(b)** Determination by flow cytometry of the number of Rh D fetal cells in maternal blood using fluorescent-label of antibody to Rh D, the mother being Rhdd. (Courtesy of Dr W. Erber.)

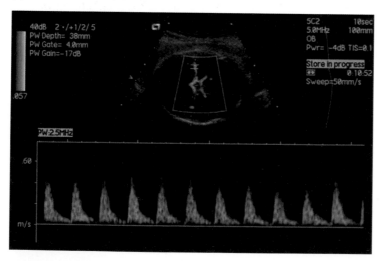

Figure 30.6 Doppler ultrasonography of the circle of Willis in a fetus. The cursor is placed over the middle cerebral artery and an increased blood velocity correlates with anaemia. (From Kumar S. and Regan F. (2005) *BMJ* **330**, 1255–8, with permission.)

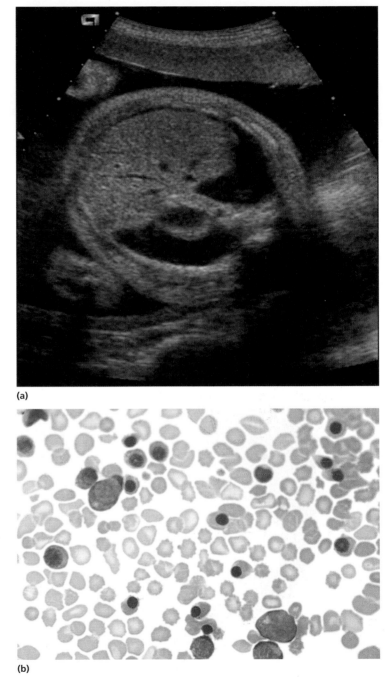

(a)

(b)

Figure 30.7 **(a)** Ultrasound features of hydrops fetalis showing skin oedema, hepatomegaly and ascites. (From Kumar S. and Regan F. (2005) *BMJ* **330**, 1255–8, with permission.) **(b)** Rh haemolytic disease of the newborn (erythroblastosis fetalis): peripheral blood film showing large numbers of erythroblasts, polychromasia and crenated cells.

Clinical features of HDN

1 *Severe disease* Intrauterine death from hydrops fetalis (Fig. 30.7a).
2 *Moderate disease* The baby is born with anaemia and jaundice and may show pallor, tachycardia, oedema and hepatosplenomegaly. If the unconjugated bilirubin is not controlled and reaches levels exceeding 250 μmol/L, bile pigment deposition in the basal ganglia may lead to **kernicterus** – central nervous system damage with generalized spasticity and possible subsequent mental deficiency, deafness and epilepsy. This problem becomes acute after birth as maternal clearance of fetal bilirubin ceases and conjugation of bilirubin by the neonatal liver has not yet reached full activity.
3 *Mild disease* Mild anaemia with or without jaundice.

Investigations will reveal variable anaemia with a high reticulocyte count; the baby is Rh D-positive, the direct antiglobulin test is positive and the serum bilirubin raised. In moderate and severe cases, many erythroblasts are seen in the blood film (Fig. 30.7b) and this is known as **erythroblastosis fetalis**.

Treatment

Exchange transfusion may be necessary; the indications for this include severe anaemia (Hb <10 g/dL at birth) and severe or rapidly rising hyperbilirubinaemia. More than one exchange transfusion may be required and 500 mL is usually sufficient for each exchange. The donor blood should be less than 5 days old, CMV-negative, irradiated and Rh D-negative and ABO compatible with the baby's and mother's serum. Phototherapy (exposure of the infant to bright light of appropriate wavelength) degrades bilirubin and reduces the likelihood of kernicterus.

ABO haemolytic disease of the newborn

In 20% of births, a mother is ABO incompatible with the fetus. Group A and group B mothers usually have only IgM ABO antibodies. The majority of cases of ABO HDN are caused by 'immune' IgG antibodies in group O mothers. Although 15% of pregnancies in white people involve a group O mother with a group A or group B fetus, most mothers do not produce IgG anti-A or anti-B and very few babies have severe enough haemolytic disease to require treatment. Exchange transfusions are needed in only 1 in 3000 infants. The mild course of ABO HDN is partly explained by the A and B antigens not being fully developed at birth and by partial neutralization of maternal IgG antibodies by A and B antigens on other cells, in the plasma and tissue fluids.

In contrast to Rh HDN, ABO disease may be found in the first pregnancy and may or may not affect subsequent pregnancies. The direct antiglobulin test on the infant's cells may be negative or only weakly positive. Examination of the blood film shows autoagglutination and spherocytosis, polychromasia and erythroblastosis.

SUMMARY

- Pregnancy results in changes in the haematological systems.
- There is a fall in haemoglobin because of an increased plasma volume that is proportionally greater than a 25% increase in red cell mass.
- Iron deficiency is frequent; folate deficiency is associated with maternal anaemia and with neural tube defects (NTDs) in the fetus.

- Serum vitamin B_{12} levels fall in pregnancy but deficiency is rare. Platelets counts also fall on average by 10%, but in some women this physiological fall may be severe or may be caused by immune thrombocytopenia.
- Pregnancy is a hypercoagulable state with increased levels of coagulation factors and risk of thrombosis or disseminated intravascular coagulation.

- Neonates have higher haemoglobin levels than adults. Anaemia at birth is usually caused by haemorrhage or immune haemolysis.
- Haemolytic disease of the newborn is brought about by RhD antibodies made by a RhD-negative mother crossing the placenta. It may cause death of the fetus (hydrops fetalis) or haemolytic anaemia. It is now rare because of administration of Rh anti-D to RhD-negative mothers at the time of exposure to RhD-positive fetal cells or blood products.
- ABO haemolytic disease of the newborn is now more frequent. It is usually mild and may occur in the first pregnancy. It is most frequently caused by group O mothers making immune IgG antibodies (which cross the placenta) against a group A or B fetus.

Now visit www.wiley.com/go/essentialhaematology to test yourself on this chapter.

Normal values

Essential Haematology, 6th Edition. © A. V. Hoffbrand and P. A. H. Moss. Published 2011 by Blackwell Publishing Ltd.

	Males	Females	Males and females
Haemoglobin	13.5–17.5 g/Dl	11.5–15.5 g/dL	
Red cells (erythrocytes)	$4.5–6.5 \times 10^{12}$/L	$3.9–5.6 \times 10^{12}$/L	
PCV (haematocrit)	40–52%	36–48%	
MCV			80–95 fL
MCH			27–34 pg
MCHC			20–35 g/dL
White cells (leucocytes)			
total			$4.0–11.0 \times 10^9$/L
neutrophils			$2.5–7.5 \times 10^9$/L
lymphocytes			$1.5–3.5 \times 10^9$/L
monocytes			$0.2–0.8 \times 10^9$/L
eosinophils			$0.04–0.44 \times 10^9$/L
basophils			$0.01–0.1 \times 10^9$/L
Platelets			$150–400 \times 10^9$/L
Red cell mass	30 ± 5 mL/kg	27 ± 5 mL/kg	
Plasma volume	45 ± 5 mL/kg	45 ± 5 mL/kg	
Serum iron			10–30 µmol/L
Total iron-binding capacity			40–75 µmol/L (2.0–4.0 g/L as transferrin)
Serum ferritin*	40–340 µg/L	14–150 µg/L	
Serum vitamin B_{12}*			160–925 ng/L (20–680 pmol/L)
Serum folate*			3.0–15.0 µg/L (4–30 nmol/L)
Red cell folate*			160–640 µg/L (360–1460 nmol/L)

MCH, mean corpuscular haemoglobin; MCHC, mean corpuscular haemoglobin concentration; MCV, mean corpuscular volume; PCV, packed cell volume.
* Normal ranges differ with different commercial kits.

World Health Organization classification of tumours of the haematopoietic and lymphoid tissues

Essential Haematology, 6th Edition. © A. V. Hoffbrand and P. A. H. Moss. Published 2011 by Blackwell Publishing Ltd.

Myeloproliferative neoplasms

Chronic myelogenous leukaemia, *BCR–ABL1* positive
Chronic neutrophilic leukaemia
Polycythaemia vera
Primary myelofibrosis
Essential thrombocythaemia
Chronic eosinophilic leukaemia, not otherwise specified
Mastocytosis
  Cutaneous mastocytosis
  Systemic mastocytosis
  Mast cell leukaemia
  Mast cell sarcoma
  Extracutaneous mastocytoma
Myeloproliferative neoplasms, unclassifiable
Myeloid and lymphoid neoplasms associated with eosinophilia and abnormalities of *PDGFRA*, *PDGFRB* or *FGFR1*
  Myeloid and lymphoid neoplasms associated with *PDGFRA* rearrangement
  Myeloid neoplasms associated with *PDGFRB* rearrangement
  Myeloid and lymphoid neoplasms with *FGFR1* abnormalities

Myelodysplastic/ myeloproliferative neoplasms

Chronic myelomonocytic leukaemia
Atypical chronic myeloid leukaemia, *BCR–ABL1* negative
Juvenile myelomonocytic leukaemia
Myelodysplastic/myeloproliferative neoplasms, unclassifiable
Refractory anaemia with ringed sideroblasts (RARS) associated with marked thrombocytosis*

---

*These represent provisional entities or provisional subtypes of other neoplasms. They are provisional because there are insufficient data to support their being a definite entity, significant controversies about their defining features and/or uncertainty about whether they are unique or closely related to other definite entities.

Myelodysplastic syndromes

Refractory cytopenia with unilineage dysplasia
  Refractory anaemia
  Refractory neutropenia
  Refractory thrombocytopenia
Refractory anaemia with ring sideroblasts
Refractory cytopenia with multilineage dysplasia
Refractory anaemia with excess blasts
Myelodysplastic syndromes associated with isolated del(5q)
Myelodysplastic syndromes, unclassifiable
Myelodysplastic syndromes in children

Acute myeloid leukaemia

Acute myeloid leukaemia (AML) with recurrent genetic abnormalities
AML with t(8; 21)(q22; q22), *RUNX1–RUNX1T1*
AML with inv(16)(p13.1q22) or t(16; 16) (p13.1; q22), *CBFB–MYH11*
Acute promyelocytic leukaemia with t(15; 17) (q22; q11–12), *PML–RARA*
AML with t(9; 11)(p22; q23), *MLLT3–MLL*
AML with t(6; 9)(p23; q34), *DEK–NUP214*
AML with inv(3)(q21q26.2) or t(3; 3)(q21; q26.2), *RPN1–EVI1*
AML (megakaryoblastic) with t(1; 22)(p13; q13), *RBM15–MKL1*
AML with mutated *NPM1**
AML with mutated *CEBPA**
AML with myelodysplasia-related changes
Therapy-related myeloid neoplasms
AML, not otherwise categorized
  AML with minimal differentiation
  AML without maturation
  AML with maturation
Acute myelomonocytic leukaemia
Acute monoblastic and monocytic leukaemia
Acute erythroid leukaemia
  Acute erythroid leukaemia, erythroid/myeloid
  Acute pure erythroid leukaemia
Acute megakaryoblastic leukaemia
Acute basophilic leukaemia
Acute panmyelosis with myelofibrosis
Myeloid sarcoma

Myeloid proliferations related to Down's
  syndrome
 Transient abnormal myelopoiesis
 AML associated with Down's syndrome
Blastic plasmacytoid dendritic cell neoplasm
Acute leukaemias of ambiguous lineage
 Acute undifferentiated leukaemia
 Acute biphenotypic leukaemia

Precursor lymphoid neoplasms

B-lymphoblastic leukaemia/lymphoma
B-lymphoblastic leukaemia/lymphoma, not
  otherwise specified
B-lymphoblastic leukaemia/lymphoma with
  recurrent cytogenetic/molecular genetic
  abnormalities
B-lymphoblastic leukaemia/lymphoma with t(9;
  22)(q34; q11.2), *BCR–ABL1*
B-lymphoblastic leukaemia/lymphoma with
  t(11q23), *MLL* rearranged
B-lymphoblastic leukaemia/lymphoma with t(12;
  21)(p13; q22), *TEL–AML1* (*ETV6–RUNX1*)
B-lymphoblastic leukaemia/lymphoma with
  hyperdiploidy
B-lymphoblastic leukaemia/lymphoma with
  hypodiploidy (hypodiploid ALL)
B-lymphoblastic leukaemia/lymphoma with t(5;
  14)(q31; q32), *IL3–IGH*
B-lymphoblastic leukaemia/lymphoma with t(1;
  19)(q23; p13.3), *E2A–PBX1* (*TCF3–PBX1*)
T-lymphoblastic leukaemia/lymphoma

Mature B-cell neoplasms

Chronic lymphocytic leukaemia/small
  lymphocytic lymphoma
B-cell prolymphocytic leukaemia
Splenic marginal zone lymphoma
Hairy cell leukaemia
Splenic lymphoma/leukaemia, unclassifiable
 Splenic diffuse red pulp small B-cell lymphoma*
 Hairy cell leukaemia variant*
Lymphoplasmacytic lymphoma
 Waldenström's macroglobulinaemia
Heavy-chain diseases
 α Heavy-chain disease
 γ Heavy-chain disease
 μ Heavy-chain disease

Plasma cell myeloma
Solitary plasmacytoma of bone
Extraosseous plasmacytoma
Extranodal marginal zone B-cell lymphoma of
  mucosa-associated lymphoid tissue (MALT
  lymphoma)
Nodal marginal zone B-cell lymphoma
 Paediatric type nodal marginal zone lymphoma
Follicular lymphoma
 Paediatric type follicular lymphoma
Primary cutaneous follicle centre lymphoma
Mantle cell lymphoma
Diffuse large B-cell lymphoma (DLBCL), not
  otherwise specified
 T-cell/histiocyte-rich large B-cell lymphoma
 DLBCL associated with chronic inflammation
 Epstein–Barr virus (EBV)-positive DLBCL of
  the elderly
Lymphomatoid granulomatosis
Primary mediastinal (thymic) large B-cell
  lymphoma
Intravascular large B-cell lymphoma
Primary cutaneous DLBCL, leg type
Anaplastic lymphoma kinase (ALK) positive large
  B-cell lymphoma
Plasmablastic lymphoma
Primary effusion lymphoma
Large B-cell lymphoma arising in HHV8-
  associated multicentric Castleman disease
Burkitt lymphoma
B-cell lymphoma, unclassifiable, with features
  intermediate between DLBCL and Burkitt
  lymphoma
B-cell lymphoma, unclassifiable, with features
  intermediate between DLBCL and classic
  Hodgkin lymphoma

Mature T-cell and NK-cell neoplasms

T-cell prolymphocytic leukaemia
T-cell large granular lymphocytic leukaemia
Aggressive natural killer (NK) cell leukaemia
Systemic EBV-positive T-cell lymphoproliferative
  disease of childhood (associated with chronic
  active EBV infection)
Hydroa vaccineforme-like lymphoma
Adult T-cell leukaemia/lymphoma

Extranodal NK/T-cell lymphoma, nasal type
Enteropathy-associated T-cell lymphoma
Hepatosplenic T-cell lymphoma
Subcutaneous panniculitis-like T-cell lymphoma
Mycosis fungoides
Sézary syndrome
Primary cutaneous anaplastic large-cell lymphoma
Primary cutaneous aggressive epidermotropic
    CD8-positive cytotoxic T-cell lymphoma*
Primary cutaneous γδ T-cell lymphoma
Primary cutaneous small/medium CD4-positive
    T-cell lymphoma*
Peripheral T-cell lymphoma, not otherwise
    specified
Angioimmunoblastic T-cell lymphoma
Anaplastic large-cell lymphoma, ALK positive
Anaplastic large-cell lymphoma, ALK negative*

Hodgkin lymphoma

Nodular lymphocyte-predominant Hodgkin
    lymphoma
Classic Hodgkin lymphoma
  Nodular sclerosis classic Hodgkin lymphoma
  Lymphocyte-rich classic Hodgkin lymphoma
  Mixed cellularity classic Hodgkin lymphoma
  Lymphocyte-depleted classic Hodgkin lymphoma

Histiocytic and dendritic cell neoplasms

Histiocytic sarcoma
Langerhans cell histiocytosis
Langerhans cell sarcoma
Interdigitating dendritic cell sarcoma
Follicular dendritic cell sarcoma
Dendritic cell tumour, not otherwise specified
Indeterminate dendritic cell tumour
Fibroblastic reticular cell tumour

Post-transplant lymphoproliferative disorders

Early lesions
  Reactive plasmacytic hyperplasia
  Infectious mononucleosis-like
Polymorphic post-transplant lymphoproliferative
    disorder
Monomorphic post-transplant lymphoproliferative
    disorder (B and T/NK cell types)*
Classic Hodgkin lymphoma-type post-transplant
    lymphoproliferative disorder

Index

Note: page numbers in *italics* refer to figures, those in **bold** refer to tables